ATLAS
of Histology

ATLAS
of Histology

Everett E. Dodd, Ph.D.

Professor of Biology
Saint Mary's College
of California

McGraw-Hill
Book Company

New York   St. Louis   San Francisco
Auckland   Bogotá   Düsseldorf
Johannesburg   London   Madrid   Mexico
Montreal   New Delhi   Panama
Paris   São Paulo   Singapore
Sydney   Tokyo   Toronto

ATLAS
of Histology

1 2 3 4 5 6 7 8 9 0   RABP   7 8 3 2 1 0 9

Library of Congress Cataloging in Publication Data

Dodd, Everett E
    Atlas of histology.

    Bibliography: p.
    Includes index.
    1.   Histology—Atlases.   I.   Title.
QM557.D63   596'.08'240222   78-14449
ISBN 0-07-017230-7

This book was set in Caledonia by Monotype Composition Company, Inc.
The editors were Alice Macnow and Henry C. De Leo;
the designer was Barbara Ellwood;
the production supervisor was Milton J. Heiberg.
The printer was Rae Publishing Co., Inc.; the binder, The Book Press, Inc.

I wish to dedicate this atlas to my wife, *Gloria*,
and our daughters, *Marlane and Melinda*.

Contents

Preface

This atlas has been written for students in undergraduate or professional school courses of histology. It is a visual teaching aid designed to help the student identify cells and tissues by using labeled color photomicrographs. Although the atlas deals only with structures seen at the level of the light microscope, it may be used as a supplement to any histology textbook.

The first part of the atlas pertains to cytology and general histology, while the remaining chapters emphasize organ histology. A good student of histology must know more about a tissue than just its morphology. Therefore, in addition to the histological descriptions of an organ or tissue, I have incorporated some gross and subgross anatomy, embryology, and physiology wherever possible. These brief accounts will also enable the student to relate laboratory specimens to the more extensive literature in the textbooks.

My illustrations are intended to complement and elucidate the more difficult concepts presented in the text. The histological descriptions of a structure are correlated with and located near an appropriately labeled color photomicrograph. Each photomicrograph slide emphasizes the visual characteristics of routinely stained tissues found in most student slide sets. Most of my photomicrographs are of hematoxylin and eosin (H&E) stained human tissues, however other stains and tissues from lower vertebrate animals were photographed, especially if certain structures could be seen more advantageously. Major histological structures in the text have been emphasized by the use of italics, indentions, and capital letters.

I wish to express my appreciation to Professors Milton Hildebrand and Lauren E. Rosenberg who kindled my interest in anatomy and histology in my early years as a graduate student. I am grateful to Professor Leon Weiss who reviewed the manuscript and photomicrographs, and to Professor Allan Hansell and Dr. Dennis Caselli who reviewed portions of the manuscript. My thanks to Dr. Gloria Dodd who contributed to the atlas and reviewed and typed the manuscript. Also, I wish to acknowledge Mr. W. H. Hartmann and the employees of the Technical Instrument Company of San Francisco for their kind assistance in helping me solve some problems concerning photomicrography. Special thanks go to Mr. Peter Karsten, formerly with McGraw-Hill, Ms. Alice Macnow, Mr. Henry De Leo, Mr. Milton Heiberg, and others of the McGraw-Hill Book Company for their encouragement and cooperation.

During my work on this atlas I have received valuable suggestions and comments from my students. I shall continue to value suggestions and corrections from those who may find errors or may experience difficulty while working with the atlas.

EVERETT E. DODD

ATLAS
Of *Histology*

Introduction to Cytology and Histology 1

The science of anatomy is concerned with the structural and functional organization of the organism. It is composed of several academic fields, each concerned with specific levels of organization. *Gross anatomy* pertains to the study of the parts of the specimen which can be dissected and observed with the naked eye. *Histology* is that portion of the science of anatomy concerned with the study of tissues, which are aggregates of cells sharing common structural and functional characteristics. *Cytology* is the study of cells making up the tissues. The successful study of both cells and tissues is dependent on several factors: (1) well-prepared specimens; (2) correct use of the microscope; (3) a systematic approach to the examination of a specimen.

Preparation of tissues

Tiny pieces of organs are killed and preserved by placing them in a chemical fixative. The fixative will prevent deterioration of most of the morphologic details present in the cells and tissues. Some fixatives preserve certain structures better than others, and some work better with certain stains. The selection of a particular fixative and stain, therefore, determines which structures are most prominently demonstrated in a section. Although some fixatives may result in the coagulation or precipitation of organic compounds, others may chemically combine with these compounds.

After fixation, the tissues are washed to remove any excess fixative and then dehydrated. Dehydration is important in maintaining the state of preservation and in preparing the tissue for embedding in paraffin or celloidin. Since the tissues are usually opaque after dehydration, they must be "cleared" or made transparent by soaking them in a clearing agent, e.g., xylol or cedarwood oil.

The cleared tissues are placed into an embedding medium, such as paraffin, where they are infiltrated and made rigid enough for sectioning. The rigid tissue is then sectioned on a microtome, usually between 1.5 to 10 μm in thickness. Next, the slices of embedded tissue are attached to glass slides, the paraffin is dissolved from the tissue, and the sections are stained. If these procedures are not properly carried out, the result may be poorly prepared tissues with many *artifacts* (abnormal features). You should select another slide of the same tissue if you find many severe artifacts. Artifacts may occur as *wrinkles* (the section has not been thoroughly infiltrated with paraffin); *splits or scratches* (the microtome blade may have had nicks on its cutting edge); *many randomly scattered granules* (certain fixatives, e.g., formol, have been imperfectly removed); *spaces or clefts* (tissues have not been completely dehydrated and have undergone shrinkage); and *small cracks* (the embedding paraffin may have been overheated).

Once the sections of tissue have been fixed on the slides and their paraffin removed, they are stained. The tissues contain a variety of components which have the ability to combine with and retain colored dyes.

Some dyes, the *cationic* dyes, are basic and carry a positive charge. These dyes react with negatively charged molecules within the fixed tissues and usually form electrostatic bonds. Although hematoxylin is essentially a basic dye, it does not react like the simple basic dyes because it forms covalent rather than electrostatic bonds. Actually hematoxylin is a complex of electronegative hematin chelated to an electropositive mordant such as iron or aluminum. This complex is called a *lake* and carries a positive charge. Certain structures, such as nuclei, react only with basic dyes and are designated as *basophilic*. Other dyes, the *anionic* dyes, such as eosin, are acidic and carry a negative charge. These dyes react with positively charged molecules within the tissue and usually form electrostatic bonds. Structures such as the cytoplasm readily stain with anionic dyes and are designated as *acidophilic*.

If the staining procedure is improperly performed, optimal contrast, visibility, and sharpness of the cytological structures will be lacking. *You should select a slide which has a uniform, moderately intense, stained section of tissue showing a high contrast between structures.*

Microscope

Since it is assumed that students of histology understand the basic function and use of the microscope, only certain points pertaining to microscopy shall be emphasized.

1 Take care in following the few simple steps in setting up your microscope, as outlined by your instructor. You should have Köhler illumination for proper illumination and maximum resolution. The microscope should have the following objectives: scanning, ×3; low power, ×10; high power, ×40; and oil immersion, ×100.

2 All exposed optical surfaces must be clean. Lens paper may be used for this purpose, but for small lenses cotton swabs may also be used. To see the clean lens, unscrew the objective from the revolving nosepiece and examine the lens with a reversed ocular. Never use solvents, such as xylol, on lenses because they may dissolve the cement holding the lens in position. If a lens becomes so dirty that a dry cotton swab is ineffective, a small amount of a commercial lens cleaner may be used with the swab. Oil can be removed from the oil immersion lens by using several cotton swabs. If lens paper only is used, streaks of oil, which are invisible to the naked eye, may remain on the lens.

3 When using the oil immersion lens, place a small drop of immersion oil on the coverslip of the slide. Slowly lower the lens into the oil, *watching from the side* as you slowly turn the adjustment knobs down. When the lens almost touches the slide, focus up with the fine adjustment knob and watch for the image to appear in the ocular. Since immersion oil is nondrying, you can leave a film on your lens while you continue your work, using other lenses. But at the close of your study, you must completely clean the lens (see above). Wipe the slide clean of oil before you study it with a ×40 objective; otherwise you may contaminate the lens when you switch powers. All slides should be cleaned before they are returned to the slide boxes.

A good histologist is like a detective. Histologists work with a number of clues to help in the identification of cells and tissues; the more clues the better. It may be helpful to consider the following points as you study your sections of tissues.

1 Pay attention to and remember the information on the label of the slide. It will identify the specimen, and sometimes the stain and fixative.

2 Examine the section under a dissecting microscope or a reversed ocular. This will tell you something about the subgross anatomy of the organ; its shape, general histological and anatomical organization, and unique macroscopic structures. At this time you should be thinking about structure and functional relationships, as well as the general physiology of the organ.

3 Start your microscopical study by first examining the entire area of a section under the ×3 objective. This will help you become more familiar with prominent landmarks and the distribution of tissues. Now is the time to determine if the slide is poorly stained or has too many serious artifacts. Next, switch to the ×10 objective. The types of tissue can now be distinguished, and their distribution should be noted. The ×40 objective is useful for a more critical study of limited regions. One can now substantiate the identification of a particular tissue, and identify cell types. Most histology requires the use of the ×3, ×10, and ×40 lenses, but where cytological detail is important in the identification of a cell, the oil immersion lens must be used.

4 During your analysis of a tissue, it is important to scan many fields to "get a feeling" for the tissues and stain. The morphology of tissues may be influenced by age or disease, and so they may appear somewhat different in various sections. To identify a tissue you should concentrate on the arrangement and relationship of its component parts. In most cases your observations will correlate with those learned earlier for a particular tissue.

5 Since morphology is more important than color, a good practice is for you to alter the color of your tissues occasionally by placing a colored piece of glass or cellophane over the light source. Also try to examine similar sections of tissue, each stained with a different stain.

Cytology

Cells are the microscopic protoplasmic building units of a tissue, and can assume one of several possible shapes. The cell is organized into a nucleus, which is surrounded by cytoplasm. The nucleus and cytoplasm contain small protoplasmic structures, the *organelles*, which contribute to the overall physiological processes and cell maintenance. In addition, nonliving metabolic products called *inclusions* may be temporarily stored in the cell's cytoplasm.

NUCLEUS. The nucleus may be spherical, elongate, or irregularly shaped. There is usually one to a cell, but some cells (liver) are binucleate, and some (skeletal muscle) are multinucleate. Nuclei contain the following organelles. **Plate 1, Fig. 1.**

Nuclear membrane. This is a dark-stained, thin membrane surrounding the nucleus. At the ultrastructural level it appears as a double-layered fenestrated membrane. The *fenestrae* or holes allow for the passage of molecules between the nucleus and cytoplasm. The interior of the nucleus is filled with nucleoplasm (nuclear sap or karyoplasm). Nucleoplasm is a nonstaining, semifluid colloidal suspension containing chromatin and the nucleolus. It is a medium which facilitates the diffusion of metabolites between the nucleus and cytoplasm. **Plate 1, Fig. 1.**

PLATE 1 _____

Nucleus
Nucleolus
Nuclear membrane
Chromatin
Nucleoplasm
Cytoplasm
Cell membrane
Nuclei of follicle cells
Connective tissue

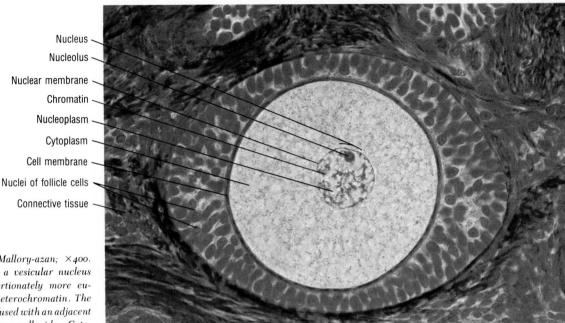

FIGURE 1.
Oocyte; rabbit; Mallory-azan; ×400.
Note that this is a vesicular nucleus
containing proportionately more eu-
chromatin than heterochromatin. The
cell membrane is fused with an adjacent
structure, the zona pellucida. Cyto-
plasm contains vacuoles and granules.

Nucleolus. In the nucleus there may be one or several prominent basophilic *nucleoli*, which are spherical or irregularly shaped. Each nucleolus is composed of ribonucleoprotein and some chromatin. They are attached to specific nucleolar organizing sites along certain chromosomes. Molecules of ribosomal RNA are synthesized in the nucleolus and then moved into the cytoplasm where they are further synthesized into ribosomes. Nucleoli are present in cells actively synthesizing protein, but inactive cells may lack them. Also, nucleoli disappear during cell division, but reappear in the nuclei of daughter cells. **Plate 1, Fig. 1.**

Chromosomes. Chromosomes carry genetic information and control specific metabolic functions of the cell. They are composed of *chromatin*, a complex of protein and deoxyribonucleic acid (DNA). Two types of chromatin are present in the interphase nucleus, *heterochromatin* and *euchromatin*, each of which has distinct morphologic and physiologic characteristics. Heterochromatin is physiologically inactive and is represented by densely coiled segments of chromosomes. These segments appear as irregular basophilic clumps which are scattered throughout the nucleoplasm and persist in the interphase nucleus. Euchromatin, by contrast, is the active component of chromatin. It is less dense, unstained, and widely distributed throughout the nucleoplasm. Euchromatin is important in the regulation of protein synthesis and other processes of cell metabolism. In general, the nucleus of an active cell, such as a mesenchyme cell, is pale and vesicular because it contains proportionately more euchromatin than heterochromatin. In inactive fibroblasts, the nuclei contain proportionately more heterochromatin than euchromatin and are therefore moderately dense and darkly stained. Dead or dying cells, or those preparing to extrude their nuclei such as the normoblasts (see Chap. 8), have very dense, deeply stained *pycnotic* nuclei with abundant heterochromatin and little or no euchromatin. **Plate 1, Fig. 1.**

CYTOPLASM. The cytoplasm is under the regulatory control of the nucleus and is the secretory and major synthesizing center of the cell. With the light microscope the cytoplasm may appear fibrous, granular, or vacuolated, or as an amorphous and homogeneous mass surrounding the nucleus. It is a complex structure composed of living protoplasmic organelles and nonliving inclusions. The inclusions are metabolic substances produced by the cytoplasm. They are pigment and secretory granules, glycogen particles, lipids, and crystals, all of which are stored within the cytoplasm. Although the ultrastructure for these organelles and inclusions has been established, an emphasis will be given to their appearance with the light microscope. **Plate 1, Fig. 1.**

Organelles. Of the numerous organelles, only the following can usually be seen with the light microscope: ergastoplasm, Golgi apparatus, mitochondria, centrioles, and microtubules during mitosis.

CELL MEMBRANE. The surface of the cytoplasm is covered by a thin cell membrane or *plasmalemma*. It is not visible with the light microscope, but because of associated substances lying on its surface the entire complex may be seen as a thin, dark line. The ultrastructure of the cell membrane, as determined with the electron microscope, is similar to that of internal cytoplasmic membranes. It appears as a trilaminar structure about 75 Å thick, and is composed of phospholipids and proteins. The surface of most cell membranes is covered with a cell coat or glycocalyx composed of sialic acid and glycoproteins, a portion of which is incorporated into the cell membrane. The glycocalyx probably filters molecules which reach the cell membrane, contributes to the adhesive properties between cells, and is important in cellular interactions. The cell membrane maintains the structural integrity of the cell, and because of its semipermeable nature will allow only certain molecules and ions to pass between the cytoplasm and extracellular environment. It plays an active role in specific cell functions, such as phagocytosis, pinocytosis, and exocytosis. **Plate 1, Fig. 1.**

ENDOPLASMIC RETICULUM (ergastoplasm). This is an extensive internal network of membranes extending from the nuclear membrane to the cell membrane; it forms a labyrinth of fluid-filled spaces. The endoplasmic reticulum is a trilaminar membrane (see above) and may or may not have tiny basophilic particles or ribonucleoproteins, *ribosomes*, attached to its surface. If the ribosomes are attached, the endoplasmic reticulum is designated as granular, and because of the numerous ribosomes the cytoplasm is basophilic. If the ribosomes are relatively few in number and unattached, the endoplasmic reticulum is of the smooth type and the cytoplasm is usually acidophilic. Ribosomes are sites of protein synthesis; therefore an abundant granular endoplasmic reticulum is indicative of high levels of metabolic activities within the cell. All cells have free ribosomes within their cytoplasm which may be important for the synthesis of proteins to be used by the cells. The attached ribosomes are probably concerned with producing proteins to be secreted by the cells.

GOLGI APPARATUS. This structure is not visible in routinely stained preparations and may appear as a nonstained area in the cytoplasm. With silver impregnation techniques it usually appears as a network of canals and elongated vacuoles adjacent to the nucleus (e.g., pancreatic cells). In some cells (neurons) the Golgi apparatus is distributed throughout the cytoplasm. The Golgi apparatus is quite elaborate in secretory cells, but is usually poorly represented or absent in inactive nonsecretory cells. The Golgi apparatus accumulates and concentrates secretions synthesized in the cytoplasm. These substances are enclosed or "packaged" within membranes provided by the Golgi apparatus, and then released into the cytoplasm as protein-rich secretory granules, pigment granules, lysosomes containing hydrolytic enzymes,

PLATE 1 *continued*

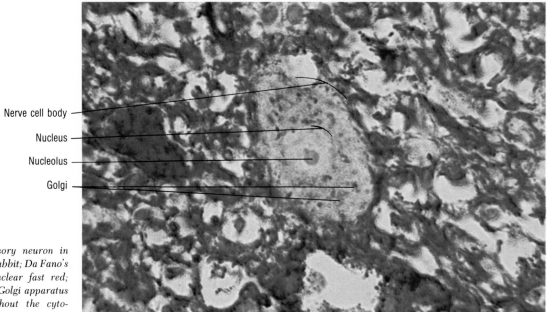

Nerve cell body —

Nucleus —

Nucleolus —

Golgi —

FIGURE 2.
Golgi apparatus; sensory neuron in
dorsal root ganglion; rabbit; Da Fano's
silver method and nuclear fast red;
×1000. Note that the Golgi apparatus
is distributed throughout the cyto-
plasm.

hormones, or lipid-filled vacuoles. These membrane-enclosed parcels may eventually migrate to the surface of the cell, where, as their membranes fuse with the plasma membrane, their contents are released (e.g., secretory granules), or they may remain within the cytoplasm (e.g., lysosomes). The Golgi apparatus is also concerned with the synthesis of glycoproteins which may coat the surface of the cell membrane as the *glycocalyx*, or form a component of mucus. **Plate 1, Fig. 2**.

MITOCHONDRIA. These are tiny, about 2.5 μm, organelles which are granular, or spheroidal in appearance. They can be demonstrated only with special stains, such as iron hematoxylin. Their numbers vary directly with the degree of metabolic activity, and they may be concentrated in regions within the cell where metabolic activity is the greatest. Studies with the electron microscope indicate that each mitochondrion is a hollow structure filled with an amorphous fluid, the matrix, and surrounded by two trilaminar membranes (unit membranes). The innermost membrane is folded to form a number of shelflike cristae which project into the interior of the mitochondrion. The matrix contains some DNA, RNA, and ribonucleoproteins. Most important, it contains enzymes of the *Krebs*, or *citric acid, cycle* as well as enzymes instrumental in protein and lipid synthesis. The surface of the inner membrane has *respiratory* and *phosphorylating enzymes* attached to its inner surface. The prime function of the mitochondria is to synthesize and release energy-rich adenosine triphosphate (ATP) molecules which can be used by the cell for a source of energy to do chemical and physical work. Mitochondria are self-replicating and

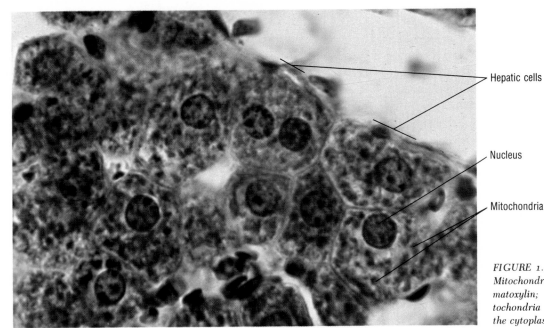

Hepatic cells

Nucleus

Mitochondria

FIGURE 1.
Mitochondria; liver cells; rat; iron he-
matoxylin; ×1000. Note that the mi-
tochondria appear as dark clumps in
the cytoplasm.

can synthesize limited types of proteins by tiny ribonucleoprotein particles (similar to cytoplasmic ribosomes) within the matrix. **Plate 2, Fig. 1.**

CENTRIOLES. Although these structures are paired short rods (the diplosome), in ordinary preparations they may appear as a dark-stained dot. The centrioles are usually located near the nucleus and sandwiched between it and the Golgi apparatus. They are surrounded by a pale-stained area of amorphous substance, the centrosphere. The centrioles plus the centrosphere are designated as the *centrosome* or *cell center*, which indicates the polarity and symmetry of the cell. In epithelial cells, the centrosome is located at the apical end of the cytoplasm or apical pole of the nucleus. The cell axis is determined by a line running through the nucleus and centrosome. Each centriole undergoes self-replication in the early stages of mitosis (prophase) to produce a daughter centriole. Each pair of centrioles then separate and migrate to the poles of the cell. During their migration they organize the production of aster fibers which grow into the cytoplasm (see below). At the conclusion of mitosis each daughter cell contains a pair of centrioles. See **Plate 4, Fig. 1.**

Tiny basal granules, which give rise to the axial filaments of cilia and flagella, may or may not be derived from preexisting centrioles. Some may develop de novo from fibrogranular substances in the cytoplasm or from the self-replication of preexisting centrioles.

MICROTUBULES. Single microtubules are elongate, tubular protein structures which cannot be resolved with the light microscope. During mitosis, however, many microtubules form bundles which can be seen as aster fibers in mitotic spindles. These fibers are important in separating replicated chromosomes during mitosis. The microtubules may also function to enhance intracellular transport and movement of metabolites, inclusions, and organelles. See **Plate 4, Fig. 1.**

OTHER ORGANELLES. Lysosomes, microsomes, and filaments represent more organelles which are usually not visually conspicuous in cells. *Lysosomes* are membrane-bound vacuoles of hydrolytic enzymes which carry out intracellular digestion. They are classified as primary or secondary according to their functional and morphological characteristics. Primary lysosomes are formed by the combined activities of the endoplasmic reticulum and Golgi apparatus. They are inactive and may appear as tiny spherical membrane-bound vesicles in the cytoplasm. Secondary lysosomes are formed as primary lysosomes coalesce with particle-containing vacuoles in the cytoplasm. These vacuoles are produced by phagocytosis or pinocytosis, and their contents are either partially or completely digested by the lysosomal enzymes. The secondary lysosomes may be morphologically distinct as a multivesicular structure usually containing undigested residues.

Microbodies (peroxisomes) are tiny (about 0.3 μm), dense membrane-bound granules containing several oxidative enzymes and catalase. The microbodies are probably formed in the granular endoplasmic reticulum and may be important in the conversion of fats to carbohydrates.

Filaments are long strands of proteins. They are usually below the limits of resolution with the light microscope, but small bundles of filaments (fibrils) may be observed. Some filaments, for example, tonofilaments (tonofibrils) in stratified squamous epithelium (see Chap. 11), may support and strengthen a tissue. Others, actin and myosin, participate in the contraction of the myofibrils in muscle cells (Chap. 5). Still others, such as neurofilaments (neurofibrils) in neurons, facilitate the transportation of metabolites (see Chap. 6).

Inclusions. Inclusions are the nonliving substances produced by and stored within the cytoplasm. They may be visible with the light microscope, but usually can only be seen with special stains.

PIGMENT GRANULES. There are several types of pigment granules, all of which can easily be seen regardless of the type of the stain used. *Melanin* is a black or brown pigment stored in granules or melanosomes (see Chap. 11).

Lipofuscin is a light yellowish brown or tan pigment and represents undigested residues of lysosomal digestion (see above). It becomes abundant in certain cells of older individuals (see Chap. 16). *Hemosiderin* is a deep golden-brown iron-containing pigment which may be found in the macrophages of the spleen and liver and abnormally in the lungs. This pigment is produced by the degradation of hemoglobin as aged erythrocytes are removed from the circulation and digested by macrophages (see Chap. 13).

GLYCOGEN. Glycogen is a polysaccharide and represents a form of carbohydrate storage within animal cells. In cells stained for glycogen (e.g., by Best's carmine method), glycogen may appear as tiny red particles or coarse clumps scattered throughout the cytoplasm. In routine preparations, glycogen will be removed by aqueous solvents, leaving only irregularly stained networks of cytoplasmic strands. **Plate 2, Fig. 2.**

SECRETORY GRANULES. These are usually tiny, dense, spherical membrane-enclosed bodies of protein seen just at the limits of resolution with the light microscope. Unlike glycogen, they are visible with routine stains. They are produced by the combined activities of the endoplasmic reticulum and Golgi apparatus and are especially prominent in the secretory cells of the pancreas (see Chap. 12).

_____ PLATE 2 *continued*

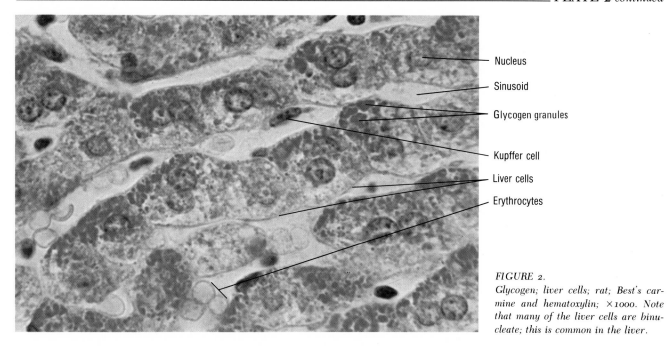

— Nucleus

— Sinusoid

— Glycogen granules

— Kupffer cell

— Liver cells

— Erythrocytes

FIGURE 2.
Glycogen; liver cells; rat; Best's car-
mine and hematoxylin; ×1000. Note
that many of the liver cells are binu-
cleate; this is common in the liver.

LIPID VACUOLES. Vacuoles containing lipids of various size are found in the cytoplasm of certain cells. They are produced by the agranular endoplasmic reticulum and Golgi apparatus. The membrane-enclosed vacuoles contain neutral fats, fatty acids, and cholesterol. As tiny lipid-filled vacuoles are produced, they may become larger by coalescing with other vacuoles. Since fats are removed by solvents used in routine preparations of tissues, the cytoplasm will appear to have holes of various size. Lipids can be localized in the vacuoles by using special fat-soluble dyes (e.g., Sudan black), or by special fixation techniques (using formalin, freezing, or osmic acid).

CRYSTALS. In some cells, such as the Sertoli and interstitial cells of the testis, proteinaceous crystals or crystalloids may be stored in the cytoplasm. They appear as irregular and massive, or thin and elongate, unstained bodies which lack a surrounding membrane (see Chap. 16).

Cell division

At some time during their existence, either frequently or infrequently, cells leave their resting or interphase stage and divide. Some adult cells, however, such as muscle and nerve cells, do not divide. Division is influenced by many varied interrelated factors such as genetics, cellular environment, and nucleocytoplasmic ratios. Somatic cells reproduce mitotically, while sex cells, oocytes and spermatocytes, reproduce meiotically.

During oogenesis and spermatogenesis, diploid germinal cells, primary oocytes and spermatocytes, undergo a first and second meiotic division (reduction divisions), whereby there is a halving of the total number of chromosomes. The resulting

PLATE 3

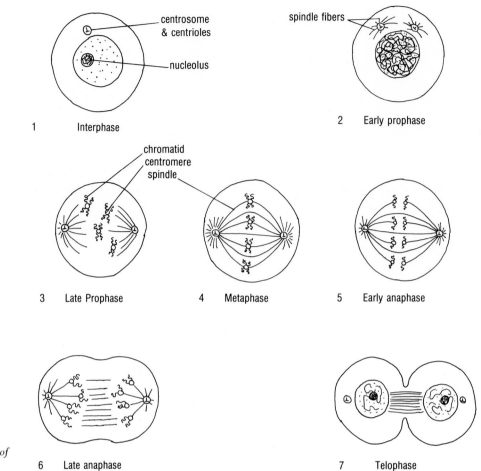

FIGURES 1–7.
Drawing of the sequential stages of mitosis.

haploid ootids and spermatids contain one-half the number of chromosomes as the primary cells.

Each diploid somatic cell divides mitotically, giving rise to two daughter cells having the same number and type of chromosomes as the parental cell. The process of mitosis involves the division of the nucleus (karyokinesis) and the division of the cytoplasm (cytokinesis). During middle interphase the DNA is doubled and the chromosomes are replicated. Mitosis is a physical separation and distribution of the chromosomes into two equal daughter cells, and the process occurs in a series of stages: *prophase, metaphase, anaphase,* and *telophase.* **Plate 3, Figs. 1 to 7.**

Interphase. Although separate chromosomes are not visible at interphase, their chromatin is widely scattered and may appear as granules or clumps of heterochromatin within the nucleus. The nuclear membrane is intact and prominent nucleoli can be seen. A pair of centrioles may be seen adjacent to the nucleus. At middle interphase there is a doubling of DNA, and the chromosomes are *replicated.* Each chromosome forms a pair of chromatin strands, *chromatids,* held together by a *centromere.* Just before the next stage, or prophase, the chromatids coil and become condensed. **Plate 3, Fig. 1; Plate 4, Fig. 1.**

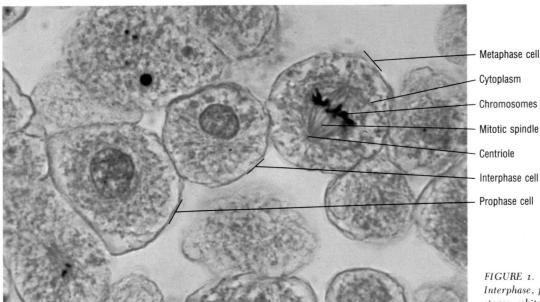

Metaphase cell

Cytoplasm

Chromosomes

Mitotic spindle

Centriole

Interphase cell

Prophase cell

FIGURE 1.
Interphase, prophase, and metaphase
stages; whitefish blastula; iron hema-
toxylin and orange G; ×1000.

Prophase. As a result of chromatid coiling and thickening, the chromosomes first appear as thin strands, so the nucleus appears somewhat like a "ball of yarn." The centrioles undergo self-replication, and each pair will organize the formation of microtubules (spindle fibers) as they migrate to opposite poles of the cell. In late prophase, with continued coiling and condensation, the separate chromosomes become distinct. The nucleolus will disappear as the nucleolar substance becomes attached to the chromatids. At the conclusion of prophase the nuclear membrane disintegrates and disappears, so that the nuclear and cytoplasmic regions of the cell are no longer separated. **Plate 3, Figs. 2 and 3; Plate 4, Fig. 1.**

Metaphase. As the microtubules are synthesized under the organizing influence of the centrioles, they radiate away from the centrioles as they grow toward the *equatorial plate* in the middle of the cell. A few bundles of microtubules, the *continuous fibers*, extend across the entire cell to the opposite pole, while others, the *spindle fibers*, terminate at the equatorial plate of the cell. The centromere of each chromosome is attached to the spindle fibers, coming from opposite poles. The cell will appear to have a fibrous *mitotic spindle* stretching between the polar centrioles and attached to chromosomes lying in the equatorial plate. Although the centromeres are in the equatorial plate, the chromosomal arms may extend irregularly into the cytoplasm. The mitotic spindle will ensure the precise distribution of the replicated chromosomes, so that each daughter cell will receive the same number and type of chromosomes. **Plate 3, Fig. 4; Plate 4, Fig. 1.**

Anaphase. The centromeres of each chromosome duplicate, so that each chromatid or daughter chromosome is attached to one pole of the cell by its own centromere. In late anaphase, by a shortening of the spindle fibers, an elongation of the continuous fibers pushing the poles apart, or by both processes occurring simultaneously, the

PLATE 4 *continued*

Anaphase cell

Telophase cell

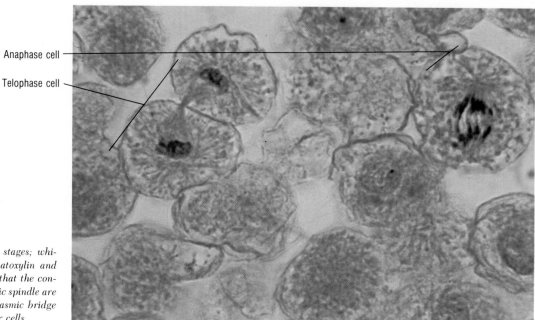

FIGURE 2.
Anaphase and telophase stages; whitefish blastula; iron hematoxylin and orange G; × 1000. Note that the continuous fibers of the mitotic spindle are still present in the cytoplasmic bridge between the two daughter cells.

daughter chromosomes are separated and pulled to opposite poles of the cell by their centromeres. During their migration through the cytoplasm, the "chromosomal arms" trail behind the centromeres which are attached to the spindle fibers. At the conclusion of anaphase, a cytoplasmic *cleavage furrow* appears on the surface of the cell and forms a peripheral girdle encircling the equatorial plate. The cytoplasm, chromosomes, and other organelles are evenly distributed on either side of the furrow. The cleavage furrow represents the place where the cell will ultimately divide, and it becomes deeper in telophase. **Plate 3, Figs. 5 and 6; Plate 4, Fig. 2.**

Telophase. This is the last stage of mitosis. It is characterized by the division of the cell (cytokinesis) into two equal daughter cells. The nuclear membrane and nucleolus reappear during telophase. The chromosomes uncoil and are once again distributed throughout the nucleoplasm as euchromatin and stained clumps of heterochromatin. In late telophase, as the cleavage furrow deepens, the cytoplasm becomes a constricted, thin intercellular bridge connecting the two halves of the cell. The continuous fibers of the spindle persist for a short period in the cytoplasmic bridge. At their midpoint, where they will eventually break apart, they are condensed and surrounded by a mass of dense amorphous substance. This condensed region of fibers appears as a dark-stained dot, the *midbody*, in the middle of the cytoplasmic bridge. As the fibers separate, the bridge is broken, thereby separating the two daughter cells. **Plate 3, Fig. 7; Plate 4, Fig. 2.**

Epithelium and Exocrine Glands 2

Epithelium is a tissue composed of a tightly bound aggregation of one or several cell types lining internal or external body surfaces, and may be one or several layers in thickness. The upper surface is exposed to gases, liquids, or semisolids, while the lower surface is bound to underlying tissues by a basement membrane. Multilayered epithelia are usually protective, and single-layered epithelia absorb, excrete, or secrete. With few exceptions, epithelia are avascular, but they are supplied by capillaries in adjacent connective tissue beds.

All epithelia are anchored to underlying tissues by a *basement membrane*, composed of an upper basal lamina and lower layer of reticular fibers. The basal lamina is an amorphous matrix containing proteins and glycoproteins produced by the epithelial cells. This lamina stains with Schiff's reagent reaction. Fibers of the reticular layer and its ground substance are produced by fibroblasts in connective tissue. These fibers stain black with silver stains. The basement membrane appears as a distinct structure if a special stain has been used, and in routinely stained sections if there is a thick reticular layer. In this atlas the basement membrane usually will be indicated only when it is visible with the light microscope.

Specializations of the cell surfaces, such as terminal bars, desmosomes, microvilli, and cilia, play an important role in epithelial function and may be seen with the light microscope. *Terminal bars* are fused plasma membranes of adjacent cells, forming a girdle around each cell just below the luminal surface. They are prominent on cells lining the intestine and gall bladder. They function to prevent substances from passing directly from the lumen to intercellular spaces and also provide strength to the epithelium. In specially stained and sectioned tissues, terminal bars appear as dark spots between the upper parts of adjacent cells. *Microvilli* are tiny (about 0.5 μm to 1 μm long), narrow, nonmotile cytoplasmic extensions on the apical ends of primarily absorptive cells. They increase the surface area and may appear as a uniform, refractile, striated border (intestinal epithelium), or an irregular brush border (epithelium of proximal convoluted tubules in the kidney). Extremely long microvilli, organized into clumps, are *stereocilia*. They are prominent on epithelial cells in the epididymis and may be both absorptive and secretory in function. Desmosomes are dense, fusiform points of attachment between adjacent plasma membranes. They are attached to the cell's cytoskeleton by cytoplasmic fibers and tonofibrils. Desmosomes provide extra binding strength between cells, and are prominent in the epithelium of skin. Some epithelia have cilia (see below), which function to move fluids and mucus over their surfaces.

Other tissues, derived from epithelium but with different morphological characteristics, are specialized as *glands* (exocrine and endocrine), *sense receptors,* or *pigmented tissue.* Since most of these specialized tissues are presented in other chapters, only the exocrine glands will be considered with epithelium.

Epithelium may be histologically classified by the number of its layers and the morphology of cells on its free surface. Although there are standard descriptions for given cell shapes, the appearance may vary according to physiological activity. For example, for any one cell type, active cells are usually taller or larger than inactive ones. In most cases the plasma membranes of many epithelial cells are difficult to observe, and thus the nuclei become important diagnostic features. Also, a student may not have enough visual information to identify a particular epithelium and should therefore examine several fields to find a suitable specimen. The classification of epithelium is based on the following nomenclature.

Number of cell layers (in section).

Simple epithelium. Single layer of cells.

Stratified epithelium. More than one layer of cells.

Pseudostratified epithelium. Single layer of cells appearing multilayered.

Transitional epithelium. Several layers of cells, but thickness varying with contraction and stretching.

Shape of surface cells (in section).

Squamous. The cell is elongate and thin and has a flat nucleus.

Cuboidal. The cell is as wide as it is tall and has a spherical nucleus.

Columnar. The cell is taller than wide and has an oval nucleus.

Simple squamous epithelium

This tissue is a single layer of squamous cells. It lines lung alveoli and, in the kidney, Bowman's capsule and the thin segment of the loop of Henle. It also lines the body cavities, as *mesothelium,* and the lumina of blood vessels, as *endothelium.*

MORPHOLOGY. In section the cytoplasm of each cell usually appears as a thin, platelike structure, but in H&E-stained tissues it may be indistinct. The nucleus is centrally located and spindle-shaped, and bulges into the lumen of an organ lined by the tissue. From a surface view, the cells have irregular outlines and form a mosaic. **Plate 1, Fig. 1.**

Simple cuboidal epithelium

The epithelium is a single layer of cuboidal cells and may be found lining renal tubules, thyroid gland follicles, ducts of glands, and the choroid plexus.

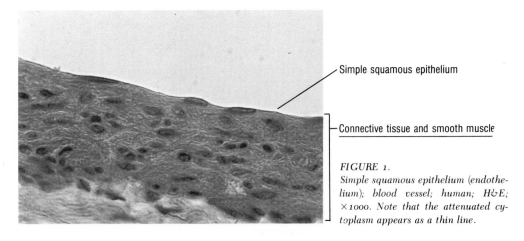

— Simple squamous epithelium

— Connective tissue and smooth muscle

FIGURE 1.
Simple squamous epithelium (endothelium); blood vessel; human; H&E; ×1000. Note that the attenuated cytoplasm appears as a thin line.

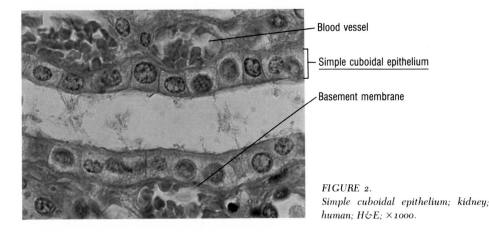

— Blood vessel

— Simple cuboidal epithelium

— Basement membrane

FIGURE 2.
Simple cuboidal epithelium; kidney; human; H&E; ×1000.

MORPHOLOGY. In sectioned tissue, the cells are as wide as they are tall, with a centrally placed spherical nucleus. The nuclei usually appear as a uniform, evenly spaced row. Viewed from the surface, the cells form a mosaic of hexagonal polygons. **Plate 1, Fig. 2.**

Simple columnar epithelium

An epithelium of this type is composed of a single layer of columnar cells. The tissue lines the stomach, intestine, gall bladder, and excretory ducts of many glands. Cilia may be present as small, uniform, hairlike structures on the apical ends of the cells. In living cells they are motile and aid in transporting substances along the free surface of the epithelium. Ciliated simple columnar epithelium is present in the uterus, oviducts, and small bronchi of the lungs.

PLATE 1 *continued*

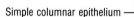
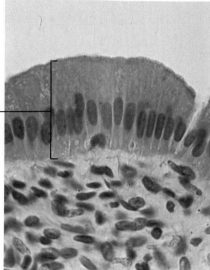

Simple columnar epithelium

FIGURE 3.
Simple columnar epithelium; gall blad-
der; human; H&E; ×1000.

MORPHOLOGY. The cells of simple columnar epithelium are taller than wide. The oval nuclei appear at about the same level, below the middle of the cells, but they may be staggered. On their free surface the cells appear much like cuboidal cells—a mosaic of hexagons—but with smaller diameters. **Plate 1, Fig. 3.**

Stratified squamous epithelium

This tissue is composed of several layers of cells, the outermost of which is squamous. If the epithelium is on a dry surface, such as skin, it is designated as *keratinized stratified squamous epithelium,* since the outer cells contain keratin, a water-impervious, fibrous protein. If the epithelium lines a wet surface, such as the vagina or esophagus, it is a *nonkeratinized stratified squamous epithelium* and the cells lack keratin.

MORPHOLOGY. The lower layer of cells rest on a basement membrane and may be cuboidal or columnar; the intermediate layers are polyhedral; and the upper layers are always squamous. The keratinized squamous cells appear as anucleate, fibrous, scalelike structures. Nonkeratinized cells do not resemble scales and are nucleated. **Plate 2, Figs. 1 and 2.**

Stratified cuboidal epithelium

This epithelium is characterized by a few layers of tissue with an outer layer of cuboidal cells. It is limited in its distribution, but can be found lining sweat gland ducts and Graafian follicles in the ovaries.

MORPHOLOGY. The basal layer is composed of small polyhedron-shaped cells. The intermediate layer, if one is present, has larger polyhedral cells lying above the basal layer. The free surface of the epithelium has cuboidal cells. **Plate 2, Fig. 3.**

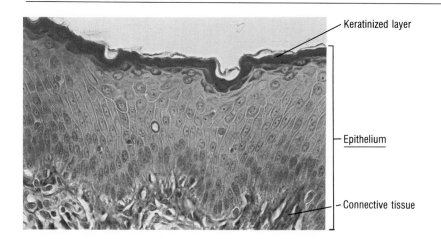

Keratinized layer

Epithelium

Connective tissue

FIGURE 1.
Stratified squamous keratinized epithelium; human scrotum; Mallory-azan; ×400. Note the tonofibrils and desquamation of anucleate squamous cells from the heavy keratinized layers.

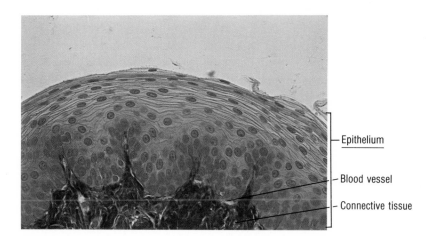

Epithelium

Blood vessel

Connective tissue

FIGURE 2.
Stratified squamous nonkeratinized epithelium; human esophagus; Mallory-azan ×400. Note that the surface squamous cells are nucleated and lack keratin.

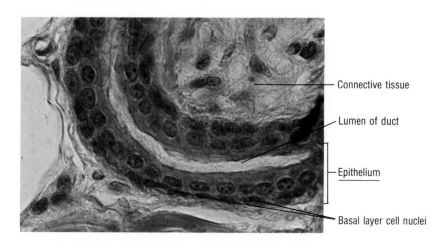

Connective tissue

Lumen of duct

Epithelium

Basal layer cell nuclei

FIGURE 3.
Stratified cuboidal epithelium; excretory duct of sweat gland; human; iron hematoxylin–methyl green; ×1000.

PLATE 3——

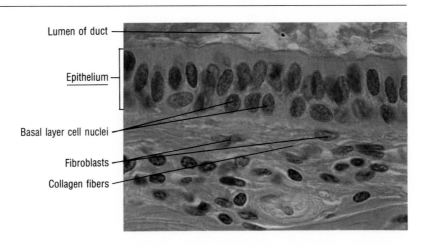

Lumen of duct

Epithelium

Basal layer cell nuclei

Fibroblasts

Collagen fibers

FIGURE 1.
Stratified columnar epithelium; excretory duct of a submaxillary gland; human; H&E; ×1000. Note that the nuclei come relatively close to the free edge of the epithelium. Compare with pseudostratified columnar epithelium (**Plate 3, Fig. 2**).

Stratified columnar epithelium

A surface layer of columnar cells rests on one or several layers of cells in this type of epithelium. This tissue is found in areas where there is a transition from pseudostratified columnar to stratified squamous epithelium. These intermediate areas are located in the pharynx, large ducts of the pancreas, and salivary and mammary glands. Stratified columnar epithelium is ciliated on the nasal surface of the soft palate and part of the larynx.

MORPHOLOGY. Stratified columnar epithelium has a basal layer of cuboidal cells; intermediate layers, if present, of polyhedral cells; and a surface layer of columnar cells. The oval, dark-stained nuclei occupy about 80 percent of the epithelium, and thus appear quite close to the free edge. This is an important diagnostic feature in distinguishing this epithelium from pseudostratified columnar epithelium (see below). **Plate 3, Fig. 1.**

Pseudostratified columnar epithelium

Although this tissue appears to be stratified, with several layers of columnar and basal cells lying at different levels, each cell is attached to a basement membrane. The tissue lines the epididymis, male urethra, and portions of excretory ducts draining the parotid glands. Pseudostratified columnar ciliated epithelium is present in the trachea, large bronchi, parts of the nasal cavity, and pharynx.

MORPHOLOGY. This tissue resembles stratified columnar epithelium (see above), and depending on the section it may be impossible to distinguish between the two. The following are generally true of pseudostratified columnar epithelium: (1) A prominent basement membrane is usually visible. (2) The nuclei are more varied; they are smaller and darker at the base of the epithelium and larger and lighter near the surface. (3) The nuclei occupy about 60 percent of the epithelium and do not come close to the free edge. (4) Careful focusing will reveal that most nuclei are usually not in the same focal plane. **Plate 3, Fig. 2.**

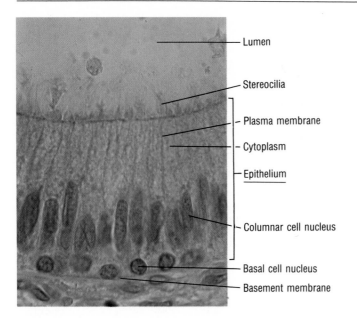

Lumen

Stereocilia

Plasma membrane

Cytoplasm

Epithelium

Columnar cell nucleus

Basal cell nucleus

Basement membrane

FIGURE 2.
Pseudostratified columnar epithelium;
human epididymis; H&E; ×1000. Note
that the nuclei do not come close to the
free edge of the epithelium; compare
with stratified columnar epithelium
(**Plate 3, Fig. 1**).

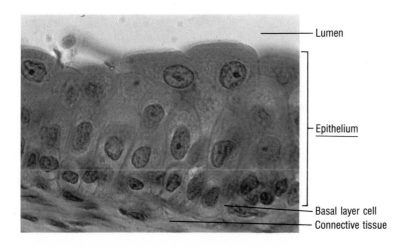

Lumen

Epithelium

Basal layer cell
Connective tissue

FIGURE 3.
Transitional epithelium; urinary blad-
der (relaxed); rhesus monkey; H&E;
×1000. Note the large, rounded cells
bulging into the lumen.

Transitional epithelium

This tissue is composed of several layers of cells, but its thickness is influenced by stretching or contraction of organs lined by it. These organs are the renal pelvis, urinary bladder, and ureters.

MORPHOLOGY. In the contracted state the epithelium is many layers thick. There is a basal layer of cuboidal or low columnar cells, an intermediate layer of polyhedral cells, and a surface layer with large rounded cells bulging into a lumen. If the epithelium is in the stretched or distended state, the upper cells become extensively flattened and the entire tissue appears to be one thin (two to five layers thick) stratified squamous layer. A typical stratified squamous epithelium, however, usually has more than 5 layers. **Plate 3, Fig. 3.**

Glandular epithelium

Exocrine glands are derived from epithelial tissue and function to secrete a variety of substances transformed from blood plasma. The secretions are dumped directly onto an epithelial surface via ducts rather than into the vascular system. The glands may be single cells located in an epithelium, or multicelled structures lying below an epithelium and connected to the surface by nonsecretory excretory ducts.

Exocrine glands may be composed of (1) *serous cells*, which secrete an aqueous albuminous substance, usually rich in enzymes; (2) *mucous cells*, which secrete a viscous mucus, an effective lubricant; (3) *seromucous cells*, which secrete both serous and mucous substances; or (4) a combination of both serous and mucous cells. Glands of the latter two categories are termed mixed glands. Exocrine glands release their secretions by one of three physical principles: in *holocrine* glands, the entire cell becomes part of the secretion; in *apocrine* glands, the apical ends of the cells' cytoplasm becomes part of the secretion; in *merocrine* glands there is no loss of the cytoplasm and secretions are released by exocytosis.

Cell morphology

MUCOUS CELLS. These cells may be found in the mucosal lining of the alimentary canal and respiratory system, either in the epithelium or glands within the lamina propria. They are also abundant in the submandibular and sublingual salivary glands. Mucous cells are relatively large, and are columnar, pyramidal, or goblet-shaped. Active mucous cells, stained with H&E, have a sparse basophilic cytoplasm filled with a colorless or pale-stained vacuolated mucigen; a flattened nucleus lies at the base of the cell. Inactive mucous cells resemble serous cells, except they lack basal striations (see below).

Mucigen is a glycoprotein, and as it is released from the apical end of the cell, it becomes a hydrated mucin. As mucin acquires water, inorganic salts, desquamated cells, and leucocytes, it becomes mucus, an effective lubricant. **Plate 4, Fig. 1.**

SEROUS CELLS. Among the various exocrine glands, serous cells are prominent in the pancreas and parotid salivary glands. They are smaller than mucous cells, they are pyramid-shaped, and the plasma membranes usually are not easily observed. The nuclei are spherical and may be eccentric or near the base of the cell. The cytoplasm is basophilic, and the base of the cell is stained darker than the apex. Concentrations of mitochondria, ribosomes, and ergastoplasm may appear as dark vertical striations at the base of the cell. Secretory granules (preenzyme zymogen granules in some cells) are located in the cytoplasm. The cells secrete a watery substance, usually rich in enzymes. **Plate 4, Fig. 2.**

SEROMUCOUS CELLS. These cells are present in the duodenal glands of Brunner, and are the mucous neck cells in the gastric glands of the stomach. Their products are intermediate between mucous and serous secretions. Cytologically they cannot be distinguished from mucous cells (see Chap. 12).

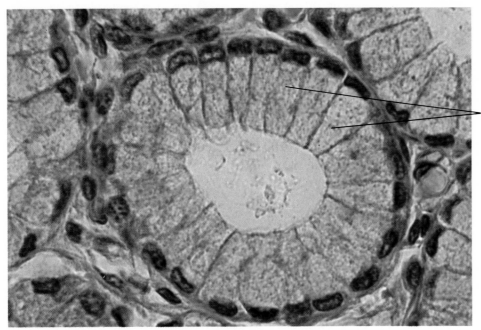

Mucous cells

FIGURE 1.
Mucous cells; submandibular gland; human; iron hematoxylin–methyl green; ×1000. Note the flat nuclei and the large lumen.

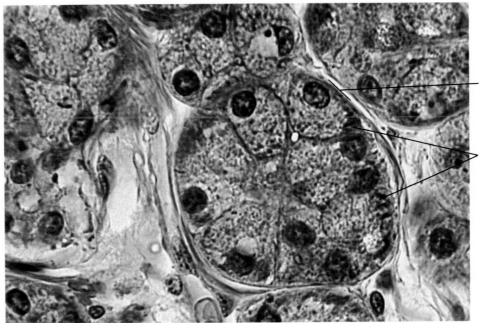

Serous cell

Basal striations

FIGURE 2.
Serous cells; submandibular gland; human; iron hematoxylin–methyl green; ×1000. Note the spherical nuclei, granular cytoplasm, and basal striations.

Exocrine gland morphology

UNICELLULAR EXOCRINE GLANDS (goblet cells). These are present as single cells in the simple epithelium of the oviduct, small intestine, and colon, and in the pseudostratified epithelium of the bronchi. They are goblet-shaped, mucus-secreting cells. The stem of the goblet rests on a basement membrane, and the upper, expanded portion is filled with mucigen. The flattened nucleus lies at the base of the cell and is surrounded by a deeply stained basophilic cytoplasm. (Refer to mucous cells). **Plate 5, Fig. 1.**

MULTICELLULAR EXOCRINE GLANDS. These may be an epithelial sheet of secreting cells; a localized concentration of mucous cells within an epithelial sheet and secreting into a common lumen (intraepithelial gland); or deep glands extending into underlying connective tissue but attached to the surface by excretory ducts. The *ducts* are lined by nonsecretory epithelium lying on a basal lamina. The epithelium is usually simple cuboidal, low columnar, or squamous in the small ducts but becomes pseudostratified to stratified in the larger ducts.

The *secretory portion or endpiece* of the gland may be tubular or saclike. The secretory epithelium rests on a basal lamina and lines the lumen of the gland. Secretions are released directly into the lumen from the apical ends of the cells, or indirectly by intercellular canaliculi. The canaliculi are formed by plasma membranes of adjacent cells and extend from the basal lamina to the lumen of the gland. They cannot be seen in routine histologic preparations.

If the secretory endpiece is composed of all mucous cells, the lumen will be large, but if only serous cells are present, the lumen is small. If the endpiece is mixed, containing both mucous and serous cells, the lumen will be relatively large and the ratios and distribution of the two cell types will vary according to the type of gland. In some mixed glands, where the mucous cells are most abundant, the serous cells are located at the end of the gland and may form small, peripheral, flattened, cresent-shaped caps, called *serous demilunes,* on the mucous cells. Secretions of the demilune cells reach the lumen of the gland through intercellular canaliculi. **Plate 5, Fig. 2.**

Classification of the deep exocrine glands is based on the architectural design of both the excretory ducts and secretory endpieces (see below).

Excretory ducts

Simple glands. An unbranched excretory duct connects the secretory endpieces to the epithelial surface.

Compound glands. The excretory duct branches as it connects many endpieces to the surface.

Secretory endpieces

Tubular. Secretory cells form a tubule, closed at one end, which may be unbranched, branched, or coiled.

Alveolar. Secretory cells form a hollow, spherical, saclike structure which may be branched or unbranched.

Tubuloalveolar. Secretory cells form both tubules and alveoli.

Using this nomenclature, the following types of glands may be identified:

Simple tubular (crypt of Lieberkühn). No excretory duct; secretory tubule opens directly onto the surface. **Plate 6, Fig. 1.**

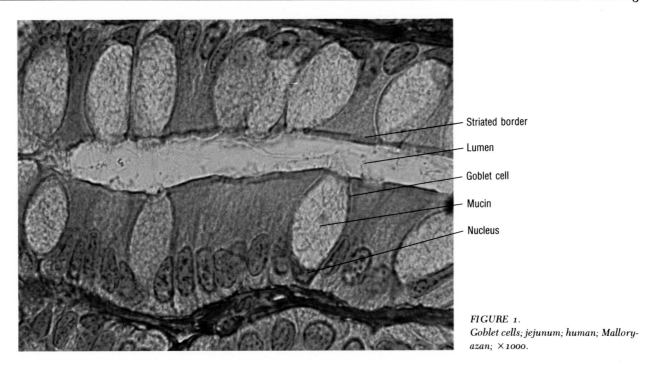

Striated border

Lumen

Goblet cell

Mucin

Nucleus

FIGURE 1.
Goblet cells; jejunum; human; Mallory-azan; ×1000.

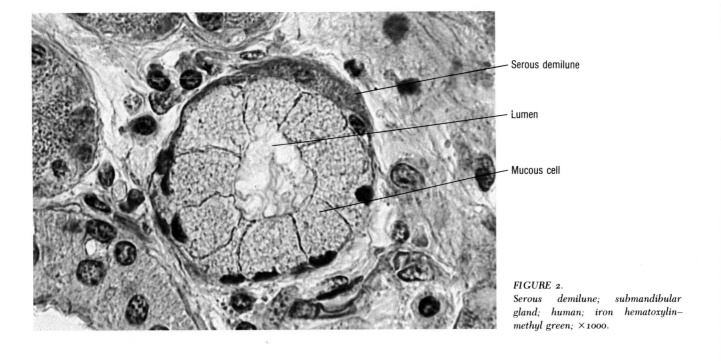

Serous demilune

Lumen

Mucous cell

FIGURE 2.
Serous demilune; submandibular gland; human; iron hematoxylin-methyl green; ×1000.

PLATE 6 _____

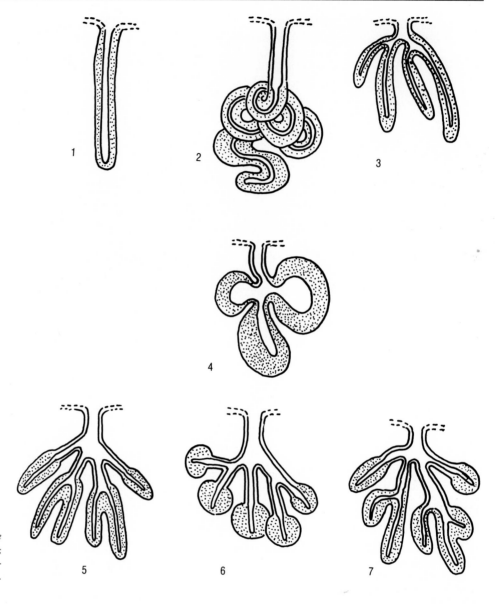

FIGURES 1–7.
Diagram of deep multicellular exocrine glands. Secretory portion is stippled; excretory ducts are unstippled; epithelial surface indicated by broken lines.

Simple coiled tubular (sweat gland). Long excretory duct; long coiled secretory tubule. **Plate 6, Fig. 2.**

Simple branched tubular (uterus, esophagus). Excretory duct short or absent; branched secretory tubules. **Plate 6, Fig. 3.**

Simple branched alveolar (sebaceous gland). Short excretory duct; several secretory alveoli. **Plate 6, Fig. 4.**

Compound tubular (testis). Long branched excretory duct; branched secretory tubules. **Plate 6, Fig. 5.**

Compound alveolar (respiratory tract). Branched excretory duct; many spherical alveoli. **Plate 6, Fig. 6.**

Compound tubuloalveolar (salivary glands, pancreas). Long branched excretory duct; irregularly branched secretory tubules connected with many alveoli. **Plate 6, Fig. 7.**

Connective Tissue 3

Connective tissues support and bind other tissues together. They may also store metabolic substances or repair damaged tissues. Unlike the specialized connective tissues of bone and cartilage, these tissues are nonrigid, relatively soft, and usually fibrous. All connective tissues contain fibers and cells embedded within a matrix of ground substance. Each tissue can be classified according to the concentration and arrangement of the types of fibers, the presence of few or many cell types, and the relative abundance of ground substance. Since classification is directly related to the identification of these components, their description shall precede the description of the types of connective tissue.

Cell types

MESENCHYME CELLS. These cells are fusiform or star-shaped (stellate), and the sparse cytoplasm is agranular and slightly basophilic. The cytoplasmic processes of adjacent cells touch to form a delicate network. The pale nucleus is very large and oval and contains small chromatin granules; one or two nucleoli are present. These are primitive cells with a multipotential to differentiate into other cell types. They are present in embryonic and some adult tissues. In the latter, mesenchyme cells usually occur along the walls of blood vessels and resemble fibroblasts, but they are smaller and the cytoplasm lacks granules (see below). **Plate 1, Fig. 1.**

PLATE 1

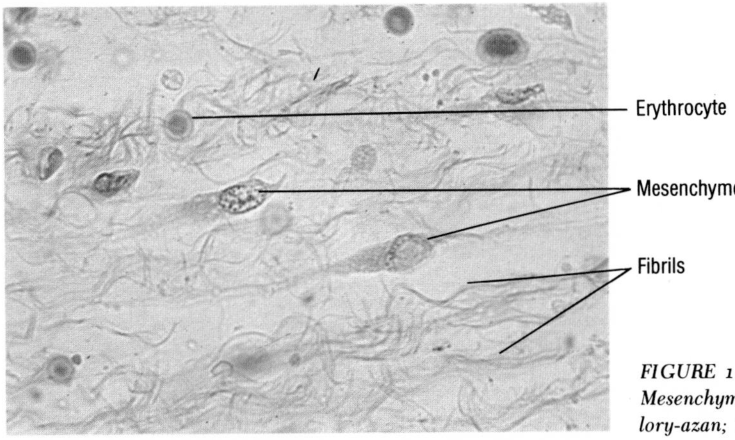

— Erythrocyte

— Mesenchyme cells

— Fibrils

FIGURE 1.
Mesenchyme cells; human fetus; Mallory-azan; ×1000.

PLATE 1 *continued*

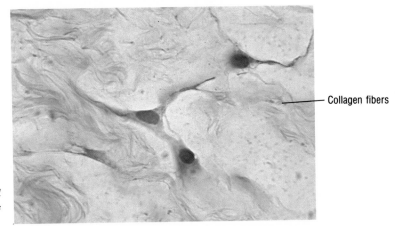

Collagen fibers

FIGURE 2.
Fibroblasts (active); human umbilical cord; H&E; ×1000. Note the granules in the cytoplasm of the fibroblasts.

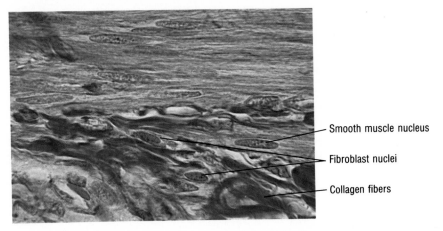

Smooth muscle nucleus

Fibroblast nuclei

Collagen fibers

FIGURE 3.
Fibroblasts (inactive); human scrotum; Mallory-azan; ×1000.

FIBROBLASTS. Young and active fibroblasts are large fusiform or attenuated cells with branched cytoplasmic processes. The abundant cytoplasm is basophilic and may be granular. The large, oval, pale-stained nucleus contains fine granules of chromatin and one or two nucleoli. The chromatin may be evenly distributed throughout the nucleoplasm. Fibroblasts are derived from mesenchymal cells (see above). They produce collagen fibers, ground substance, and probably elastic fibers. In growing or healing tissues, fibroblasts are active and capable of division, and can migrate through connective tissues. **Plate 1, Fig. 2.**

Inactive fibroblasts, designated as *fibrocytes* by some authors, are present in resting, nongrowing tissues. They are long, thin, flattened cells with an agranular, sparse cytoplasm which is clear or pale acidophilic. Since the cytoplasm usually is indistinct in a sectioned tissue, the cell may be identified only by a long, flat, dark-stained nucleus lying on a collagen fiber. **Plate 1, Fig. 3.**

RETICULAR CELLS. These cells resemble mesenchyme cells, from which they are derived. They may be stellate, flattened, or fusiform. The active cells have an abundant, moderately basophilic cytoplasm surrounding a large, oval, pale-stained vesicular nucleus. The inactive cells have a sparse and slightly acidophilic cytoplasm surrounding a somewhat flattened, elongate nucleus. Nucleoli are present in both active and inactive cells. The reticular cells may produce reticular fibers or, if stimulated, become somewhat phagocytic. They are abundant in lymphoid tissues and may be found lying along reticular fibers (see below). **Plate 2, Fig. 1.**

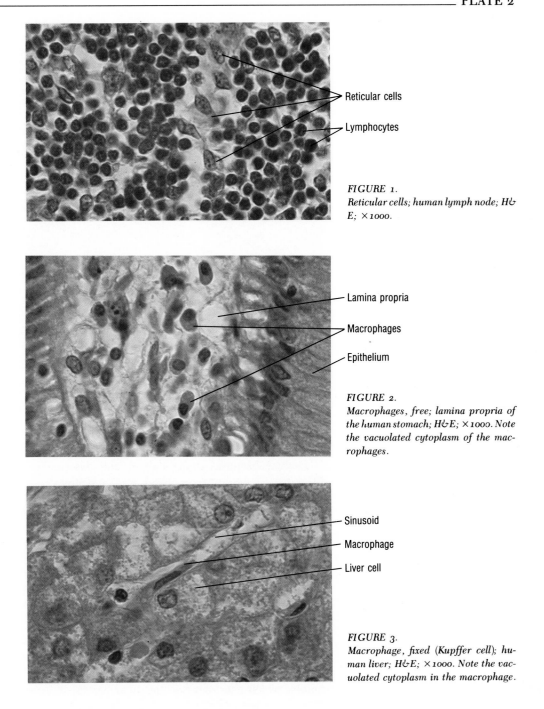

FIGURE 1.
Reticular cells; human lymph node; H&
E; ×1000.

FIGURE 2.
Macrophages, free; lamina propria of
the human stomach; H&E; ×1000. Note
the vacuolated cytoplasm of the mac-
rophages.

FIGURE 3.
Macrophage, fixed (Kupffer cell); hu-
man liver; H&E; ×1000. Note the vac-
uolated cytoplasm in the macrophage.

MACROPHAGES. These cells may be classified either as fixed (nonmigratory) or free (migratory) macrophages. *Fixed macrophages* (histiocytes) are fusiform, are usually stretched along fibers, and tend to resemble fibroblasts. The cytoplasm is basophilic and usually filled with granules, vacuoles, and debris because of the phagocytic nature of the cells. Short, blunt pseudopods are present, but are usually not visible in histological sections. The dark-stained, oval nucleus is of small to moderate size, indented on one side, and filled with clumps of heterochromatin; nucleoli are present, but not conspicuous. *Free macrophages* are cytologically similar to the fixed ones, but because they migrate through tissues and are not attached to fibers, they appear rounded rather than elongate (see Chap. 8). **Plate 2, Figs. 2 and 3.**

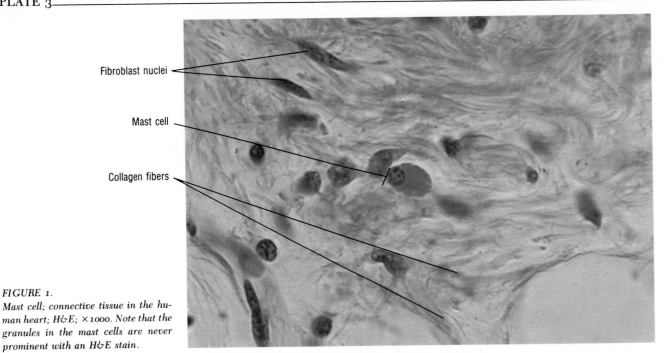

Fibroblast nuclei

Mast cell

Collagen fibers

FIGURE 1.
Mast cell; connective tissue in the human heart; H&E; ×1000. Note that the granules in the mast cells are never prominent with an H&E stain.

Under certain conditions, such as inflammation or tissue damage, fixed macrophages may be stimulated to become free macrophages. Although both types phagocytize bacteria, tissue debris, and dead cells, free macrophages are more efficient scavengers. Macrophages also contribute to the immunologic processes by phagocytizing and processing antigens in preparation for immunologic responses by lymphocytes and plasma cells (see Chaps. 7, 8).

Macrophages may be derived from preexisting macrophages or from monocytes, which in turn are derived from promonocyte precursors in bone marrow. Macrophages are the phagocytic cells of the *reticuloendothelial*, or *macrophage*, *system* which lines the sinusoids and sinuses in certain organs. They are the *Kupffer cells* in the liver sinusoids, *alveolar macrophages* in the alveoli of lungs, and *microglial cells* in the central nervous system.

MAST CELLS. These are large cells, about 15 μm in diameter, which are oval, round, or irregularly shaped. The cytoplasm is filled with prominent basophilic granules which may obscure the relatively small, round nucleus. The granules are not prominent in H&E–stained preparations because they do not stain well with hematoxylin and are water soluble. They are quite visible and appear purplish red with metachromatic dyes such as toluidine blue. The granules contain heparin (an anticoagulant), histamine (a vasodilator which also increases capillary permeability), and serotonin (a vasoconstrictor). Although mast cells may be designated as "tissue basophils" because they resemble basophil leucocytes, their origin and relationship to the basophil leucocytes are unknown. **Plate 3, Fig. 1.**

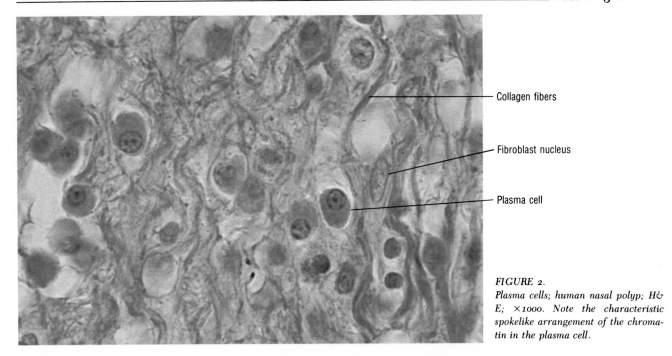

— Collagen fibers

— Fibroblast nucleus

— Plasma cell

FIGURE 2.
Plasma cells; human nasal polyp; H&
E; ×1000. Note the characteristic
spokelike arrangement of the chroma-
tin in the plasma cell.

LEUCOCYTES (neutrophils, eosinophils, lymphocytes, and monocytes). These leucocytes may be present as additional cell types in connective tissue. Their detailed morphology and function will be found in Chaps. 7 and 8. Leucocytes migrate into connective tissues from adjacent blood and lymphatic vessels, but only the lymphocytes and monocytes can reproduce in these regions.

PLASMA CELLS. These cells are normally present in the lamina propria of the alimentary canal, lymphoid tissue, or in any connective tissue with a chronic inflammation. They are derived from large lymphocytes (lymphoblasts, which in turn are derived from antigen-stimulated B lymphocytes) and produce immunoglobulins. The cells are oval-shaped and have a deeply stained basophilic cytoplasm, except for a pale region adjacent to the nucleus. The small, round, eccentric nucleus usually has coarse chromatin arranged like spokes on a wheel. Further morphology and function of these cells are described in Chap. 8. **Plate 3, Fig. 2.**

ADIPOSE CELLS (fat cells). There are two types of fat cells, white and brown. *Brown fat cells* are common to brown adipose tissue and have limited distribution (see below). They are relatively small polygon-shaped cells. The spherical nucleus is usually eccentrically positioned in an extensive granular cytoplasm filled with many lipid droplets and particles of glycogen. In the living animal the cells may appear brown or tan, probably because of a high concentration of pigmented cytochromes within the numerous large mitochondria. **Plate 4, Fig. 1.** *White fat cells* are large spherical or polygon-shaped cells, appearing either in clusters or singly in loose

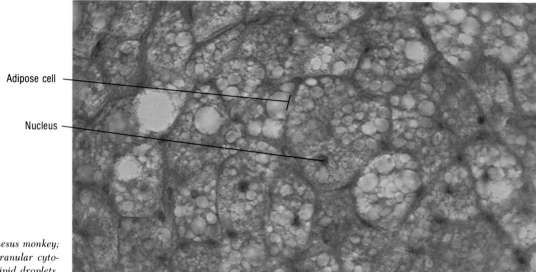

Adipose cell

Nucleus

FIGURE 1.
Adipose cells (brown); rhesus monkey; H&E; ×400. Note the granular cytoplasm containing many lipid droplets.

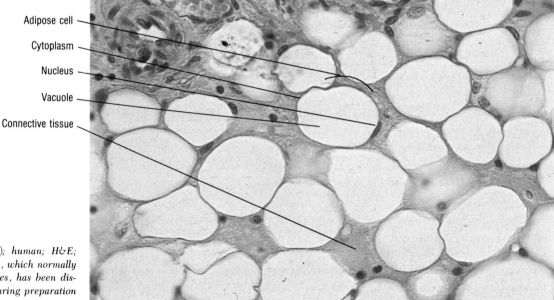

Adipose cell

Cytoplasm

Nucleus

Vacuole

Connective tissue

FIGURE 2.
Adipose cells (white); human; H&E; ×1000. Note that fat, which normally fills the large vacuoles, has been dissolved by solvents during preparation of the tissue.

connective tissue (see below). They are widespread and form the major component in white adipose tissue (see below). The cytoplasm forms a thin ring around a single large vacuole filled with fat. The flattened nucleus is located in the peripheral ring of cytoplasm and forms a slight bulge. Since the fat is dissolved by solvents during the preparation of routine sections, the cell appears as a thin, pale-stained ring of cytoplasm surrounding an empty vacuole. White fat cells are nonmitotic; therefore new cells differentiate from mesenchymal cells. The fusiform-shaped mesenchyme cells first produce many small lipid droplets in their cytoplasm, but eventually the droplets coalesce to become the single large, fat-filled vacuole. **Plate 4, Fig. 2.**

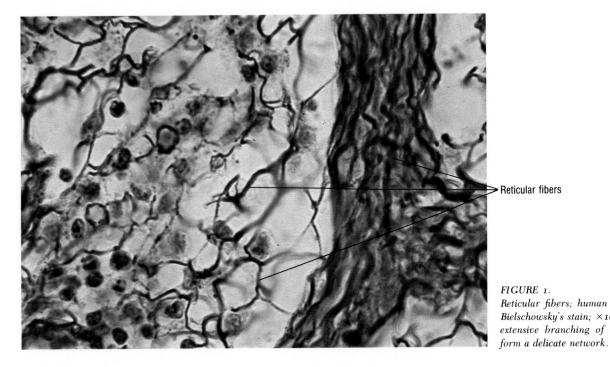

Reticular fibers

FIGURE 1.
Reticular fibers; human lymph node; Bielschowsky's stain; × 1000. Note the extensive branching of the fibers to form a delicate network.

Ground substance

GROUND SUBSTANCE. Fibers and cells are embedded within an amorphous jellylike ground substance. Ground substance will stain metachromatically with certain stains (toluidine), but since it is easily removed by fixatives, it will not be visible in routinely fixed and stained sections. Ground substance contains water, inorganic compounds, proteins, and high concentrations of glycosaminoglycans (polysaccharides containing amino sugars). The latter are in the form of (1) hyaluronic acid, which functions as a lubricant and shock absorber; and (2) chondroitin sulfates A, B, and C, and keratosulfate, which provides resiliency to the ground substance. In addition to the functions already indicated, the glycosaminoglycans are directly related to the viscosity of the ground substance and will vary in proportions according to the type of connective tissue.

Fibers

RETICULAR FIBERS. These are delicate collagen fibers, about 0.5 to 1.0 μm in diameter. Unlike the thicker collagen fibers, reticular fibers branch freely and anastomose to form a delicate network or reticulum; they are also covered by a thin coat of glycosaminoglycans. The fibers do not stain well with H&E, but since the coat will appear black by reacting with silver stains, they are designated as argyrophilic fibers. Reticular fibers may precede collagen fibers during development or healing of wounds. They provide strength and support for delicate tissues. **Plate 5, Fig. 1.**

PLATE 5 *continued*

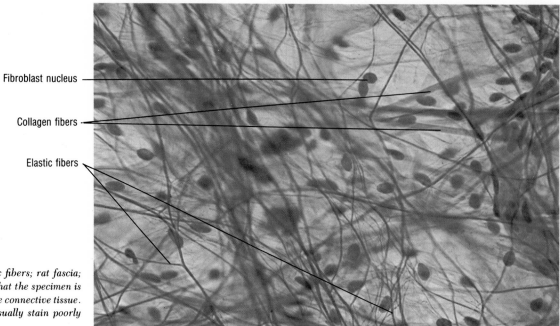

Fibroblast nucleus

Collagen fibers

Elastic fibers

FIGURE 2.
*Collagen and elastic fibers; rat fascia;
H&E; ×400. Note that the specimen is
an example of a loose connective tissue.
The elastic fibers usually stain poorly
with H&E.*

COLLAGEN FIBERS. These are thick (1 to 12 μm in diameter), wavy, longitudinal bundles of many thin fibrils of tropocollagen, bound together by an organic cement. The fibrils are about 0.4 μm in diameter, unbranched, and have a periodic banding along their length. The bands, however, are not visible with the light microscope. The fibers frequently branch and anastomose to form a coarse network. They have a high tensile strength and are common in areas where tension forces are exerted on tissues. In H&E–stained sections, the fibers appear pink and either delicately striated or homogeneous. **Plate 5, Fig. 2.**

ELASTIC FIBERS. These coiled and higly branched fibers are thinner than collagen fibers. They form an elastic network of many fused fibers. Although the proteinaceous elastic fibers are composed of microfibrils embedded within an amorphous elastin matrix, they appear homogeneous with the light microscope. The fibers are synthesized by fibroblasts and smooth muscle cells. Elastin usually stains pale pink or not at all with H&E, but appears dark brown with selective stains, such as the Taenzer-Unna orcein elastic stain. Elastic fibers may be stretched but will return to their original length when the tension is released. **Plate 5, Fig. 2.**

Types of connective tissue

The classification of connective tissue may be based on the relative proportions of cells and fiber types, and the abundance of ground substance. From these criteria the following classifications may be considered.

1 *Loose connective tissue.* Low density of fibers, high density of cells with an abundant ground substance; many different cell and fiber types.

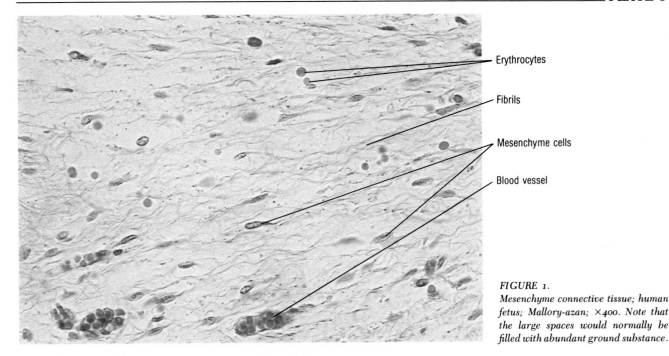

Erythrocytes

Fibrils

Mesenchyme cells

Blood vessel

FIGURE 1.
Mesenchyme connective tissue; human fetus; Mallory-azan; ×400. Note that the large spaces would normally be filled with abundant ground substance.

2 *Dense connective tissue.* High density of fibers, low density of cells with a relatively small amount of ground substance; different fiber and cell types are limited. Depending on the type of fibers and their arrangement, *regular* (orderly and almost parallel) or *irregular* (random and nonparallel), the dense connective tissue may be further classified into four categories: *dense, regular collagenous; dense, irregular collagenous; dense, regular elastic; dense, irregular elastic.*

3 *Reticular tissue.* Reticular fibers and reticular cells within an abundant ground substance.

4 *Adipose tissue.* A high density of adipose cells and a low density of reticular fibers within a small amount of ground substance.

5 *Mesenchyme tissue.* A low density of mesenchyme cells and an abundant ground substance. The early embryonic tissue has no fibers, but in older tissue a few scattered, delicate fibrils are present.

6 *Mucous tissue.* A low density of fibroblasts and collagen fibers within an abundant ground substance.

MESENCHYME TISSUE. The components are an abundant fluidlike ground substance containing mesenchyme cells; delicate fibrils may be present (see above). The tissue is present in early embryos, filling the spaces between organs and other tissues. Although the tissue appears as a delicate reticulum, the adjacent cytoplasmic processes of the mesenchyme cells touch but are not fused. Mesenchyme cells are multipotential and can differentiate during later development to give rise to cells of various types: blood, muscle, adipose, mast, sheath of Schwann, fibroblasts, reticular cells, osteoblasts, and chondroblasts. Mesenchyme cells retain some of their multipotential characteristics in the adult and are occasionally present in loose connective tissue associated with capillaries. **Plate 6, Fig. 1.**

PLATE 6 continued

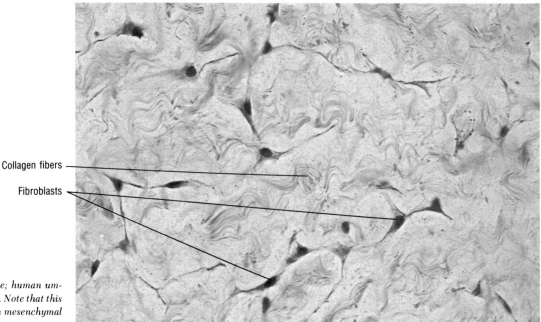

Collagen fibers

Fibroblasts

FIGURE 2.
Mucous connective tissue; human umbilical cord; H&E; ×400. Note that this tissue is more dense than mesenchymal connective tissue.

MUCOUS TISSUE. The major components are an abundant ground substance, some fibroblast cells, and collagen fibers. The fibroblasts are stellate cells with cytoplasmic processes which may form a delicate reticulum. Although fibroblasts are the common cell type, macrophages and lymphocytes may also be present (see above for their descriptions). During development of the embryo, mucous tissue is derived from an earlier mesenchymal connective tissue. It represents an intermediate stage of connective tissue development. Although it contains relatively few fibers in the early developmental stages, it will become more fibrous in later development. Mucous connective tissue is abundant under embryonic skin and packs the umbilical cord as *Wharton's jelly*. Normally, it is absent in the adult *Homo sapiens*. **Plate 6, Fig. 2.**

RETICULAR TISSUE. The components of this tissue are reticular cells, reticular fibers, and an abundant ground substance. The tissue is a delicate, branching network of reticular fibers with reticular cells lying along the fibers. It forms a framework to support bone marrow, lymphoid tissues, lymphoid nodules, and lymphoid organs (spleen, tonsils, and lymph nodes). **Plate 7, Fig. 1.**

LOOSE (AREOLAR) CONNECTIVE TISSUE. The major components are collagen fibers, fibroblasts, macrophages, and ground substance. In addition, to a lesser degree, there are also elastic fibers, reticular fibers, and reticular and mesenchyme cells. Other cell types, such as adipose cells, mast cells, neutrophils, eosinophils, monocytes, lymphocytes, and plasma cells, may also be present. This tissue is characterized by an irregular network of relatively few thin fibers containing large spaces filled with an abundant ground substance and many cells. It provides support, binds tissues together, and allows some degree of flexibility in organs. Although loose connective tissue is widespread, it is abundant in the subcutaneous layer of the skin and lamina propria of the alimentary canal and respiratory system. Loose

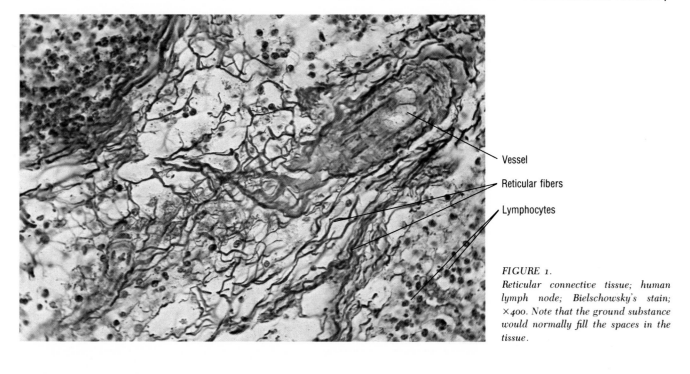

Vessel

Reticular fibers

Lymphocytes

FIGURE 1.
Reticular connective tissue; human lymph node; Bielschowsky's stain; ×400. Note that the ground substance would normally fill the spaces in the tissue.

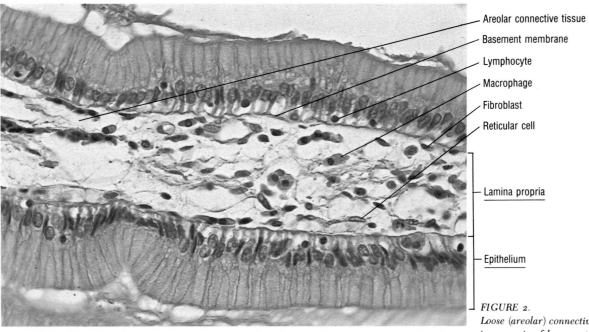

Areolar connective tissue

Basement membrane

Lymphocyte

Macrophage

Fibroblast

Reticular cell

Lamina propria

Epithelium

FIGURE 2.
Loose (areolar) connective tissue; lamina propria of human stomach; H&E; ×400. Note that the specimen is a fold of the cardiac mucosa of the stomach, separating two gastric pits. Note the many spaces and numerous cell types in this connective tissue.

connective tissue also forms the stroma of various organs and surrounds blood vessels and nerves. **Plate 7, Fig. 2.**

DENSE, IRREGULAR COLLAGENOUS CONNECTIVE TISSUE. The major components are collagen fibers and fibroblasts. The tissue is a dense, irregular network of coarse collagen bundles within a moderately abundant ground substance. Compared to loose connective tissue, the interspaces of the network are tiny and the fibroblasts

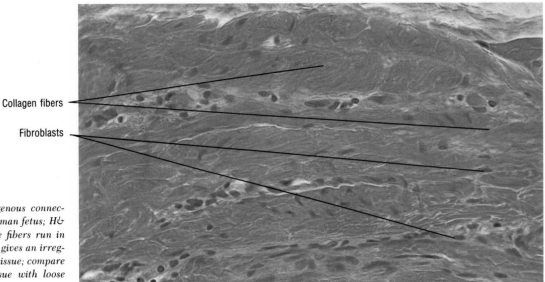

Collagen fibers —

Fibroblasts —

FIGURE 1.
Dense, irregular collagenous connec-
tive tissue; dermis of human fetus; H&
E; ×400. Note that the fibers run in
many directions, which gives an irreg-
ular appearance to the tissue; compare
the density of this tissue with loose
connective tissue.

are flattened. The tissue is present in the dermis, capsules of certain organs, periosteum, and other structures which resist tension stresses in any direction. **Plate 8, Fig. 1.**

DENSE, REGULAR COLLAGENOUS CONNECTIVE TISSUE. The major components are collagen fibers and fibroblasts. This tissue is a tightly packed concentration of parallel collagen fibers. Ground substance is scarce, and the cells may only be seen flattened in spaces between the fibers. This tissue is organized to resist tension stresses in one direction and is characteristic of tendons, ligaments, and aponeuroses. In *tendons* (**Plate 8, Fig. 2**), coarse fibers, about 35 μm in diameter, are separated from others by delicate networks of elastic tissue. The fibroblasts appear as rows of flattened, rod-shaped cells, *tendon cells*, lying between the fibers. Several fibers are organized into bundles or fasciculi by thin strands of loose connective tissue, the *endotendineum*. In the larger tendons groups of fasciculi are held together, but separated from other groups, by thick septa of loose connective tissue, the *peritendineum*. The entire tendon is covered by a fibrous sheath of dense, irregular collagenous connective tissue, the *epitendineum*. Blood vessels and nerves are carried throughout the tendon within these connective tissue sheaths, but do not enter the fasciculi. *Aponeuroses* are similar to tendons, except they are flat sheets of tissue subdivided into several layers. The fibers of one layer run in a direction that is different from fibers of adjacent layers. This type of organization contributes to the strength of the aponeurosis. *Ligaments* are also similar to tendons, except the fibers tend to be thicker and more irregularly arranged. The fibroblasts are less numerous than in the tendon, and they also appear irregularly arranged as they lie between the fibers.

DENSE, IRREGULAR ELASTIC CONNECTIVE TISSUE. This tissue is a dense, irregular network of elastic fibers and fibroblasts embedded within a sparse ground substance. This type of tissue is present in the walls of large arteries as spiral fenestrated membranes. It is also present in Scarpa's fascia, a supporting superficial layer on the lower part of the abdominal wall. Elastic tissue functions to return organs to their original shape after they have been stretched. **Plate 9, Figs. 1 and 2.**

PLATE 8 *continued*

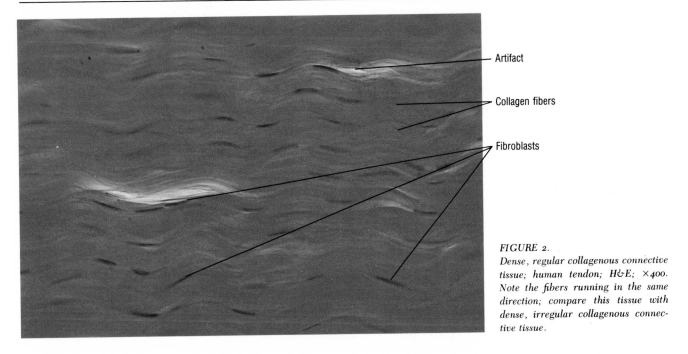

Artifact

Collagen fibers

Fibroblasts

FIGURE 2.
Dense, regular collagenous connective tissue; human tendon; H&E; ×400. Note the fibers running in the same direction; compare this tissue with dense, irregular collagenous connective tissue.

PLATE 9

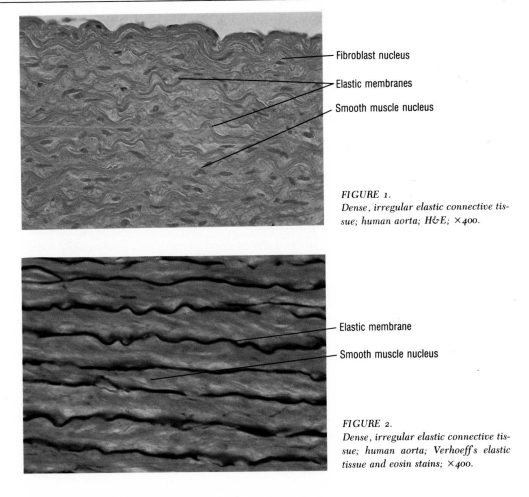

Fibroblast nucleus

Elastic membranes

Smooth muscle nucleus

FIGURE 1.
Dense, irregular elastic connective tissue; human aorta; H&E; ×400.

Elastic membrane

Smooth muscle nucleus

FIGURE 2.
Dense, irregular elastic connective tissue; human aorta; Verhoeff's elastic tissue and eosin stains; ×400.

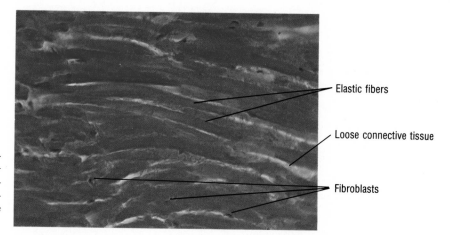

Elastic fibers

Loose connective tissue

Fibroblasts

FIGURE 3.
Dense, regular elastic connective tissue; ligamentum nuchae of a cow; H&E; ×400. Note that the fibers are relatively straight and not "wavy"; compare with dense, regular collagenous connective tissue.

DENSE, REGULAR ELASTIC CONNECTIVE TISSUE. The components are elastic fibers, fibroblasts, and sparse ground substance. The fibers are thick and somewhat regularly arranged, but unlike collagenous tissue, they are not wavy, may form acute branches which fuse with branches of other fibers, and have relatively few fibroblasts. The fibers are surrounded by a delicate reticulum of loose connective tissue which may bind them into bundles. The loose connective tissue may be seen in spaces between the fibers and bundles. Dense, regular elastic connective tissue is found in the ligamenta flava of the vertebral column, in the vocal cords, and in the ligamentum nuchae of quadrupeds. These structures can be stretched but will return to their resting positions because of their elasticity. **Plate 9, Fig. 3.**

ADIPOSE TISSUE. There are two types of adipose tissue which occur in the human: brown and white. *Brown adipose tissue* (**Plate 10, Fig. 1**) is abundant in the fetus and present in young individuals, but is scarce or may be absent in the adult. In the adult it may be present in the axillae, near the thyroid gland, or within the renal hilus. The tissue is lobulated, pigmented, richly vascularized, and it may appear somewhat glandular. The cells are multilocular with many small vacuoles of fat in the cytoplasm (see above). They are surrounded by a delicate network of reticular and collagen fibers. This tissue, unlike white adipose tissue, is not easily influenced by changes in fat metabolism or nutritional states. Its function in the human is questionable.

In H&S–stained preparations *white adipose tissue* (**Plate 10, Fig. 2**) appears as a tightly packed group of polygonal or rounded, thin-walled cells of various sizes which once contained lipid. Although adipose cells are supported mostly by reticular fibers, these fibers usually are not visible in routine preparations. Capillaries, other cells (fibroblasts and macrophages), and collagen and elastic fibers may also be present in the relatively scarce ground substance.

Although loose connective tissue has various amounts of adipose cells, a typical adipose tissue is characterized by a high concentration of these cells. The tissue is a storage depot for fat, provides a degree of mechanical protection, and is an excellent insulator against changes in environmental temperature. White adipose tissue is widespread and can be found in the mesenteries, omentum, and subcutaneous layer as the panniculus adiposus. It also surrounds the gonads and kidneys.

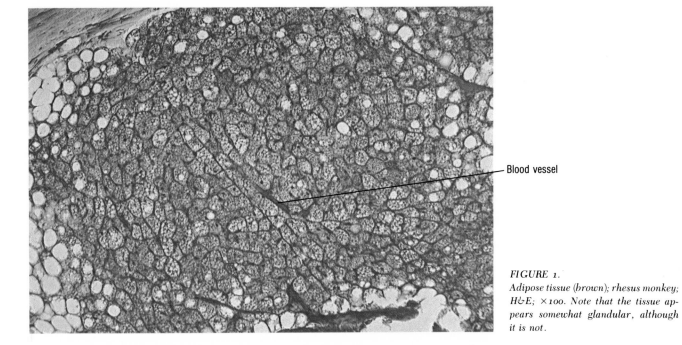

Blood vessel

FIGURE 1.
Adipose tissue (brown); rhesus monkey;
H&E; ×100. Note that the tissue ap-
pears somewhat glandular, although
it is not.

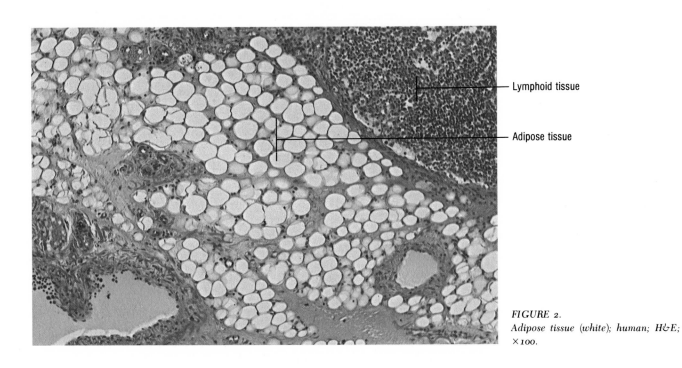

Lymphoid tissue

Adipose tissue

FIGURE 2.
Adipose tissue (white); human; H&E;
×100.

Cartilage and Bone 4

Cartilage and bone are specialized rigid or semirigid connective tissues which provide structural support to other tissues. Although they are somewhat resilient, both resist tensile, compression, and shearing forces. They are similar to other connective tissues in that they have a cell-filled amorphous matrix composed of ground substance and fibers. Unlike cartilage and the general connective tissues, bone is hard because of the presence of inorganic salts in its matrix.

Cartilage

There are three types of cartilage: *hyaline*, *fibrocartilage*, and *elastic*. Each is classified by the amount and types of fibers within the matrix. Most cartilages have a basic organization of a fibrous *perichondrium* surrounding a matrix filled with cells, the *chondrocytes*. Fibrocartilage and articular hyaline cartilage, however, lack a perichondrium. All cartilages are avascular, and so nutrients, oxygen, and wastes must diffuse between blood vessels in the perichondrium and chondrocytes in the matrix. Cartilage grows as chondrocytes produce new cartilage within the interior of the mass (interstitial growth), and chondroblasts (immature chondrocytes) produce cartilage on the surface (appositional growth).

PERICHONDRIUM. This is a thin, fibrous layer surrounding the matrix. It is divided into an inner and outer region. Its inner region, next to the matrix, is chondrogenic and contains mesenchyme cells which can differentiate into chondroblasts. The mesenchyme cells are irregular in shape, have scanty basophilic cytoplasm, and have a large, pale, oval-shaped nucleus with several nucleoli. This inner region may not be prominent in adult cartilage, but does retain its chondrogenic potential. The outer region does not contribute to cartilage growth. It is composed of a dense layer of irregular collagenous fibers and fibroblasts. **Plate 1, Figs. 1** and **2**.

MATRIX. This is a prominent component of cartilage, appearing as a homogeneous substance, filled with *lacunae* (holes) containing chondrocytes. It is composed of an organic ground substance and collagen or elastic fibers. The ground substance

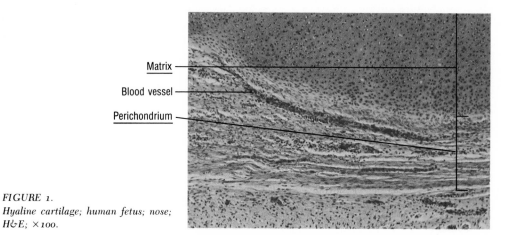

Matrix
Blood vessel
Perichondrium

FIGURE 1.
Hyaline cartilage; human fetus; nose;
H&E; ×100.

contains basophilic chondromucoprotein (a copolymer of mucoprotein plus acidic chondroitin sulfates A and C). The fibers form dense, anastomosing networks in the matrix, but are usually inconspicuous in an H&E preparation. Depending on age, growth, or regeneration, the matrix may be either acidophilic or basophilic. In nonactive or young regions of cartilage the matrix may be acidophilic or slightly basophilic. This is due to low concentrations of chondromucoprotein which reveal acidophilic fibers. Also, in adult cartilage, the accumulation of a basic albuminoid substance adds to the acidophilic characteristic of the matrix. In growing or regenerating cartilage, the matrix is basophilic because of high concentrations of chondromucoprotein. The regions of matrix immediately surrounding the lacunae, the *capsules*, are deeply stained because they represent the newest cartilage produced by the chondrocytes. **Plate 1, Figs. 1, 2** and **3.**

CHONDROBLASTS. These are immature chondrocytes. They are prominent and functional during appositional growth of fetal cartilage or regeneration in adult cartilage. Chondroblasts lie just below the perichondrium. They are derived from mesenchyme cells and will differentiate into chondrocytes. They are rounded or somewhat flattened and smaller than the mesenchymal cells. The large, pale, oval or round nucleus contains nucleoli and is surrounded by pale basophilic cytoplasm. The cells secrete a thin, pale-stained matrix with inconspicuous lacunae. **Plate 1, Fig. 2.**

CHONDROCYTES. These cells, like chondroblasts, are matrix-producing cells. They may appear in one of several forms depending on their maturity and position in the cartilage. Young cells may be found under the chondroblast layer in fetal cartilage or under active perichondrium of adult cartilage. They are small, slightly flattened cells with prominent lacunae. The cells may be embedded within a pale acidophilic or basophilic matrix. The cytoplasm is slightly acidophilic, and surrounds a relatively small, dense nucleus containing one or more nucleoli. As young chondrocytes mature, they become larger (approximately up to 34 μm) and more spherical, and lie deeper within the matrix. The cytoplasm will become more acidophilic and vacuolated with fat and glycogen. Mature chondrocytes may also appear flattened, especially in cartilage on articulating surfaces, such as joints. Unfortunately, because of dehydration optimal chondrocyte morphology is lacking in routine H&E sections.

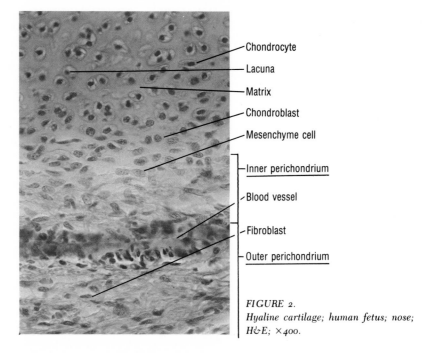

Chondrocyte

Lacuna

Matrix

Chondroblast

Mesenchyme cell

Inner perichondrium

Blood vessel

Fibroblast

Outer perichondrium

FIGURE 2.
Hyaline cartilage; human fetus; nose;
H&E; ×400.

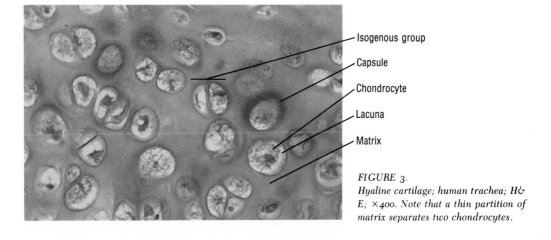

Isogenous group

Capsule

Chondrocyte

Lacuna

Matrix

FIGURE 3.
Hyaline cartilage; human trachea; H&
E; ×400. Note that a thin partition of
matrix separates two chondrocytes.

The chondrocytes usually appear as shrunken, distorted, stellate structures lying within partially filled lacunae. **Plate 1, Figs. 2 and 3.**

Interstitial growth occurs only in young cartilage having a pliable matrix with a low collagen content and prolific matrix-producing chondrocytes. Only in the most mature chondrocytes (hypertrophied cells), are these chondrogenic abilities lost. During interstitial growth a dividing chondrocyte may form a small group of daughter cells, an *isogenous group*, within one lacuna. Each cell is quickly separated from others in the group by secreting thin partitions of intercellular matrix. In the early stages of development the isogenous group is surrounded by a common *capsule*, but as matrix is secreted and the chondrocytes move apart, the capsule is lost. Each chondrocyte will develop its own capsule as it continues to produce matrix. **Plate 1, Fig. 3.**

PLATE 2 _____

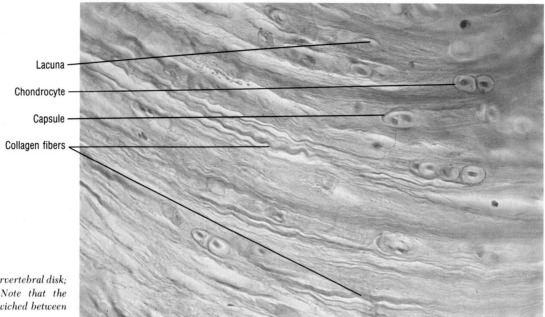

Lacuna ———
Chondrocyte ———
Capsule ———
Collagen fibers ———

FIGURE 1.
Fibrocartilage; rat; intervertebral disk;
Mallory-azan; ×400. Note that the
chondrocytes are sandwiched between
collagen fibers.

HYALINE CARTILAGE. This is the most widespread type of cartilage in both the embryo and adult. It reduces friction between articulating bones and provides a temporary model on which endochondral bones develop. Hyaline cartilage is present in the larger respiratory tubes, costal cartilages, articular ends of long bones, and developing endochondral bones.

Morphology. The matrix is a basophilic or acidophilic homogeneous structure containing lacunae, capsules, and chondrocytes. Although collagen fibers are present in the abundant ground substance, they usually are not visible. Except for articular surfaces, all hyaline cartilages have a perichondrium. **Plate 1, Figs. 1, 2,** and **3.**

FIBROCARTILAGE. This is a unique tissue, sharing characteristics of both hyaline cartilage and collagenous connective tissue. Therefore it is usually located in transitional regions between these two tissue types. Fibrocartilage has many parallel collagen fibers which are structurally suited to resist tension forces. It is present in public symphyses, intervertebral disks, and especially around joints where tendons insert onto bone.

Morphology. At first the tissue resembles dense, irregular collagenous connective tissue because of the prominent fibrous bundles, but matrix and chondrocytes are inconspicuously sandwiched between these bundles. The chondrocytes, within their lacunae and surrounding capsules, may appear separately or be organized into rows. A perichondrium is lacking. **Plate 2, Fig. 1.**

ELASTIC CARTILAGE. As the name implies, elastic cartilage is quite flexible. It is important in providing support to organs which can return to their original shape

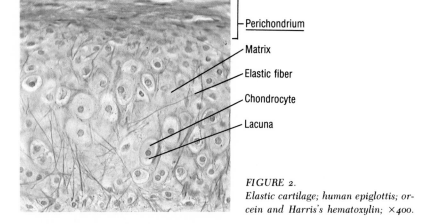

- Perichondrium
- Matrix
- Elastic fiber
- Chondrocyte
- Lacuna

FIGURE 2.
Elastic cartilage; human epiglottis; orcein and Harris's hematoxylin; ×400.

after being stretched; for example, the larynx, epiglottis, eustachian tube, and pinna. It is built on the same plan as hyaline cartilage, but the major difference is that elastic fibers are in the ground substance.

Morphology. Chondrocytes, lacunae, and capsules are well defined in peripheral regions of elastic cartilage, but within the interior they may be hidden by dense elastic fibers. Elastic fibers are highly branched, coiled strands of irregular diameter which form a dense network around the capsules. They course randomly in the ground substance and invade the perichondrium. The fibers appear dark brown with Taenzer-Unna orcein stain and black with Weigert's elastic stain. With general stains such as H&E, they stain poorly (pale pink), or not at all. **Plate 2, Fig. 2.**

Bone

Bone is the most rigid and hardest of all the supporting tissues in the body. It is adapted to resist tension, compression, and shearing forces more effectively than cartilage because its ground substance is impregnated with inorganic salts. Apart from hardness, marrow cavities, blood vessels, and nerves, bone otherwise resembles cartilage. It has a fibrous layer, the periosteum, which surrounds a matrix containing cells, the osteocytes.

There are two major types of bone development in the body: *endochondral* (intracartilaginous) and *intramembranous*. In endochondral bones (all bones of the skeleton except the roof of the skull, clavicle, and sesamoid bones), a hyaline cartilage model precedes development, but is eventually replaced by ossified tissue. Intramembranous or membrane bones, on the other hand, first appear as ossified spicules in a condensed bed of mesenchyme. Later, these spicules fuse into a definitive bone; examples are the clavicle, roof of the skull, and anterior part of the mandible.

The development, growth, and maintenance of cartilage and bone are under the combined influence of hormones and vitamins: *somatotropin* (regulates cartilage growth and chondrocyte metabolism); *thyroxine* (regulates normal skeletal development); *cortisone* (retards maturation of cartilage); *estrogen* (promotes fibrillogenesis in cartilage); *testosterone* (influences cartilage anabolism and maturation); *parathor-mone* and *calcitonin* (regulates normal bone resorption); *vitamin D* (promotes calcification of bone and cartilage and aids calcium absorption from the digestive tract); *vitamin C* (important for the synthesis of collagen and ground substance); *vitamin A* (promotes normal skeletal growth by maintaining epiphyseal cartilage plates, see below).

Bones may develop from one or more centers of ossification. If a bone has multiple centers, such as the tibia, a *primary center* is the first to appear. It will be active in the long growth of bone and ossification of the shaft (diaphysis). *Secondary centers* usually appear after birth and are responsible for the ossification of the ends of bone (epiphyses). In a long bone (tibia) there are three distinct morphological areas:

1 *Epiphyses* (singular, epiphysis). These are the ends of the bone. In early development they are separated from the shaft by cartilage. Later they fuse to the shaft and become part of the larger bone. It is at this cartilaginous junction that growth in length of the bone occurs.

2 *Diaphysis*. This corresponds to the shaft of the long bone.

3 *Metaphysis*. This is a region of the diaphysis just below the line of junction of the epiphysis.

Histogenesis of endochondral bone

PRIMARY CENTER OF OSSIFICATION. At the onset of osteogenesis, chondrocytes, deep within the middle third of a preformed hyaline cartilage model, hypertrophy, absorb matrix, and leave irregular spicules of cartilage. These spicules later calcify and become deeply basophilic as the chondrocytes die and degenerate.

While calcified cartilage spicules form within the interior of the model, mesenchyme cells (or, according to some, osteoprogenitor cells), located in the inner region of the perichondrium, differentiate into osteoblasts. The osteoblasts will produce a tube of *periosteal bone* encircling the middle third of the cartilage model. This bone is formed in a manner similar to intramembranous ossification (see below). As osteoblasts become embedded within the bony matrix, they differentiate into nonosteogenic osteocytes. Periosteal bone first appears below the *periosteum* (the old perichondrium) as a fenestrated, nonlamellated bony mass of tissue (woven bone), but eventually it will fill in to become compact lamellated bone. The diaphysis will increase in diameter by appositional growth.

Coincident with periosteal bone formation, an osteogenic bud composed of mesenchyme cells, osteoblasts, and blood vessels, forms in the periosteum. The bud then migrates through holes in the periosteal bone and invades the field of calcified cartilage spicules within the bone's interior. There it proliferates as *primary marrow*. Osteoblasts cover the surface of the spicules and secrete layers of a soft and uncalcified osteoid matrix, which later becomes calcified. As the spicules become encased in bone, new osteoblasts remain on their surface, being formed by a continued differentiation of mesenchyme cells. The older osteoblasts become embedded within the bone and transform into osteocytes. The bone-covered spicules of calcified cartilage may now be designated as *trabeculae*, large beamlike structures.

As periosteal bone continues to be deposited on the surface, there is a cessation of bone production within the interior and the trabeculae are resorbed to form a large primary marrow cavity. Bone resorption is under the influence of hormones (parathormone and calcitonin) and osteoclasts (large multinucleate cells).

EXPANSION OF THE PRIMARY CENTER OF OSSIFICATION. As the bone increases its size by appositional and interstitial growth, the primary center of ossification expands toward the two epiphyses as adjacent cartilage regions become osteogenic. These regions ossify in a manner similar to that described above, but the morphological pattern of ossification is different and characteristic of an expanding center. This pattern is seen as four morphological zones representing different stages of osteogenic activity. As the bone grows in length, chondrocytes continuously proliferate in the youngest zone (nearer the epiphysis) and are replaced by bone in the oldest zone (nearer the diaphysis). There is a continued erosion, remodeling, and lengthening of periosteal bone to keep up with this internal expansion. The result is a lengthening of the diaphysis, diaphyseal bone, and marrow cavity. **Plate 3, Fig. 1.**

The four zones are perpendicular to the length of the bone and extend across its width. They are composed of parallel columns of cartilage cells separated by partitions of cartilage. The zones are described below, going from the youngest to the oldest (epiphysis towards the diaphysis).

1 *Zone of resting cartilage.* This zone may be expansive or restricted. Small, immature chondrocytes are evenly scattered throughout the matrix. **Plate 3, Fig. 1; Plate 4, Fig. 1.**

2 *Zone of proliferation.* Interstitial growth occurs in this zone as the bone increases its length. Small, flat, mitotically active chondrocytes are stacked into prominent, long, parallel columns. **Plate 3, Fig. 1; Plate 4, Fig. 1.**

3 *Zone of maturation.* Although this zone is narrower than the zone of proliferation, it also contributes to interstitial growth by cell enlargement rather than by cell proliferation. As nonmitotic chondrocytes undergo maturation, they gradually hypertrophy and absorb some matrix. This activity enlarges the lacunae and eventually forms spicules of matrix. The cells accumulate vacuoles of glycogen and lipids in the cytoplasm and begin to secrete alkaline phosphatase. This enzyme is important in the formation of calcified cartilage spicules. As organic phosphates are split, this causes a supersaturation of calcium phosphate, which precipitates as crystals of hydroxyapatite in the matrix.

The youngest cells in this zone are adjacent to the zone of proliferation. They are relatively large, cuboidal or polygonal cells with a small nucleus and an abundant pale acidophilic cytoplasm. The lacunae are prominent. The oldest cells (considered by some as a distinct zone of hypertrophy) lie in large, sometimes confluent, lacunae. These chondrocytes are quite large, with a small nucleus surrounded by an extensively vacuolated acidophilic cytoplasm. **Plate 3, Fig. 1; Plate 4, Figs. 1 and 2.**

4 *Zone of calcification (zone of degeneration).* As the old, hypertrophied cells become surrounded by calcified cartilage, they can no longer be nourished and die. This zone, then, is characterized by dead and dying chondrocytes, with pycnotic nuclei and fragmented cytoplasm. These cells lie in large, irregular cavities between dark basophilic spicules of calcified cartilage. Trabeculae are formed as osteoblasts secrete bone onto the surfaces of the calcified cartilage spicules. They project into the marrow cavity, but their ends are continually being reabsorbed under the influence of osteoclasts and hormones. **Plate 3, Figs. 1 and 2; Plate 4, Figs. 1 and 2.**

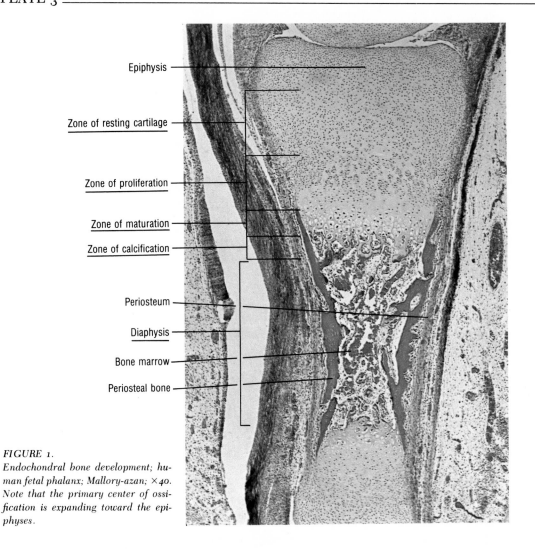

Epiphysis

Zone of resting cartilage

Zone of proliferation

Zone of maturation

Zone of calcification

Periosteum

Diaphysis

Bone marrow

Periosteal bone

FIGURE 1.
Endochondral bone development; human fetal phalanx; Mallory-azan; ×40. Note that the primary center of ossification is expanding toward the epiphyses.

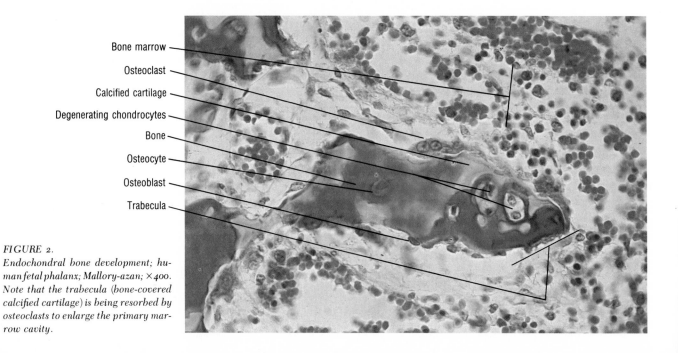

Bone marrow

Osteoclast

Calcified cartilage

Degenerating chondrocytes

Bone

Osteocyte

Osteoblast

Trabecula

FIGURE 2.
Endochondral bone development; human fetal phalanx; Mallory-azan; ×400. Note that the trabecula (bone-covered calcified cartilage) is being resorbed by osteoclasts to enlarge the primary marrow cavity.

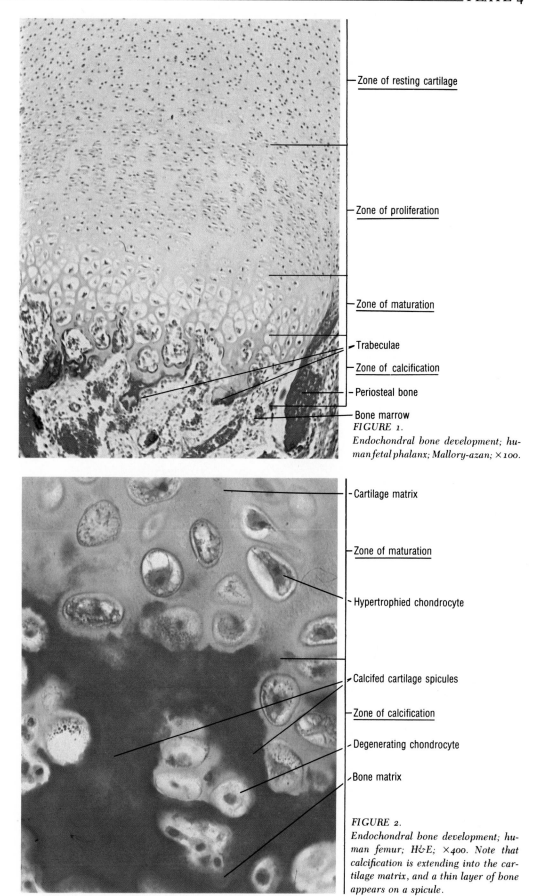

Zone of resting cartilage

Zone of proliferation

Zone of maturation

Trabeculae

Zone of calcification

Periosteal bone

Bone marrow

FIGURE 1.
Endochondral bone development; human fetal phalanx; Mallory-azan; ×100.

Cartilage matrix

Zone of maturation

Hypertrophied chondrocyte

Calcifed cartilage spicules

Zone of calcification

Degenerating chondrocyte

Bone matrix

FIGURE 2.
Endochondral bone development; human femur; H&E; ×400. Note that calcification is extending into the cartilage matrix, and a thin layer of bone appears on a spicule.

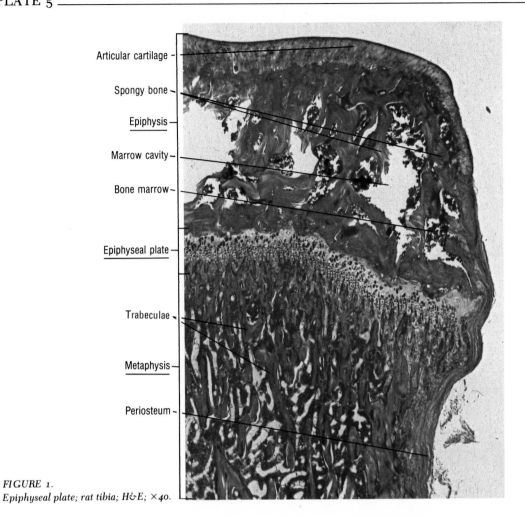

Articular cartilage –

Spongy bone –

Epiphysis –

Marrow cavity –

Bone marrow –

Epiphyseal plate –

Trabeculae –

Metaphysis –

Periosteum –

FIGURE 1.
Epiphyseal plate; rat tibia; H&E; ×40.

SECONDARY CENTER OF OSSIFICATION. If a bone (the tibia) has secondary centers, they develop in the epiphyses after much of the diaphysis has become ossified. The secondary centers go through approximately the same sequential steps as outlined above, except that the location is different. Ossification first starts within the interior of the epiphysis, produces spongy bone (see below), and eventually spreads radially to replace all but two areas of cartilage with bone: *articular cartilage* covering joint surfaces, and the *epiphyseal plate*. The epiphyseal plate is located above the metaphysis (which is the expanded end of the diaphysis and filled with spongy bone). **Plate 5, Fig. 1.**

EPIPHYSEAL PLATE. As the secondary center of ossification develops, an osteogenic region of cartilage, the epiphyseal plate, is sandwiched between the diaphysis and epiphysis. Its osteogenic activity is similar to that described above in the section on expansion of the primary center of ossification. The plate is formed after birth and contributes to the long growth of a bone until maturity—approximately 17 years in the female and 20 years in the male. The plate also grows in diameter, appositionally, to keep up with the rest of the growing bone. It retains a uniform thickness because cartilage growth and bone replacement balance each other. When the plate becomes

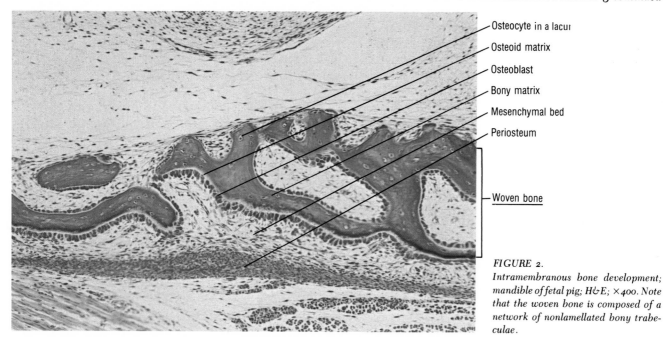

Osteocyte in a lacuı
Osteoid matrix
Osteoblast
Bony matrix
Mesenchymal bed
Periosteum

Woven bone

FIGURE 2.
Intramembranous bone development; mandible of fetal pig; H&E; ×400. Note that the woven bone is composed of a network of nonlamellated bony trabeculae.

nonfunctional it ossifies, thereby fusing the epiphysis to the diaphysis. This fusion leaves a prominent landmark, the *epiphyseal line*, which can be seen on the adult bone. **Plate 5, Fig. 1.**

Histogenesis of intramembranous bone (membrane bone)

During the development of a membrane bone, such as a flat bone in the roof of the skull, one or more ossification centers appear early in the fetus. A center may be identified as a dense, vascular region of mesenchyme cells lying within a bed of mesenchymal connective tissue. Some of the mesenchyme cells differentiate into osteoblasts as the matrix becomes more abundant. The osteoblasts secrete a noncalcified osteoid matrix on collagen fibers, which subsequently become bony, needlelike spicules as the matrix is impregnated with calcium salts. As the spicules enlarge, by appositional growth, osteoblasts become buried within the bony matrix and transform into osteocytes. New osteoblasts, derived from mesenchyme cells, continue to secrete bone on the surface of the spicules.

As the spicules lengthen, they radiate away from the ossification center. Eventually they anastomose to form a radiating network of trabeculae (little beams). This network becomes woven bone as it expands within a mesenchymal bed containing vascular and mesenchymal tissue. Woven bone continues to thicken as osteoblasts secrete bone on the trabecular surfaces. **Plate 5, Fig. 2.**

In the skull the outer layer of the mesenchymal bed becomes the fibrous pericranium, and the inner layer becomes the dura mater. Both layers surround the developing bone and contain collagen fibers, fibroblasts, mesenchyme cells, blood vessels, and nerves. They contribute to further bone growth and retain osteogenic potentialities even in the adult.

After birth, woven bone develops into lamellated spongy bone. The inner and outer surfaces of the spongy bone becomes platelike as lamellated compact bone forms in these regions. The compact bone is produced by the combined thickening of surface trabeculae and osteogenic activity of the pericranium and dura mater. In the interior of the bone trabeculae cease to thicken, leaving spaces which become filled with marrow. The result of this devleopment is a flat bone, the margins of which are adjacent to other bones in the skull. The bone has two flat layers of compact bone, the outer and inner tables, housing a spongy bony layer, the diploë.

The morphology of structures associated with embryonic and adult bone

CALCIFIED CARTILAGE SPICULES. These are irregular strands of acellular cartilage matrix. They are deeply basophilic because of the high concentrations of calcium salts. The spicules are not present in adult bone. **Plate 3, Fig. 2; Plate 4, Fig. 2**.

MESENCHYME CELLS (osteoprogenitor cells). These large cells have a sparse, pale basophilic cytoplasm surrounding a large, pale, oval nucleus. In developing bone they have the potential to differentiate into osteoblasts, osteoclasts, and possibly hematopoietic stem cells. They retain this potential wherever they are found in adult bone (haversian canals, endosteum, and periosteum). **Plate 7, Fig. 2**.

OSTEOBLAST CELLS. These appear as an epithelial-like layer of flattened, low cuboidal or columnar cells. The vesicular nucleus may be eccentrically positioned in a deep basophilic cytoplasm; a prominent nucleolus is present. The cells are present in osteogenic regions of adult and fetal bone. **Plate 3, Fig. 2; Plate 5, Fig. 2; Plate 7, Fig. 2**.

OSTEOID MATRIX. During osteogenesis, this preosseus matrix appears as a thin, homogeneous, faint acidophilic layer. It is deposited on the surface of older bone by osteoblasts. When it is first secreted, it is a soft, uncalcified, organic matrix containing collagenous fibers. Later, as the matrix becomes impregnated with calcium salts, it hardens into bone. **Plate 5, Fig. 2; Plate 7, Fig. 2**.

NONLAMELLATED AND LAMELLATED BONE. *Woven nonlamellated bone* (prenatal or healing adult bones) is distinguished from *lamellated bone* (postnatal bones) in several ways: it lacks bony lamellae, there is a random distribution of lacunae, and the collagen fibers form an irregular network. The lamellae in postnatal bone may be organized into spongy or compact layers. Regardless of age, all bone contains the following components: matrix, lacunae, and osteocytes. Woven bone: **Plate 5, Fig. 2; Plate 7, Fig. 2.** Lamellated bone: **Plate 6, Figs. 1 and 2**.

Matrix. This contains collagen fibers, inorganic salts [mainly $CaCO_3$ and $Ca_3(PO_4)_2$], and an organic ground substance of glycosaminoglycans containing chondroitin sulfate. In a decalcified, stained section, the matrix is an homogenous, dark acidophilic substance. It appears light tan in a ground bone preparation. **Plate 5, Fig. 2; Plate 6, Fig. 2**.

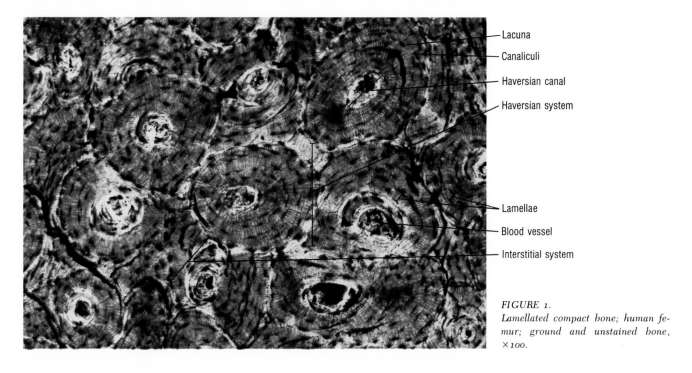

Lacuna

Canaliculi

Haversian canal

Haversian system

Lamellae

Blood vessel

Interstitial system

FIGURE 1.
Lamellated compact bone; human fe-
mur; ground and unstained bone,
×100.

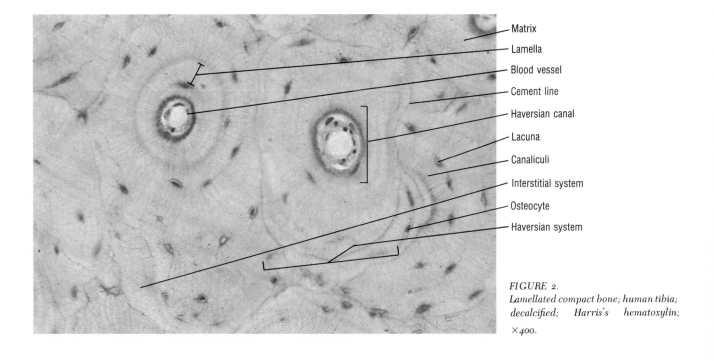

Matrix

Lamella

Blood vessel

Cement line

Haversian canal

Lacuna

Canaliculi

Interstitial system

Osteocyte

Haversian system

FIGURE 2.
Lamellated compact bone; human tibia;
decalcified;   Harris's   hematoxylin;
×400.

Lacunae. These are tiny oval holes (about 35 μm in length) within the matrix. They appear lightly stained or colorless in a decalcified, stained section of bone. In a ground bone preparation, however, they may appear light or dark, depending on the light source. They house the osteocytes, and each lacuna has many radiating canaliculi (small tubules) extending into the matrix. The canaliculi are quite visible as cobweblike structures in ground bone preparations. They are continuous with canaliculi of adjacent lacunae. **Plate 5, Fig. 2; Plate 6, Figs. 1 and 2.**

Osteocytes. These may appear as large, flat, oval or irregularly shaped cells lying within the lacunae; they are absent in ground bone preparations. The pale basophilic cytoplasm has tiny processes extending into the canaliculi, where they touch processes of adjacent osteocytes. The prominent oval nucleus is filled with a moderate amount of chromatin and contains a nucleolus. **Plate 5, Fig. 2; Plate 6, Fig. 2; Plate 7, Fig. 2.**

SPONGY BONE (cancellous or trabecular bone, substantia spongiosa). This is lamellated bone located in the interior of membrane bones (diploë), epiphyses of endochondral bones, and the interior of short bones. Although spongy bone is lamellated, it lacks the orderly pattern of lamellar distribution as seen in compact bone. Spongy bone is composed of a network of trabeculae enclosing irregular, marrow-filled spaces; it lacks haversian systems. **Plate 5, Fig. 1.**

COMPACT BONE (substantia compacta). This lamellated bone is located on the surface of both endochondral and membrane bones. The bone contains haversian systems, and the lamellae are distributed in an orderly and uniform pattern. Compact bone is relatively solid and lacks trabeculae. **Plate 6, Figs. 1 and 2.**

LAMELLAE. These are parallel layers of bony matrix, approximately 3 to 7 μm in thickness. They may be flat or circumferential. The lamellation of bone and the lamellar boundaries is due to the specific orientation of collagen fiber bundles as they spiral between adjacent lamellae. Several lamellae, which may or may not appear concentric and which lie either under the periosteum or endosteum, are designated as the *circumferential* lamellae. **Plate 6, Figs. 1 and 2.**

HAVERSIAN SYSTEMS (osteons). These are prominent, bony, branching tubes with small lumina (haversian canals) containing nerves, blood, and lymphatic vessels. The thick walls of an haversian system are composed of many (up to 20) concentric lamellae. Osteocytes, lying either within or between lamellae, are distributed in a series of concentric rings around the haversian canal. Each system is separated from other systems by a layer of cement, the *cement line*. The cement line is composed of matrix that is low in collagen fiber content and high in inorganic salts. This line may appear basophilic or refractile in stained sections, but in ground bone it is a thin tan line lacking canaliculi. A continuous canalicular system extends from the haversian canal out to the periphery of the system, but usually does not cross the cement line. **Plate 6, Figs. 1 and 2.**

INTERSTITIAL SYSTEMS. These are irregular pieces of lamellar bone which are sandwiched between haversian systems but separated from them by cement lines. They represent parts of earlier systems which were partially absorbed during the remodeling of bone. Both the interstitial and haversian systems are characteristic of postnatal compact bone. **Plate 6, Figs. 1 and 2.**

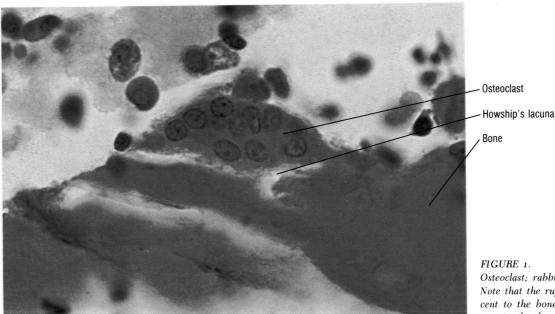

Osteoclast

Howship's lacuna

Bone

FIGURE 1.
Osteoclast; rabbit rib; H&E; ×1000.
Note that the ruffled cytoplasm adja-
cent to the bone indicates active re-
sorption by the osteoclast.

VOLKMANN'S CANALS. These large canals carry nerves, blood, and lymphatic vessels between the marrow cavity, haversian systems, and the periosteal surface of lamellated bone. They are distinguished from haversian systems because they travel perpendicularly or obliquely through the lamellae and are not surrounded by concentric lamellae.

TRABECULAE. Trabeculae are found either in endochondral centers of ossification, woven nonlamellated bone, or spongy lamellated bone. In centers of endochondral ossification trabeculae appear as irregular, mottled masses of matrix in decalcified, stained preparations; they have a basophilic core of calcified cartilage covered by acidophilic bone, **Plate 3, Fig. 2; Plate 4, Fig. 1.** In nonlamellated woven bone, **Plate 5, Fig. 2,** or lamellated spongy bone, **Plate 5, Fig. 1,** they are irregular, beamlike, acidophilic, bony structures of varying thickness.

OSTEOCLASTS. These are large, multinucleate cells, approximately 20 to 100 μm in diameter, which have a vacuolated or foamy, pale acidophilic or basophilic cytoplasm. In regions of prenatal or postnatal bone resorption, osteoclasts may be found on the surface or lying in shallow depressions of bone, *Howship's lacunae.* Osteoclasts originate from a fusion of mesenchyme cells, and although they are long-lived, there is a continual turnover of nuclei as more cells fuse with them.

As bone is resorbed, osteoclasts are probably important for the digestion of matrix, since they secrete hydrolytic enzymes. In active cells the plasma membrane appears as a ruffled border because of numerous microvilli touching the bony surface. Cell activity is influenced by parathormone and calcitonin; the former stimulates and the latter inhibits osteoclast activity. **Plate 3, Fig. 2; Plate 7, Fig. 1.**

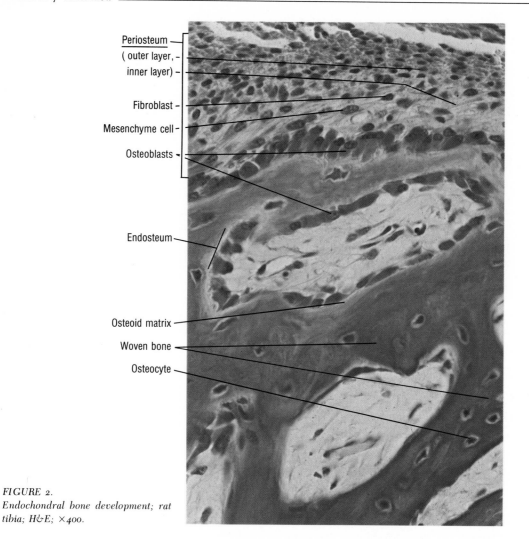

Periosteum —
(outer layer, –
inner layer) –

Fibroblast –

Mesenchyme cell –

Osteoblasts ◂

Endosteum —

Osteoid matrix —

Woven bone ◂

Osteocyte ◂

FIGURE 2.
Endochondral bone development; rat
tibia; H&E; ×400.

PERIOSTEUM. This is a moderately thick layer of collagenous fibers. Although two regions (inner and outer) are histologically distinct during bone growth or repair, they are not apparent in normal adult bone. The outer region is dense and fibrous, and the inner region is less dense, more vascular, and more cellular (containing mesenchyme cells, osteoblasts if the bone is osteogenically active, and fibroblasts). **Plate 5, Fig. 2; Plate 7, Fig. 2.**

ENDOSTEUM. This tissue lines the large cavities and canals of prenatal or postnatal bone; it represents the boundaries of bone marrow. It is a single layer of mesenchyme cells which may appear inactive and squamous (adult bone) or active and cuboidal (osteoblasts, in growing or healing bone). Endosteum functions in osteogenesis, bone resorption, healing, and remodeling throughout the life of the individual. **Plate 7, Fig. 2.**

SHARPEY'S FIBERS (perforating fibers). These are bundles of collagenous fibers which extend from the outer region of the periosteum to anchor into the interstitial systems and periosteal lamellae of postnatal bone. In decalcified, stained bone they may appear as irregular canals, and in ground bone as irregular dark lines passing perpendicular to the lamellae. Sharpey's fibers bind the periosteum to bone. They are most numerous at sites where tension forces are exerted on the periosteum, such as muscle insertions.

BONE MARROW. This tissue is osteogenic and hematopoietic. As a hematopoietic tissue (red bone marrow), it is present in the large cavities of endochondral and membrane bones of the child. During the teens it is replaced by fat cells (yellow marrow) except in spongy bone of the skull, clavicles, vertebrae, sternum, pelvis, humerus, and femur. Bone marrow has a framework of reticular tissue which supports sinusoids, blood vessels, and hematopoietic cells. **Plate 3, Fig. 1; Plate 5, Fig. 1.**

BLOOD AND LYMPHATIC VESSELS. In all but long bones the vascular pattern is relatively simple. The periosteum supplies the marrow and the spongy and compact bone with many arterioles. A venous system drains these structures with a pattern of vessels that resembles the arterial supply. In long bones there are three major arterial supplies, and each is named according to the areas that are served: diaphyseal nutrient arteries, metaphyseal arteries, and epiphyseal arteries. The nutrient artery enters the midshaft of the bone and bifurcates within the marrow cavity into ascending and descending limbs. As the branches extend to the epiphyses they (1) supply the marrow with sinusoids, (2) supply haversian systems with vessels, (3) anastomose with some branches of epiphyseal and metaphyseal arteries.

The marrow sinusoids, the remaining branches of nutrient arteries, and some regions of the epiphyses and metaphyses are drained by the central venous sinus (nutrient vein). The sinus approximates the pattern of nutrient arteries, but it may emerge at various points on the bone, near the metaphyses. Parts of the epiphyses and metaphyses are drained by veins that resemble the arterial pattern to these regions. Capillaries in the haversian systems are drained by a vascular plexus formed by a confluence of vessels in the periosteum and surrounding musculature. The plexus is drained by the systemic veins of the musculature.

Although lymphatic vessels are present in the periosteum, haversian canals, Volkmann's canals, and the marrow, they usually are more apparent in the periosteum.

NERVES. Many myelinated and nonmyelinated nerves are present in the periosteum. Small nerves accompany blood vessels into the interior of the bone, and their distribution is similar to that of the vascular system.

Muscular Tissue 5

There are three types of muscular tissue: skeletal, cardiac, and smooth. All three types are composed of muscle fibers (muscle cells), connective tissue, blood vessels, and nerves. The fibers are oriented so that their long axes are parallel to the direction of muscle contraction. Each muscle fiber has a sarcolemma (plasma membrane) surrounding a sarcoplasm (cytoplasm). The sarcoplasm of cardiac and skeletal muscle fibers is filled with threadlike myofibrils, composed of actin and myosin myofilaments, while smooth muscle only has myofilaments. Although myofibrils are composed of several proteins, actin and myosin are the most abundant ones concerned with the physical processes of contraction. Physiologically, muscle is classified either as *voluntary*, that is, under somatic motor nerve control, or *involuntary*, that is, controlled by autonomic nerves. Structurally, muscle may be striated with transversely striated myofibrils, or nonstriated and lacking cross striations.

Skeletal muscle (striated voluntary muscle)

Skeletal muscle is the axial and appendicular musculature of the body. It mainly functions to move or limit movement of the skeleton. Each muscle has its own characteristic size and dimensions, but all of them have a common structural design. They are covered by a superficial connective tissue sheath, the *epimysium* (deep fascia), containing various amounts of collagen, reticular, and elastic fibers. The epimysium is continuous with an inner sheath of connective tissue, the *perimysium*, which is more delicate than the epimysium and which organizes muscle fibers into parallel cylindrical bundles or fasciculi. The perimysium continues as a thin sheath of reticular fibers, the *endomysium*, surrounding each muscle fiber. All the sheaths are continuous, with aponeuroses or tendons of dense, regular collagenous connective tissue which anchor muscles to the periosteum of bones or other tissues. **Plate 1, Fig. 1.**

MUSCLE FIBERS. Muscle fibers are parallel to each other within a fascicle. They are elongate and cylindrical, with tapering ends which end in connective tissue of the sheaths or tendons. Their size varies from 10 to 100 μm in diameter and up to 30

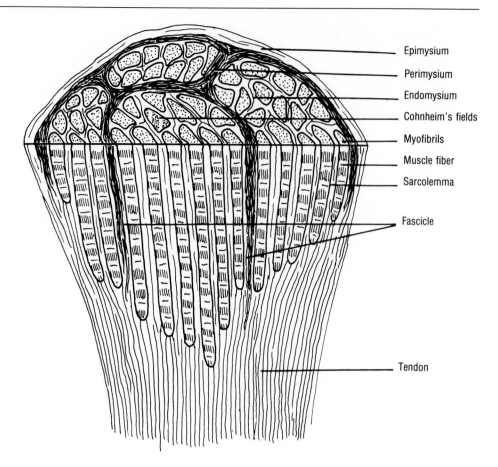

Epimysium

Perimysium

Endomysium

Cohnheim's fields

Myofibrils

Muscle fiber

Sarcolemma

Fascicle

Tendon

FIGURE 1.
Diagram of a skeletal muscle sectioned
in two planes. Nuclei are not shown.
(Modified from A. Ham, *Histology*, 3d
ed., J. B. Lippincott Co., Philadelphia,
1957.)

cm in length, and some do not extend the length of the fascicle. There are three types of fibers in mammalian muscle: red (slow-contracting), white (fast-contracting), and intermediate, but their distribution has not been extensively studied in man. Most skeletal muscles are composed of all three types of fibers, but depending on the muscle one type may predominate. The *red fibers* contain an abundant sarcoplasm and are narrow in diameter. The sarcoplasm has many mitochondria and is rich with myoglobin (a respiratory pigment), and the myofibrils have thick Z lines (see below). *White fibers* are wider than the red ones. Their scarce sarcoplasm is poor in myoglobin and mitochondria, and the myofibrils have thin Z lines. *Intermediate fibers* generally resemble red fibers, but are intermediate between the red and white ones. **Plate 1, Figs. 2** and **3.**

Sarcolemma. The sarcolemma appears as a poorly stained, thin membrane. It is a tough, elastic structure formed by the combination of the plasma membrane of the muscle fiber with a thick basal lamina. The latter is composed of glycosaminoglycans and delicate reticular fibers. **Plate 1, Figs. 1** and **2; Plate 2, Fig. 2.**

Nuclei. Each fiber has many elongate nuclei lying parallel to its long axis, just under the sarcolemma. The dark-stained nuclei have an abundant amount of chromatin and one or two nucleoli. **Plate 2, Fig. 1.**

Sarcoplasm. The sarcoplasm usually is not visible in H&E preparations. It contains typical cell organelles, myofibrils, a well-developed membrane system (sarcoplasmic reticulum), myoglobin (a respiratory pigment), glycogen granules, and lipid droplets.

PLATE 1 *continued*

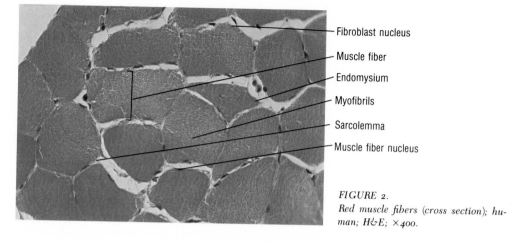

Fibroblast nucleus

Muscle fiber

Endomysium

Myofibrils

Sarcolemma

Muscle fiber nucleus

FIGURE 2.
Red muscle fibers (cross section); human; H&E; ×400.

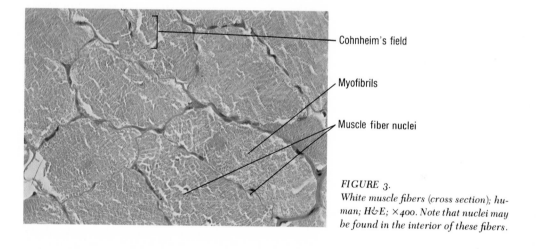

Cohnheim's field

Myofibrils

Muscle fiber nuclei

FIGURE 3.
White muscle fibers (cross section); human; H&E; ×400. Note that nuclei may be found in the interior of these fibers.

PLATE 2

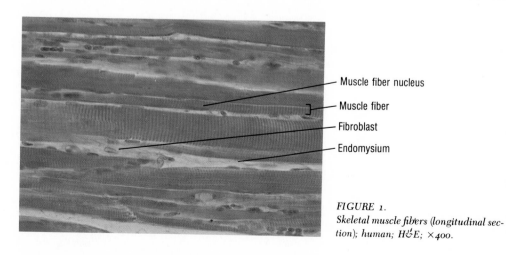

Muscle fiber nucleus

Muscle fiber

Fibroblast

Endomysium

FIGURE 1.
Skeletal muscle fibers (longitudinal section); human; H&E; ×400.

A band
I band
Fibroblast nucleus
H band
Z line
Sarcomere
Muscle fiber
Sarcolemma
Endomysium

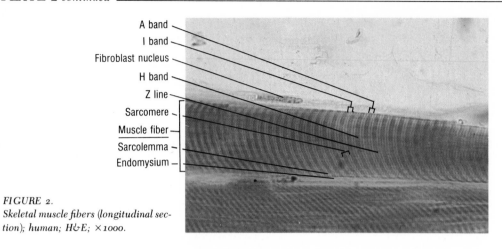

FIGURE 2.
Skeletal muscle fibers (longitudinal section); human; H&E; ×1000.

Myofibrils. These are unbranched, parallel columns, about 1.0 μm in diameter. Each column is composed of two types of myofilaments: thick myosin filaments (1.5 μm long by 100 Å in diameter), and thin actin filaments (1.0 μm long by 50 Å in diameter). Because of artifacts caused by shrinkage of the tissue during fixation, the myofibrils may be grouped into longitudinal bundles, *Koelliker's columns*, and separated by sarcoplasm. In cross section, the bundles appear as polygonal areas of myofibrils, *Cohnheim's fields*. **Plate 1, Figs. 1** and **3**. Each myofibril is transversely striated along its length by an alternation of myofilaments. These striations are visible with the light microscope and form the following structures.

A BAND (anisotropic band). This is a concentration of myosin filaments, which appear dark with an H&E stain or any cationic dye. In polarized light, however, the A band will appear bright and doubly refractive (anisotropic). Its length remains constant during contraction. **Plate 2, Fig. 2.**

I BAND (isotropic band). The actin filaments are located here and, unlike myosin, appear light and unstained with cationic dyes. The I band will be seen as a dark and singly refractive (isotropic) structure when viewed with a polarizing microscope. Its length will vary directly with different degrees of contraction or stretching. It is short or absent in contracted muscle, but long in stretched muscle. **Plate 2, Fig. 2.**

H BAND. This is a less anisotropic or lighter-stained region transversely bisecting an A band. It can be seen when the muscle is relaxed, but disappears during extreme contraction. **Plate 2, Fig. 2.**

M LINE. This is a faint line transecting the middle of the H band. It represents thickened regions of the myosin filaments and is difficult to observe in H&E stained sections.

Z LINE. This structure transversely bisects the I band, and it is visible as a thin, dark line when stained with H&E or any cationic dye. It does not extend beyond the limits of the myofibril. The Z line functions as a base to which actin filaments are attached. **Plate 2, Fig. 2.**

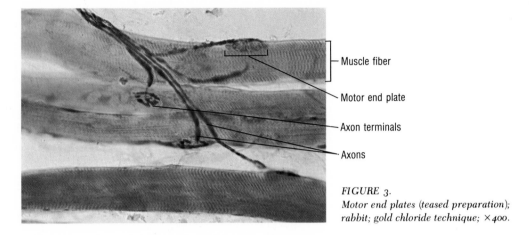

— Muscle fiber

— Motor end plate

— Axon terminals

— Axons

FIGURE 3.
Motor end plates (teased preparation);
rabbit; gold chloride technique; ×400.

SARCOMERE. This is one of many similar structural and functional units along the length of the myofibril. It is about 2.0 μm long and includes all parts of the myofibril between two successive Z lines. Its length varies directly with muscle contraction or stretching. **Plate 2, Fig. 2.**

BLOOD AND LYMPHATIC VESSELS. Arteries and veins are present in the epimysium and continue as arterioles and venules in the perimysium. Capillaries run longitudinally in the endomysium, between muscle fibers, close to the sarcolemma. They unite by transverse anastomoses to form plexuses around the muscle fibers. Lymphatic vessels are present only in the epimysium and perimysium.

NERVES

Motor end plates. Muscles are innervated by highly branched motor nerves, and each branch terminates as a motor end plate, about halfway along the length of a muscle fiber. A motor end plate consists of many axon terminals lying within some wrinkles of the sarcolemma. A concentrated sarcoplasm with many muscle nuclei also lies under these wrinkles. Nerve impulses are transmitted from the axon terminals of the motor end plate to the sarcolemma of the muscle fiber. Functionally, one motor nerve with its motor end plates, innervating several muscle fibers, is considered a motor unit. **Plate 2, Fig. 3.**

Free sensory nerve endings. Some sensory nerves branch and freely terminate on or between tendon or muscle fibers, while others form encapsulated structures, spindles (see below and refer to Chap. 18).

Muscle spindles. A muscle spindle is a bundle of delicate skeletal fibers (intrafusal fibers), about 40 mm in length. It is encapsulated by a thick connective tissue layer, which is continuous with the perimysium. The spindle is located near a tendon and is innervated by somatic motor and sensory nerves. The terminal ends of sensory

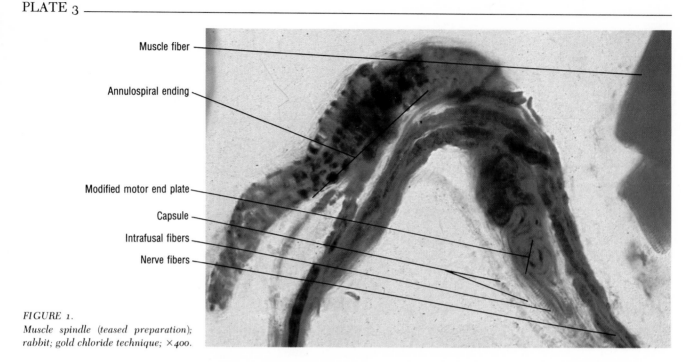

Muscle fiber

Annulospiral ending

Modified motor end plate

Capsule

Intrafusal fibers

Nerve fibers

FIGURE 1.
Muscle spindle (teased preparation);
rabbit; gold chloride technique; ×400.

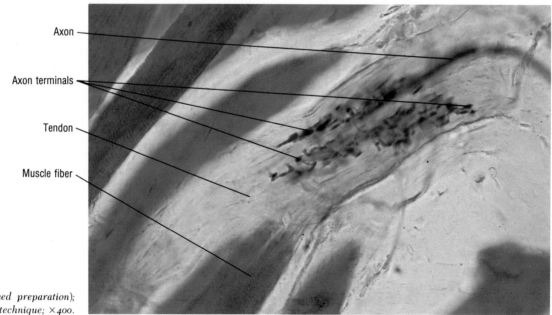

Axon

Axon terminals

Tendon

Muscle fiber

FIGURE 2.
Tendon spindle (teased preparation);
rabbit; gold chloride technique; ×400.

neurons, annulospiral endings, may spiral around the muscle fibers, but motor neurons terminate as modified motor end plates. Muscle spindles are proprioceptive receptors, and although they are abundant in muscles of the extremities, they are not present in all skeletal muscle. **Plate 3, Fig. 1.**

Tendon spindles. These are fusiform proprioceptive receptors, approximately 3.0 mm long. They are composed of club-shaped axon terminals of sensory fibers surrounding some collagen fibers of the tendon. The spindle is separated from the tendon by a thin connective tissue capsule. **Plate 3, Fig. 2.**

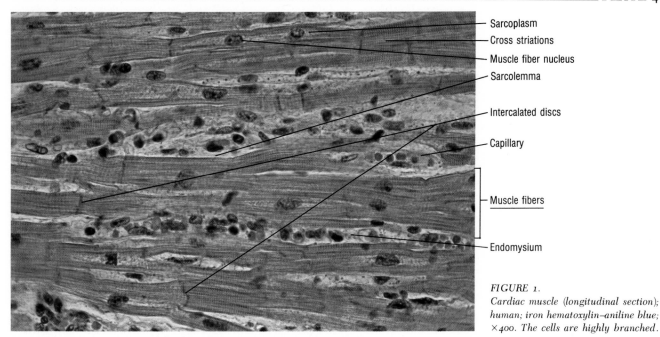

Sarcoplasm
Cross striations
Muscle fiber nucleus
Sarcolemma

Intercalated discs

Capillary

Muscle fibers

Endomysium

FIGURE 1.
Cardiac muscle (longitudinal section);
human; iron hematoxylin–aniline blue;
×400. The cells are highly branched.

Cardiac muscle (striated involuntary muscle)

Cardiac muscle is present in the myocardium of the heart. It is composed of branched and anastomosing bundles arranged in a somewhat parallel manner. Unlike skeletal muscle, these bundles are composed of many separate, branched cardiac muscle cells. Although cardiac fibers resemble a syncytium, they are separated by transverse intercalated disks between their adjacent ends. Cardiac tissue is organized into incomplete and interconnecting bundles by prominent layers of connective tissue. The bundles may vary in size from a few hundred to several thousand fibers in diameter. Endomysium is present in the interspaces between cardiac fibers. It contains collagen and reticular fibers, capillaries, lymphatics, and nerves. Modified cardiac cells, *Purkinje fibers*, are special nerve-impulse-conducting fibers and will be considered with the heart.

MUSCLE FIBERS.   The fibers are elongate and somewhat cylindrical, have truncate ends, and may or may not be branched. They are about 80 μm long by 15 μm wide. Typically, they are cross-striated, have much sarcoplasm, and have a single centrally placed nucleus. **Plate 4, Figs. 1 and 2.**

Sarcolemma. This membrane surrounds the cardiac fiber. It is similar to skeletal muscle membranes, but is thinner.

Sarcoplasm. This compares favorably with that of skeletal muscle, except it is relatively more abundant between myofibrils and around the nucleus. In addition, the sarcoplasm is rich with mitochondria, glycogen granules, and lipid vacuoles. It may contain some lipofuscin pigment in older individials. **Plate 4, Figs. 1 and 2.**

Nuclei. Each cell has one elongate, dark-stained nucleus, located at the middle of the cell and deep within the sarcoplasm. The long axis of the nucleus lies parallel to the long axis of the cell. **Plate 4, Figs. 1 and 2.**

Cross striations (A and I bands)
Endomysium
Nucleus
Nucleolus

Muscle fiber

Sarcoplasm
Sarcolemma

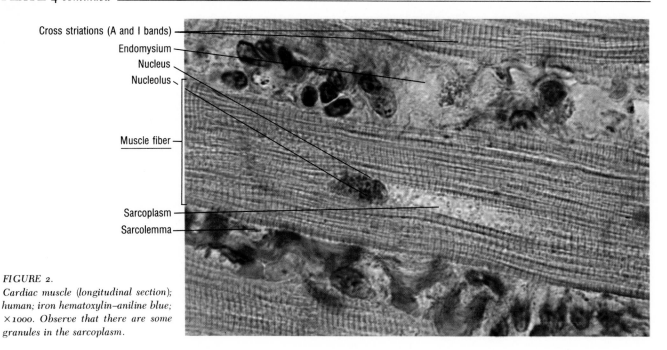

FIGURE 2.
Cardiac muscle (longitudinal section);
human; iron hematoxylin–aniline blue;
×1000. Observe that there are some
granules in the sarcoplasm.

Myofibrils. These are similar to those in skeletal muscle, but are less prominent and have faint cross striations. The A, I, and H bands and the Z and M lines are all present. **Plate 4, Figs. 1** and **2.**

Intercalated disks. The disks are thin, dark transverse lines appearing along the length of a cardiac fiber and represent points of cohesion between cells. They are a complex of cell junctions, formed by opposing sarcolemma membranes at the ends of adjacent cells. They appear either as straight or stepped lines extending transversely across the fibers. The disks are more difficult to observe with H&E–stained preparations than with certain other stains, for example, iron hematoxylin. **Plate 4, Fig. 1.**

BLOOD AND LYMPHATIC VESSELS. Coronary vessels are continuous with a rich vascular network of capillaries, lying in the endomysium, and surrounding the cardiac fibers. Lymphatics are also present in the endomysium. **Plate 4, Fig. 1.**

NERVES. Cardiac cells are closely associated with terminal ends of unmyelinated sympathetic and parasympathetic nerves. Special neuromuscular junctions, however, have not been observed.

Smooth muscle (nonstriated involuntary muscle)

Smooth muscle is widely distributed throughout the body and is abundant in organs demonstrating involuntary muscular movement, for example, the intestines, blood vessels, and trachea. The muscle fibers are usually organized into small bundles or

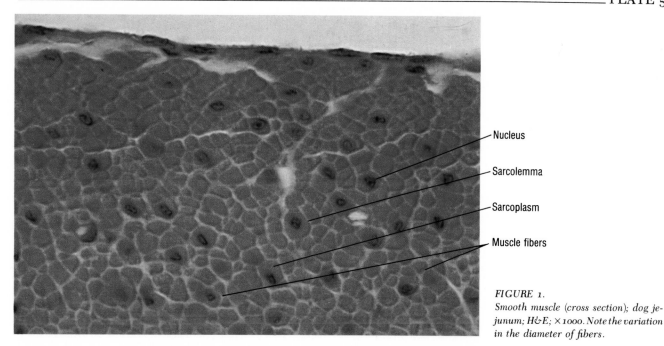

Nucleus

Sarcolemma

Sarcoplasm

Muscle fibers

FIGURE 1.
Smooth muscle (cross section); dog je-
junum; H&E; × 1000. Note the variation
in the diameter of fibers.

fasciculi by loose connective tissue. Some fibers may occur separately while others form a network. Depending on their organization, smooth muscle fibers may work independently or in concert to reduce a surface area or shorten tissue in a particular direction.

MUSCLE FIBERS. The fibers vary in length, from 15 μm to more than 500 μm. They are narrow, elongate, and spindle-shaped. Each fiber is nonstriated and has a single centrally located nucleus in the sarcoplasm. The fusiform fibers are staggered, so that adjacent thick and thin regions overlap. **Plate 5, Figs. 1 and 2.**

Sarcolemma. This is a thin membrane surrounding the cell and composed of the plasma membrane and basal lamina. The basal lamina is the only visible component in a stained section. An extensive network of delicate elastic, reticular, and collagen fibers is present between the laminae and surrounds each muscle fiber. This network of fibers is continuous with the tissue surrounding the fascicle. Together they form a system where forces of individual contractions are spread throughout the tissue. **Plate 5, Figs. 1 and 2.**

Nuclei. These may be thin and elongate in stretched fibers, or ovoid and wrinkled in contracted ones. The nuclei are centrally located in the sarcoplasm, and their long axes are parallel to the length of the fibers. They have two or more nucleoli. The moderately abundant chromatin may be distributed within the nucleoplasm or concentrated under the nuclear membrane. **Plate 5, Figs. 1 and 2.**

Sarcoplasm. This is the cytoplasm of the cell. It may appear fibrous or without texture. It contains typical cell organelles, inclusions, and contractile myofilaments.

Sarcolemma
Sarcoplasm
Nucleus
Nucleolus
Muscle fibers

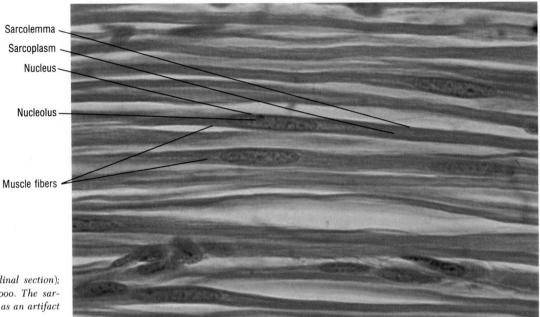

FIGURE 2.
Smooth muscle (longitudinal section); dog jejunum; H&E; ×1000. The sarcoplasm appears fibrous as an artifact of fixation.

The myofilaments are unstriated, thin filaments parallel to the length of the fiber. They are composed of action and myosin proteins. Myofilaments are readily seen with the electron microscope, but may appear as artifacts of clumped filaments in H&E–stained tissues. **Plate 5, Figs. 1** and **2.**

BLOOD AND LYMPHATIC VESSELS. While blood vessels and lymphatic capillaries are present in connective tissue surrounding the fasciculi, smooth muscle fibers are not directly supplied with these vessels.

NERVES. Unmyelinated motor nerves from sympathetic and parasympathetic divisions of the autonomic nervous system are present in the interfascicular connective tissue. Branches of these nerves extend between the muscle fibers and may terminate on the surface of one or more of them. Most of the fibers are not directly innervated, but they may receive stimuli by transmission of impulses from fiber to fiber.

Nervous Tissue 6

Anatomically the nervous system may be arbitrarily separated into three major divisions: central nervous system (CNS) (brain and spinal cord); peripheral nervous system (PNS) (spinal and cranial nerves, including their ganglia); and autonomic nervous systems (ANS) (visceral sensory nerves, ganglia, sympathetic and parasympathetic nerves). The CNS and PNS divisions are concerned more with conscious voluntary control over the function of certain organs (e.g., skeletal muscle), while the ANS provides an unconscious involuntary control to visceral organs, vessels, and glands.

Neurons

The neuron is the basic cell type of nervous tissue. It is an irritable cell modified to transmit a nerve impulse. Physiologically neurons may be classified as follows: *afferent* or *sensory*, conveying impulses from innervated sensory receptors toward the CNS; *efferent* or *motor*, transmitting impulses from the CNS to peripheral organs; and *internuncial* or *association*, which are interposed between afferent and efferent neurons and also connect different parts of the CNS.

Neurons have an enlarged cytoplasmic nerve cell body containing the nucleus. The cytoplasm is drawn out into threadlike peripheral structures, the axon and dendrites. Although neurons have only one axon, one or more dendrites may be present. Moreover, their position on the cell body will characterize one of three possible morphological types of neurons: (1) *multipolar* neurons have many dendrites; (2) *bipolar* neurons have one dendrite antipodal to the axon; (3) *unipolar* neurons have one dendrite joined with the axon to form a common stem with the nerve cell body. In unipolar neurons the axon and dendrites appear morphologically similar and can only be distinguished physiologically. Generally, axons carry impulses away from nerve cell bodies and dendrites carry impulses toward them, but in unipolar sensory neurons the peripheral processes carrying impulses toward the nerve cell body may be designated as axons.

PLATE 1

Neuropil —

Dendrite —

Nissl substance —

Nucleolus —

Nucleus —

Nerve cell body —

Blood vessel —

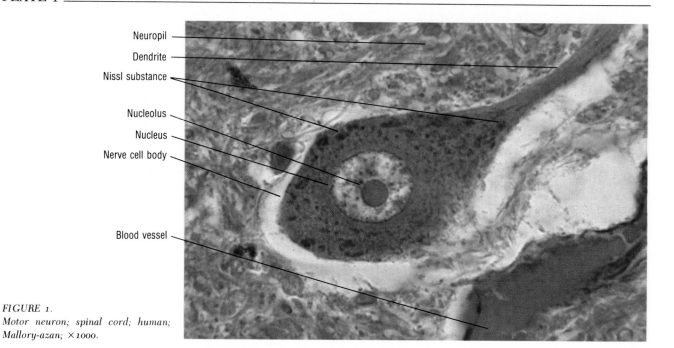

FIGURE 1.
Motor neuron; spinal cord; human;
Mallory-azan; ×1000.

NERVE CELL BODY (perikaryon). This is an abundant mass of basophilic cytoplasm or neuroplasm. It contains a prominent, centrally placed, pale-stained *nucleus* with a sparse chromatin network and a large, round nucleolus. In addition to the usual cell organelles, it contains randomly oriented, proteinaceous, threadlike structures, *neurofibrils*, which are best seen in silver-stained preparations. These are composed of smaller neurofilaments and neurotubules which can only be seen with the electron microscope. Although evidence is inconclusive, various functions of the neurofibrils have been suggested; they may support the neuroplasm or possibly transport metabolites. *Pigment* granules, such as melanin or lipofuscin, may be present in the neuroplasm. Melanin is present in those neurons located only in certain regions of the CNS (e.g., substantia nigra, a nucleus in the mesencephalon), and some ganglia of the PNS and ANS. The yellowish lipofuscin granules are either concentrated or scattered in many large neurons of the adult. They may also be present in ganglion cells. Both pigments are lacking in neurons of the newborn, but they eventually appear in the child and increase in concentration until puberty. Only lipofuscin continues to increase after puberty and into old age. Vacuoles of lipids may also be present in the neuroplasm. A chromophil substance, *Nissl substance*, readily stains with basic aniline dyes (cresyl violet) and appears as irregular dark basophilic clumps scattered throughout the cell body. The size and abundance of the clumps usually vary directly with the cell size, and they are larger in motor neurons than in sensory neurons. Nissl substance is composed of condensed granular endoplasmic reticulum, which is important in the synthesis of cytoplasmic proteins. **Plate 1, Figs. 1** and **2.**

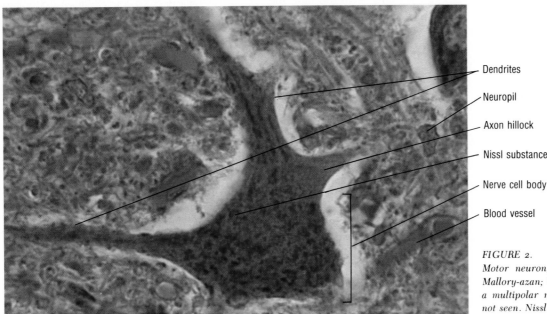

Dendrites

Neuropil

Axon hillock

Nissl substance

Nerve cell body

Blood vessel

FIGURE 2.
Motor neuron; spinal cord; human;
Mallory-azan; ×1000. Note that this is
a multipolar neuron. The nucleus is
not seen. Nissl substance is present in
the dentrites, but not the axon hillock.

DENDRITES (dendrons). These are usually highly branched, thin cytoplasmic structures located close to the nerve cell body; they carry small spiny processes. These processes synapse with telodendria or endings of axons. Cytoplasmic organelles and inclusions of the nerve cell body are usually present in the dendritic neuroplasm (dendroplasm). In a section of tissue the dendrites are difficult to distinguish from unmyelinated axons (see below), except they do not form tracts, have no sheaths, and may contain Nissl substance (small dendrites lack Nissl substance). **Plate 1, Figs. 1** and **2.**

AXON (axis cylinder). Neurons have only a single, usually long, thin axon extending from the axon hillock, an elevated region on the nerve cell body. The axon may have small branches, collaterals, extending at approximately right angles from its longitudinal axis. The axon terminates as many small branches, telodendrons, which may form axodendritic or axosomatic synapses. In the former synapse telodendrons terminate on dendrites, and in the latter synapse telodendrons terminate on the nerve cell body of another neuron. The axonal neuroplasm (axoplasm) contains mitochondria, agranular endoplasmic reticulum, and a prominent longitudinal bundle of parallel neurofibrils. Nissl substance is lacking both in the axon and axon hillock.

The axons or nerve fibers are covered by accessory sheaths. These sheaths may be formed by glial cells in the CNS and Schwann cells in the PNS and ANS. If the cytoplasm and plasma membranes of these cells wrap around an axon several times, leaving the nucleus and some cytoplasm on the surface, the result is a lipid-filled sheath, *myelin*, surrounding the axon. The superficial cytoplasm, containing the nucleus, is the *sheath of Schwann* or *neurilemma*. These myelinated fibers are distinct from unmyelinated ones, which have only one or no wraps around the axon and lack myelin. With the light microscope, *Schwann cells* appear flat and elongate with a flattened, dark-stained nucleus. The nuclei usually appear uniformly distributed in a section of nerve tissue.

The myelin and neurilemma are interrupted by constrictions, *nodes of Ranvier*, along the length of the axon. The myelin is discontinuous at these points, while the neurilemma is incomplete and only partially covers the nodes. Periodically along the myelin sheath, a series of light clefts, *incisures of Schmidt-Lantermann*, may be seen in special preparations (teased tissues stained with osmic acid). These are imperfections in the myelin wrappings around the axon. Myelinated fibers conduct nerve impulses with a greater velocity than unmyelinated ones. The nodes, lacking an insulation of myelin, allow the nerve impulse to jump from node to node (saltatory conduction) rather than move slowly down the plasma membrane.

In H&E–stained sections of myelinated fibers the myelin may be dissolved, leaving only a vacuolated sheath with a lacy, delicate, proteinaceous network, neurokeratin. These fibers will appear as a pale gray unstained axis cylinder surrounded by a clear or pale-stained myelin sheath. Unmyelinated fibers will be more difficult to identify, but in both cases nerve fibers may be distinguished by Schwann cell nuclei and associated connective tissue. **Plate 1, Fig. 2; Plate 2, Figs. 1 and 2.**

Peripheral nervous system

This system is composed of cranial and spinal nerves and their associated ganglia, all of which lie outside the CNS. These nerves are bundles of myelinated and unmyelinated fibers which carry impulses between the CNS and peripheral organs. The ganglia are aggregations of nerve cell bodies of afferent neurons.

NERVES. Each peripheral nerve is surrounded by connective tissue sheaths of collagen and some elastic fibers. This tissue is continuous as it extends from the surface to deep within a nerve, eventually surrounding the axons. These sheaths organize the nerve into bundles or fasciculi of fibers. They carry blood and lymphatic vessels and provide structural support to the delicate nerve fibers. Depending on their anatomical location, the sheaths are designated as *epineurium, perineurium,* or *endoneurium*. The epineurium is located on the surface of a nerve and is composed of loose connective tissue. It contains large blood vessels and small nerves, *nervi nervorum*. Perineurium is located deeper in the nerve, and its dense connective tissue is concentrically organized to surround bundles or fasciculi of fibers. Endoneurium, surrounds the neurilemma of each fiber within a fascicle and is composed of a delicate loose connective tissue. **Plate 2, Fig. 3.** In general, fibers may be placed in one of three classes depending on their diameters and velocity of impulse transmission.

A class (large myelinated fibers, 4 to 20 μm in diameter). These are somatic afferent and efferent neurons; transmission speed is about 5 to 120 m/s.

B class (small myelinated fibers, 2 to 3 μm in diameter). These are visceral afferent and efferent preganglionic fibers of the autonomic nervous system (see below); transmission speed is about 3 to 15 m/s.

C class (tiny unmyelinated fibers, 0.2 to 1.5 μm in diameter). These are efferent postganglionic fibers of the autonomic nervous system, and visceral afferent fibers; transmission speed is about 0.3 to 1.6 m/s.

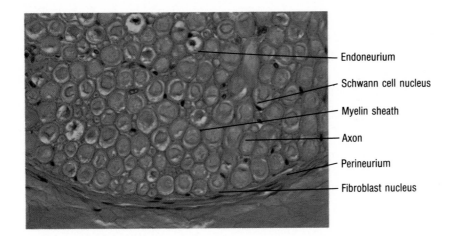

— Endoneurium

— Schwann cell nucleus

— Myelin sheath

— Axon

— Perineurium

— Fibroblast nucleus

FIGURE 1.
Myelinated axons (cross section); human; nerve; H&E; ×400. Note that this nerve is composed of many myelinated axons (nerve fibers) of various diameters.

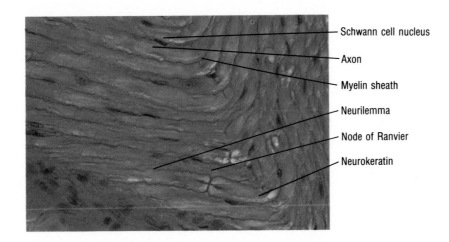

— Schwann cell nucleus

— Axon

— Myelin sheath

— Neurilemma

— Node of Ranvier

— Neurokeratin

FIGURE 2.
Myelinated axons (longitudinal section); human nerve; H&E; ×400.

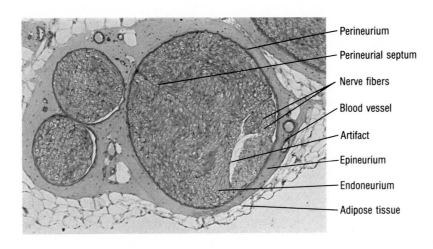

— Perineurium

— Perineurial septum

— Nerve fibers

— Blood vessel

— Artifact

— Epineurium

— Endoneurium

— Adipose tissue

FIGURE 3.
Nerve (cross section); human; H&E; ×100. Note that this is a small myelinated nerve divided into three fasciculi. The endoneurium appears as tiny strands of tissue surrounding each nerve fiber.

PLATE 3

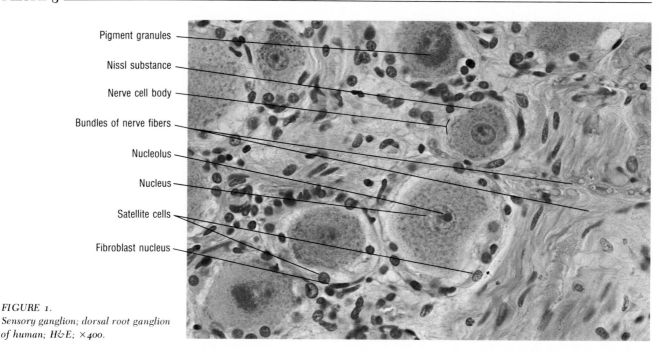

Pigment granules —
Nissl substance —
Nerve cell body —
Bundles of nerve fibers —
Nucleolus —
Nucleus —
Satellite cells —
Fibroblast nucleus —

FIGURE 1.
Sensory ganglion; dorsal root ganglion
of human; H&E; ×400.

CRANIOSPINAL GANGLIA (sensory ganglia). These are enlarged bodies on the sensory roots of the spinal nerves (dorsal root ganglia) and the following cranial nerves: trigeminal (gasserian ganglion); glossopharyngeal (superior and petrosal ganglia); vagus (jugular and nodose ganglia); vestibulocochlear (vestibular and cochlear ganglia); and facial (geniculate). These ganglia are aggregations of many cell bodies of afferent somatic nerves of the PNS and afferent visceral nerves of the ANS. The nerve cell bodies are usually separated into groups by large fasciculi of nerve fibers. Each ganglion has a capsule of dense, irregular collagenous connective tissue which is continuous with the sheaths of the nerve. Septa carrying blood and lymphatic vessels extend from the capsule to the interior of the ganglion.

Nerve cell bodies in craniospinal ganglia. The nerve cell bodies vary from 15 to 100 μm. They are unipolar neurons with an oval or tear-shaped body attached to its processes by a single stem. Although both the central and peripheral processes may be designated as axons, the peripheral process conveys the impulse toward the nerve cell body. The abundant basophilic cytoplasm contains diffuse small granules of Nissl substance and a large, centrally located, round, vesicular nucleus with a prominent round nucleolus. The afferent somatic cell bodies are usually large (25 to 100 μm in diameter) than the visceral neurons, but it is difficult to distinguish between them. **Plate 3, Fig. 1.**

Satellite cells (capsule cells). Each nerve cell body is surrounded by a thin capsule of delicate collagen fibers, fibroblasts, and satellite cells. The flattened satellite cells immediately surround the cell body and are continuous with the neurilemma of the axons. They, along with the fibrous tissue of the capsule, support the neurons and possibly regulate the exchange of metabolites between them and adjacent capillaries. The nuclei of the satellite cells are relatively dark, oval to flat, and lack prominent nucleoli. Flattened fibroblast nuclei lie more peripherally to the satellite cells. **Plate 3, Fig. 1.**

Autonomic nervous system

Visceral innervation is accomplished by the afferent and efferent fibers of the ANS. The visceral efferent fibers are divided into sympathetic (thoracolumbar) and parasympathetic (craniosacral) divisions of the ANS. Both divisions are composed of ganglia, efferent preganglionic fibers running from the CNS to a ganglion, and postganglionic efferent fibers from a ganglion to an innervated organ. These fibers travel through spinal, cranial, and visceral nerves. One anatomical difference between these divisions is the position of the ganglia: *sympathetic ganglia* may form a chain close to the vertebral column (paravertebral ganglia) or form random concentrations of cell bodies near the aorta (collateral ganglia), while the *parasympathetic ganglia* are located within or close to the structure they innervate (terminal ganglia).

The visceral afferent neurons usually accompany visceral efferent neurons through the same visceral, spinal, and cranial nerves, carrying impulses from sensory receptors in the visceral organs to the CNS. They enter sensory roots and their nerve cell bodies are located in the sensory ganglia.

VISCERAL NERVES. Visceral fibers may form parts of cranial and spinal nerves or appear as anatomically distinct nerves containing afferent and efferent visceral fibers. These small nerves have some collagenous connective tissue surrounding the fasciculi, but elaborate sheaths are absent. In an H&E–stained cross section, any unmyelinated fibers appear as small, undistinguished clusters of gray dots (axis cylinders) surrounded by Schwann cells and connective tissue; with silver stains the dots appear black. The appearance of myelinated fibers has already been described (see axons).

AUTONOMIC GANGLIA. These are concentrations of nerve cell bodies of efferent visceral neurons (postganglionic fibers). They may appear as linked segmental swellings along the length of the vertebral column, *paravertebral ganglia;* isolated nonsegmental bodies somewhat distal to the vertebral column and near the aorta, *collateral ganglia;* or in or near the walls of organs which are innervated, *terminal ganglia.* Fasciculi are not present within the autonomic ganglia, and thus there is a random mixing of nerve cell bodies with processes of visceral efferent and afferent neurons. Each ganglion is surrounded by a dense, irregular collagenous connective tissue capsule with vascularized septa extending into its interior.

Nerve cell bodies in autonomic ganglia. Nerve cell bodies are usually from 20 to 60 μm in diameter, multipolar, and stellate. The cytoplasm may contain some pigment granules, fine, granular Nissl substance, and a large, ovoid, vesicular, usually eccentrically placed nucleus. **Plate 3, Fig. 2.**

Nerve cell body —

Nissl substance —

Nerve fibers —

Satellite cells —

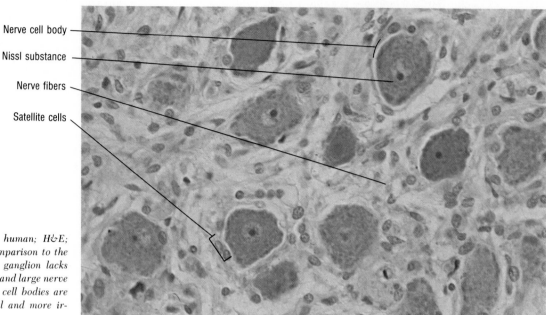

FIGURE 2.
Sympathetic ganglion; human; H&E;
×400. Note that in comparison to the
sensory ganglion, this ganglion lacks
bundles of nerve fibers and large nerve
cell bodies. The nerve cell bodies are
generally less spherical and more ir-
regular.

Satellite cells. These cells may form an incomplete membranous capsule around each ganglion cell. Refer to the sensory ganglia for their description. **Plate 3, Fig. 2.**

Central nervous system

The CNS is composed of the brain and spinal cord. Some of the characteristic histological structures associated with this system are: (1) *neuroglia*, a specialized connective tissue supporting the neurons, (2) *nuclei*, an aggregation of nerve cell bodies within the CNS; (3) *tracts*, bundles of myelinated and unmyelinated fibers running through the CNS; (4) *meninges*, protective membranes surrounding the CNS; (5) *choroid plexus*, a vascular tissue which produces cerebrospinal fluid; (6) *neuropil*, the ubiquitous fibrous bed of the CNS composed of axons, dendrites, and neuroglia; (7) *gray matter*, a tissue composed of nerve cell bodies, mainly unmyelinated fibers, and glial cells, and (8) *white matter*, a fibrous tissue composed of mainly myelinated fibers and glial cells.

NEUROGLIA (glia). This is a nonnervous, supporting tissue which contributes to the fibrous neuropil between nerve cell bodies and influences the physiology of the CNS. It is composed of ependyma and three types of neuroglia cells: *astrocytes*, *oligodendroglia*, and *microglia*. Although silver or gold staining techniques must be used to demonstrate the cytoplasmic processes of these cells, identification may be possible with an H&E preparation which stains the nucleus and some surrounding cytoplasm.

Ependyma. In the embyro, the ependyma is a stratified columnar ciliated epithelium. It lines the ventricles of the brain and central canal of the spinal cord. The bases of the lower cells form a network of long processes extending deep into the neuropil of the CNS. The ependyma influences the composition of the cerebrospinal fluid

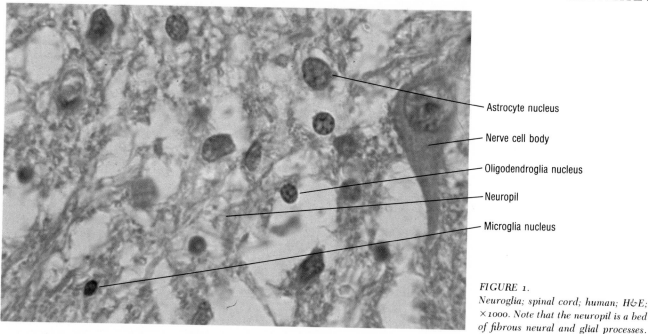

— Astrocyte nucleus

— Nerve cell body

— Oligodendroglia nucleus

— Neuropil

— Microglia nucleus

FIGURE 1.
Neuroglia; spinal cord; human; H&E;
×1000. Note that the neuropil is a bed
of fibrous neural and glial processes.

through its secretory and absorptive functions. The adult epedyma in humans is a simple, nonciliated cuboidal epithelium. The cells have reduced basal processes, but microvilli are present. The cells have a moderatly large, oval to round, dark-stained nucleus lying within a basophilic cytoplasm.

Astrocytes. These are relatively small cells, about 10 μm in diameter, but are the largest of the neuroglia cells. They have highly branched processes radiating in all directions away from a central hub. There are two types of astrocytes: fibrous and protoplasmic. The *fibrous astrocytes* are more abundant in the white matter than gray matter. They have long, thin, mainly unbranched cytoplasmic processes containing filaments. The fibrous processes support tracts of nerve fibers by forming networks around axons and nerve cell bodies; some are also attached to blood vessels. The oval, pale nucleus is smaller than the nuclei of neurons. It has moderately dense chromatin and contains no nucleoli. *Protoplasmic astrocytes* are mainly found in the gray matter of the CNS along with some fibrous types. The protoplasmic astrocytes have an abundant cytoplasm with many, thick branched processes. The processes may terminate as expanded footlike structures on blood vessels, or bind the pia mater to the CNS. The cytoplasm is vacuolated and contains many granules. Although the pale, oval nucleus is larger than the fibrous astrocyte nucleus (see above), it is difficult to distinguish between the two. These cells may selectively regulate the movement of metabolites, fluids, and gases between the blood, cerebrospinal fluid, and nervous tissue, and thus may help to establish a blood-brain barrier. **Plate 4, Fig. 1.**

Oligodendroglia. These cells are present in both the gray and white matter. They are smaller (7 μm in diameter) than astrocytes, are somewhat boxlike or pear-shaped, and usually appear in clumps or rows. The scanty cytoplasm is drawn out into a few thin, poorly branched, short, knobby processes. Compared to astrocytes, their round, eccentric nuclei are smaller, darker, and more densely packed with chromatin.

Oligodendroglia usually lie next to nerve cell bodies in the gray matter. In white matter their processes form myelin sheaths around axons. **Plate 4, Fig. 1.**

Microglia. These are not as numerous as other glial cells and are mainly located in the gray matter, near blood vessels and nerve cell bodies. They are also scattered between myelinated fibers in the white matter. Microglia are the smallest of the glial cells (about 5 μm in diameter). The nucleus is the smallest, darkest, and most irregular of the glial nuclei; it may be rod-shaped, oval and indented, or bent. The sparse cytoplasm forms a few short, twisted branches with numerous small spinelike processes. The processes extend between neurons and surround capillaries. If the CNS is injured, microglia may become amoeboid and phagocytic, and in this respect are considered macrophages. **Plate 4, Fig. 1.**

CHOROID PLEXUS. The roof of the lateral, third, and fourth ventricles is the tela choroidea. It is composed of a vascular pia mater and ependyma. The choroid plexus is a group of highly vascularized folds of the tela which extends into the lateral and third and fourth ventricles. Each fold is formed from a network of fenestrated capillaries and some nerve fibers, lying within a bed of many collagen fibers and a few elastic fibers. The surface is lined by an ependymal layer of simple cuboidal epithelium. The low cuboidal cells have a large, round nucleus, and a brush border on their apical surface. The epithelium is instrumental in the movement of ions, fluids, and organic molecules from the blood into the ventricles during the formation of cerebrospinal fluid. This fluid contains water, some proteins, inorganic salts, glucose, and a few lymphocytes. The cerebrospinal fluid bathes and cushions the neural tissues against injuries and provides a medium whereby substances can be carried to and from the cells. As the fluid is secreted, it slowly circulates through the ventricles but eventually leaves the fourth ventricle via three apertures in the roof; a median *foramen of Magendie* and a pair of lateral *foramina of Luschka*. As the cerebrospinal fluid percolates through the subarachnoid space (see below), most of it surrounds the brain, but some bathes the spinal cord. In the head, it diffuses into endocranial venous sinuses from arachnoid villi which extend into the sinuses. In the spinal cord the cerebrospinal fluid passes into dural veins, sinuses, and lymphatics surrounding the spinal nerves. Small (0.1 mm), usually round, calcified bodies (psammoma bodies) may appear in the adult choroid plexus, and their numbers may increase with age. The bodies are a series of concentric rings organized around degenerate cells of the choroid. **Plate 4, Fig. 2.**

SPINAL CORD. The spinal cord is a hollow tube, continuous with the medulla oblongata of the brain, which gives rise to 31 pairs of segmentally arranged spinal nerves. It is surrounded by the meninges (pia, arachnoid, and dura) and housed within a bony vertebral canal formed by the vertebrae. The lumen, or central canal, of the spinal cord contains circulating cerebrospinal fluid, and is lined by ependyma (see above). The interior of the spinal cord is an extensive column of gray matter surrounding the central canal, and is roughly in the form of the letter H. Peripheral to and surrounding the gray matter the remainder of the cord is composed of tracts of white matter. The ventral or anterior surface of the spinal cord is bilaterally divided by a deep *anterior median fissure*, extending about 3 mm into the cord, and contains the pia mater. Somewhat lateral to the anterior median fissure is a pair of almost inconspicuous depressions, points of attachment for the ventral roots of spinal nerves. The dorsal or posterior surface of the cord is a shallow groove, the *posterior median sulcus*, which is continuous with the *posterior median septum*, a sheet of neuroglia extending about 5 mm into the cord. Lateral to the posterior median sulcus are the prominent paired posterior lateral sulci, points of attachment for the dorsal roots of the spinal nerves. **Plate 5, Figs. 1 and 2.**

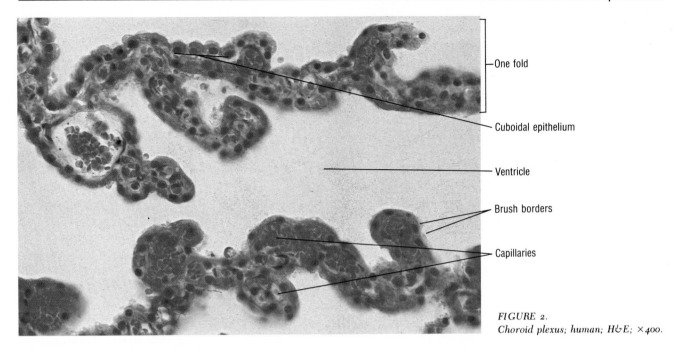

One fold

Cuboidal epithelium

Ventricle

Brush borders

Capillaries

FIGURE 2.
Choroid plexus; human; H&E; ×400.

GRAY MATTER. The gray matter is organized into the following anatomical components: anterior and posterior commissures; posterior columns (horns); anterior columns (horns); and lateral columns (horns). In addition, many nuclei are present; however, only the nucleus dorsalis shall be considered. **Plate 5, Figs. 1** and **2.**

Anterior and posterior gray commissures. The tissue forming the crossbar of the H, immediately anterior and posterior to the central canal, are the anterior and posterior commissures. These are nerve fibers connecting the lateral halves of the gray matter. **Plate 5, Figs. 1** and **2.**

Posterior columns (posterior horns). These long, narrow paired columns compose the uppermost portions of the H. They contain fibers, nerve cell bodies, and neuroglia cells. The shape of the H varies somewhat, depending on the level of the spinal cord. The columns receive direct endings or collaterals of somatic and visceral afferent fibers coming from the dorsal roots of the spinal nerves. These nerve fibers may synapse directly with motor neurons in the anterior columns or with internuncial neurons which then synapse with motor neurons. **Plate 5, Figs. 1** and **2.**

Anterior columns (anterior horns). These are the paired lower portions of the H; they are usually short and broad. Cell bodies of somatic and visceral efferent neurons are located here. The somatic efferent nerve cell bodies may be distinguished from the visceral efferent cell bodies in various ways; they are larger than the visceral bodies, are star-shaped, have a prominent central vesicular nucleus, and contain coarse Nissl substance in the neuroplasm. Telodendrons of other neurons synapse with the dendrites of these motor cells. The axons of the efferent neurons form the ventral root of the spinal nerves. **Plate 5, Figs. 1** and **2.**

Lateral columns (lateral horns). These are present in the lower cervical, thoracic, and upper lumbar regions of the spinal cord. They appear as lateral projections of the crossbar of the H, between the anterior and posterior columns. The tissue contains nerve cell bodies of the visceral efferent neurons of the sympathetic division

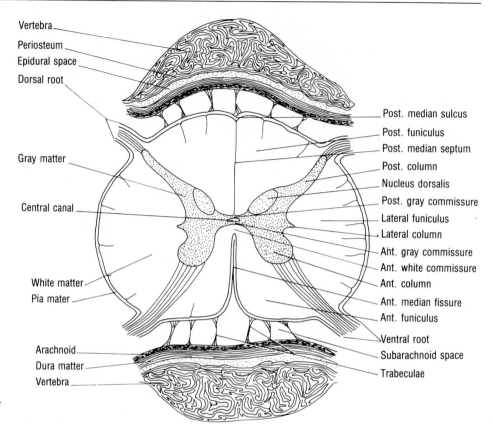

Vertebra
Periosteum
Epidural space
Dorsal root

Gray matter

Central canal

White matter
Pia mater

Arachnoid
Dura matter
Vertebra

Post. median sulcus
Post. funiculus
Post. median septum
Post. column
Nucleus dorsalis
Post. gray commissure
Lateral funiculus
Lateral column
Aht. gray commissure
Ant. white commissure
Ant. column
Ant. median fissure
Ant. funiculus
Ventral root
Subarachnoid space
Trabeculae

FIGURE 1.
Drawing of the spinal cord, thoracic
region, (cross section); human.

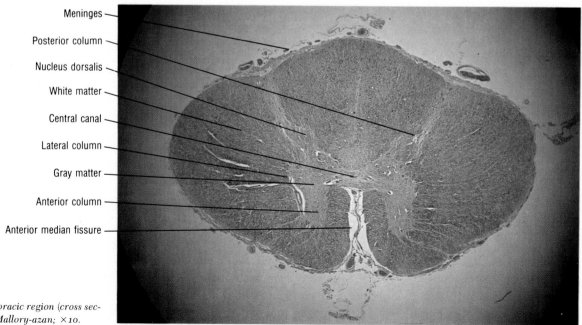

Meninges
Posterior column
Nucleus dorsalis
White matter
Central canal
Lateral column
Gray matter
Anterior column
Anterior median fissure

FIGURE 2.
Spinal cord, thoracic region (cross sec-
tion); human; Mallory-azan; ×10.

of the autonomic nervous system. The nerve cell bodies are smaller (15 to 45 μm) than the somatic motor neurons in the anterior horns. They are ovoid or fusiform and have a finer type of Nissl substance in the cytoplasm. The myelinated axons (preganglionic fibers) of these neurons leave the ventral root and enter the sympathetic ganglia via the white ramus communicans. **Plate 5, Figs. 1 and 2.**

Nucleus dorsalis (nucleus thoracicus). This is an aggregation of large, oval nerve cell bodies located at the bases of the posterior columns on their medial surfaces. It appears as a large, oval mass within the gray matter. The nucleus is prominent at the levels between the VIIIth cervical and IVth lumbar vertebrae. Neurons within the nucleus dorsalis synapse with collaterals of afferent neurons coming from the dorsal spinal roots. Their myelinated axons travel in the lateral white funiculus (see below) as the posterior spinocerebellar tract ascending to the cerebellum. **Plate 5, Figs. 1 and 2.**

WHITE MATTER. The white matter is composed of neuroglia and predominantly myelinated fibers which run the length of the spinal cord. The fibers also decussate (cross over) in the *anterior white commissure*, a region just anterior (ventral) to the anterior gray commissure. In each half of the spinal cord the white matter is organized into three longitudinal bundles or funiculi (anterior, lateral, and posterior), and each funiculus is composed of several ascending and descending fiber tracts, or *fasciculi*. The tracts are composed of fibers forming connections between the brain and all levels of the spinal cord, and between the CNS with sensory receptors or effector organs. The ascending tracts carry impulses toward the brain while descending tracts carry impulses from the brain. Although special myelin stains are needed to identify these tracts, the general anatomical regions of the funiculi can be determined. **Plate 5, Figs. 1 and 2.**

Posterior (dorsal) funiculus. This is located between the median septum and posterior gray column. The posterior funiculus extends between the levels of the Ist cervical and Ist coccygeal vertebrae. **Plate 5, Figs. 1 and 2.**

Lateral funiculus. This is lateral to the gray columns, is located between the dorsal and ventral spinal roots, and extends from the Ist thoracic to the IId lumbar vertebra. **Plate 5, Figs. 1 and 2.**

Anterior (ventral) funiculus. This is located between the anterior median fissure and the ventral root. The length of this funiculus is variable. **Plate 5, Figs. 1 and 2.**

BRAIN. The brain lies within the cranial cavity of the skull, and is surrounded by the meninges. It has twelve pairs of cranial nerves. The brain in man, as in the lower vertebrate animals, is composed of five divisions, each with specialized structures. The *telencephalon* with cerebral hemispheres; the *diencephalon* with the thalamus; the *mesencephalon* with the corpora quadrigemina; the *metencephalon* with the cerebellum; and the *myelencephalon* with the medulla oblongata. The most inferior region, the medulla oblongata, is continuous with the superior level of the spinal cord. The interior of the brain is organized into a number of interconnected cavities, or *ventricles*, filled with cerebrospinal fluid. The first and second ventricles are located in the cerebral hemispheres. They are continuous with the third ventricle in the diencephalon by the foramen of Monro. The third ventricle is confluent with the cerebral aqueduct which runs through the mesencephalon and terminates at the fourth ventricle. The fourth ventricle is located within the metencephalon and myelencephalon and is continuous with the central canal of the spinal cord. Except for the choroid plexus, the brain is composed of the same type of tissues as are found in the spinal cord, but their distribution is more complex. In the cerebellum and cerebral hemispheres, the gray matter (cortex) lies on the surface of the white matter (medulla). This is the reverse of the condition found in the spinal cord. Only the cerebellar and cerebral regions will be presented to illustrate some histology of the brain.

Cerebellum. This structure functions in the coordination of motor movements. Anatomically the cerebellum is divided into two lateral hemispheres by a median vermis. It lacks a cavity and is composed of a thin superficial cortex of gray matter covering a deeper medullary body of white matter. The cortex is folded into many parallel transverse ridges, *folia cerebelli,* by deep fissures. Each folium of folded cortex has a core, white lamina, extending from the medullary body. Several nuclei are present in the medullary body, the most prominent of which is the dentate nucleus. Fibers leave this nucleus, via the superior peduncle, to reach the lateral and ventral nuclei of the thalamus and red nucleus of the mesencephalon. Three distinct histological layers may be identified in the cortex: (1) outer molecular layer; (2) intermediate Purkinje cell layer; (3) inner granular layer next to the medullary body. **Plate 6, Figs. 1 and 2.**

MOLECULAR LAYER. This is the outermost and thickest of the three layers. It contains glial cells, dendrites, and many unmyelinated axons. Of the relatively few neurons present, the more superficial ones, outer *stellate cells,* are smaller than the deeper *basket cells.* The processes of both cell types contribute to the neuropil. These are considered to be inhibitory interneurons which, by complex interconnections, modify the activity of Purkinje cells (see below) and others in the cortex. **Plate 6, Figs. 1 and 2.**

GRANULAR LAYER. This is the innermost layer of the cortex. It is moderately thick and densely packed with nerve cell bodies of small neurons, *granule cells,* and a few large *Golgi type II* neurons (see below). Occasionally, light, irregular spaces, or *glomeruli,* appear between clumps of the cells. The glomeruli represent complex synaptic regions between neurons. The granule cells are multipolar and have a small, dark, round nucleus surrounded by a thin ring of cytoplasm; Nissl substance is lacking. They relay impulses coming from the body, carried by afferent mossy fibers, to the Purkinje cells.

The Golgi type II neurons are scattered through the upper regions of the granular layer. They are large multipolar neurons containing Nissl substance and a prominent nucleus. Their axons synapse with a complex of processes from granule cells and afferent mossy fibers. They are inhibitory neurons which modify impulses going to the Purkinje cells. Golgi type II neurons are characterized by short axons which remain in the same region as the nerve cell bodies. They differ from Golgi type I neurons which have longer axons that terminate in regions quite distant from the nerve cell body. **Plate 6, Figs. 1 and 2.**

PURKINJE LAYER. This is a single layer of large, flask-shaped cells, *Purkinje cells,* lying between the molecular and granular layers. They have a large vesicular nucleus containing a prominent nucleolus. The basophilic cytoplasm is filled with irregular, coarse clumps of Nissl substance. The Purkinje cells are multipolar neurons with a few major branched dendrites extending into the molecular layer. Their single axons leave the cortex through the granular layer and converge on deep cerebellar nuclei (globose, dentate, fastigial, and emboliform) within the medullary body. The Purkinje cells convey afferent impulses from the cerebellar cortex which play an inhibitory role on the function of these nuclei. **Plate 6, Figs. 1 and 2.**

Cerebrum. Among many complex functions, this region of the brain is concerned with memory, consciousness, intelligence, interpretation of sensations, and thinking. The cerebrum is the largest part of the brain and covers much of the inferior portions. It is divided into two large *cerebral hemispheres* by a deep longitudinal fissure, the bottom of which is bordered by a broad sheet of white matter, the *corpus callosum.* This structure allows a correlation of neurological activity on both sides of the brain.

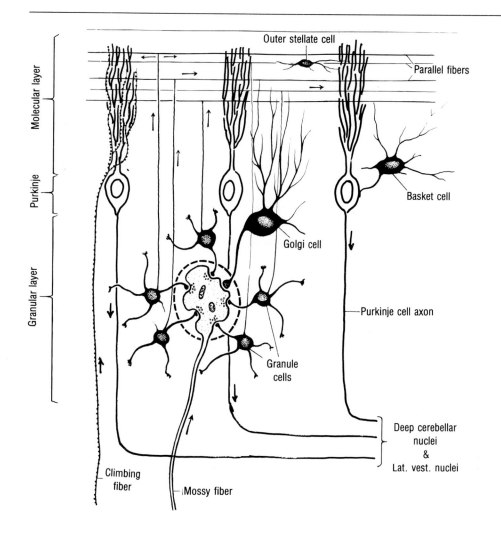

Molecular layer

Purkinje

Granular layer

Outer stellate cell

Parallel fibers

Basket cell

Golgi cell

Purkinje cell axon

Granule
cells

Deep cerebellar
nuclei
&
Lat. vest. nuclei

Climbing
fiber

Mossy fiber

FIGURE 1.
Schematic drawing of the cerebellum illustrating cell and fiber arrangement and direction of nerve impulses. (From R. C. Truex and M. B. Carpenter, Human Neuroanatomy, Williams and Wilkins, Baltimore, 1969.)

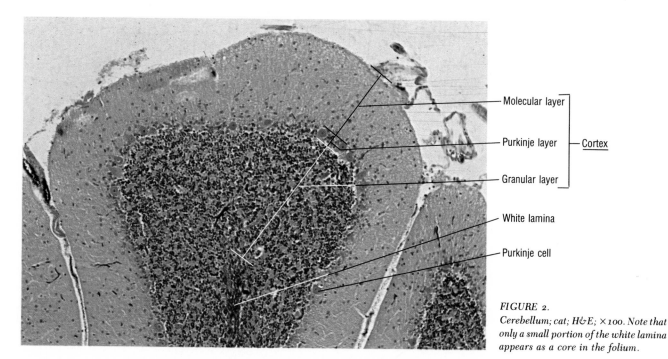

Molecular layer

Purkinje layer — Cortex

Granular layer

White lamina

Purkinje cell

FIGURE 2.
Cerebellum; cat; H&E; ×100. Note that only a small portion of the white lamina appears as a core in the folium.

PLATE 7 ——————————————————————————————————————

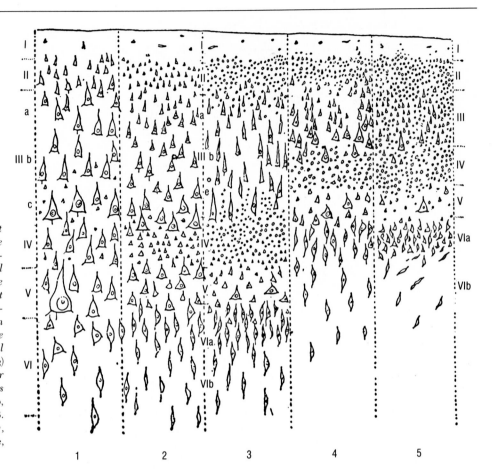

FIGURE 1.

Types of neopallial cortex. Note that 1 is designated as an agranular type of cortex because relatively few granule cells are present. The pyramidal cells are most abundant, and some are quite large. The six layers are not sharply separated, which is a characteristic of the agranular cortex. In the other types the layers are more distinct. (1) Agranular (precentral gyrus); (2) frontal (frontal lobe); (3) parietal (parietal lobe); (4) polar (occipital lobe); (5) granulous (calcarine cortex). (After von Economo, 1929. From R. C. Truex and M. B. Carpenter, Human Neuroanatomy, Williams and Wilkins, Baltimore, 1969.)

The walls of the hemispheres are composed of a deep *medulla* (white matter) covered by a superficial *cortex* (gray matter).

The medulla is composed of subcortical nuclei and tracts mainly of myelinated fibers. The fibers may be: (1) commisural, which interconnect similar areas of both hemispheres; (2) association, which interconnect cortical areas on the same hemisphere; or (3) projection, which connect the cortex with lower levels of the CNS.

The cerebral cortex is folded into a number of folds, *gyri*, separated by furrows, *sulci*. The cerebral cortex varies in histological structure and thickness, depending on the region of the hemisphere. It is thinner in the occipital region (about 1.5 mm) than in the precentral region (about 4 mm). The cortex is thickest over the crests of the gyri and thinnest in the sulci. The cerebral cortex contains glial cells and neurons with mainly unmyelinated fibers. Of the neurological regions of the cerebral cortex, only the neopallium (neocortex) has six poorly defined horizontal layers of tissue, each with characteristic types of neurons. The paleopallium (olfactory cortex) and archipallium lack these six layers. These variations are evident in the different regions of the cortex and are directly related to functional differences. The six layers of the neopallial cortex are given in sequence, going from the most superficial to the deepest level: (I) *molecular layer*, (II) *external granular layer*, (III) *pyramidal cell layer*, (IV) *internal granular layer*, (V) *ganglionic layer*, and (VI) *fusiform layer*. Thin sections with either routine or special silver stains will not show the synaptic patterns between these six cortical layers, but the cell types and their distributions can be demonstrated. Each of the six layers of the neocortex may be characterized by their types of neurons and processes. **Plate 7, Fig. 1.**

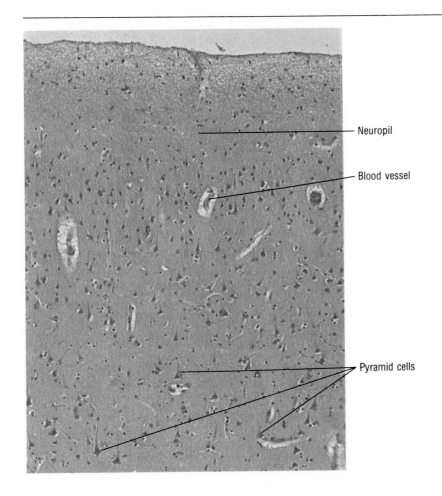

— Neuropil

— Blood vessel

— Pyramid cells

FIGURE 2.
Cerebral cortex; human; H&E; ×100.
Note that only the upper layers of the
cerebral cortex are seen. The layers
are not sharply set apart from each
other.

Molecular layer I contains many neuroglia cells, a band of myelinated fibers, and relatively few neurons of the granular and horizontal type.

External granular layer II contains small granule cells (Golgi type II) and many small pyramidal cells.

Pyramidal cell layer III contains mainly medium- and large-sized pyramidal cells, and some Martinotti and granule cells.

Internal granular layer IV contains mainly small granule cells (Golgi type II), and some small pyramidal cells. Many myelinated fibers occur in this region.

Ganglionic layer V contains mainly large pyramidal cells, and some granule and Martinotti cells. The axons of the pyramidal cells enter the medulla as projection and association fibers; some form part of the corpus callosum. In the motor cortex, the axons of the giant pyramidal cells of Betz form some of the fibers in the corticospinal tract.

Fusiform layer VI contains fusiform cells, some small granule cells (Golgi type II), large granule cells (Golgi type I), and Martinotti cells. Axons of the fusiform cells enter the medulla as projection and association fibers. Many prominent bundles of myelinated fibers, coming from and going toward the medulla, are also present in this layer.

The main types of neurons which are present in the cerebral cortex are the pyramidal cells, granular cells, and fusiform cells. Other less numerous types are the cells of Martinotti and the horizontal cells of Cajal.

PYRAMIDAL CELLS. These neurons may be small, medium, or large, and the cell bodies vary from 10 to 100 μm in size. The cell body is triangular, with its apex directed to the surface of the cerebral cortex. The basophilic cytoplasm contains prominent Nissl substance and a large, round, vesicular nucleus. A large apical dendrite extends from the apex of the cell and branches as it approaches the upper cortical level. Several basal dendrites extend horizontally from the lower portion of the cell body and usually branch immediately. The axon arises from the base of the cell and may terminate in the deep cerebral cortex or extend into the medulla. The pyramidal cells are concerned with projection and associations and are present in layers II, III, IV, and V. **Plate 7, Figs. 1 and 2; Plate 8, Fig. 1.**

GRANULE CELLS. These are mainly small, approximately 4 to 8 μm in size, round or polygonal multipolar neurons. The sparse cytoplasm contains a round, dark nucleus. Some have a short axon terminating near the cell body (Golgi type II neurons). Larger granule cells, stellate pyramidal cells, have a long axon which extends into the medulla (Golgi type I neurons). Granule cells primarily function as intracortical connections between other neurons. They are found in all layers of the cerebral cortex, but are most numerous in layer IV. **Plate 8, Fig. 1.**

FUSIFORM CELLS (spindle cells, polymorphic cells). These are small neurons. The fusiform or angular cell body contains a small, dark-stained nucleus. Dendrites extend from both ends of the fusiform cell, one going into the upper levels of the cerebral cortex and the other repeatedly branching near the cell body. The axon emerges from near the middle of the cell and runs into the underlying medulla. These cells, like the pyramidal cells, function as association and projection neurons. They are present in layer VI. **Plate 7, Fig. 1.**

HORIZONTAL CELLS. These are small, fusiform, pear-shaped multipolar neurons. Their long, thin, highly branched dendrites and axons extend horizontally through the superficial cortex. They are found only in layer I and function as intercortical connections between neurons. **Plate 8, Fig. 1.**

MARTINOTTI CELLS. These are small, triangular or polygonal multipolar neurons. Their axons run toward the surface of the cerebral cortex and may terminate in one layer or extend through several layers before terminating. They, like the horizontal cells, function as interneural connections between other neurons. The Martinotti cells are found throughout most layers of the cerebral cortex. **Plate 8, Fig. 1.**

PHYSIOLOGY AND INTRACORTICAL CIRCUITS OF THE CORTICAL NEURONS. In general, an impulse is carried by afferent fibers (projection fibers from the thalamus, or association and commisural fibers, cortico-cortico connections) mainly up to the third and fourth layers of the cerebral cortex. Here, they synapse either with efferent cortical neurons, or intercortical neurons, or both. The intercortical neurons are the granular, Martinotti, and horizontal cells. Because their axons are of the ascending, horizontal, and short variety, the impulse may spread both vertically and horizontally. The efferent cortical neurons have many axonal collaterals which also will contribute to the "spread of an impulse." The impulse may involve a large area before it leaves the cortex via efferent projection, association, or commisural fibers. These fibers mainly represent descending axons of pyramidal, fusiform, and large granule cells which enter the white matter. **Plate 8, Fig. 1.**

Meninges. The meninges are three sheaths of connective tissue which enclose the CNS to protect and nourish it. The outermost sheath is the *dura mater*, below that is the *arachnoid*, and innermost is the *pia mater*. The latter meninx, unlike the others, closely follows the contours of the CNS. The combined arachnoid and pia layers may be referred to as the leptomeninges. **Plate 5, Fig. 1.**

DURA MATER. This is a tough, nonelastic membrane of dense, irregular collagenous connective tissue, rich with blood vessels and nerves. In the *skull* the dura is

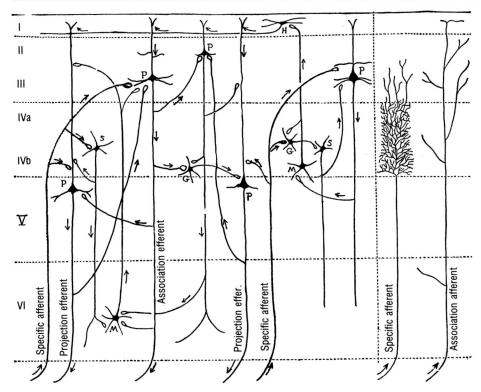

I

II

III

IVa

IVb

V

VI

Specific afferent
Projection efferent
Association efferent
Projection effer.
Specific afferent
Specific afferent
Association afferent

FIGURE 1.
Schematic diagram of some of the circuits in the cerebral cortex. Note the following: Synaptic junctions are indicated by loops; P = pyramidal cells; H = horizontal cells; M = Martinotti cells; S = stellate pyramidal cells; and G = granule cells. (From R. C. Truex and M. B. Carpenter, Human Neuroanatomy, Williams and Wilkins, Baltimore, 1969.)

composed of two layers, separated by large vascular sinuses. The outer endosteal layer is fused to the skull and represents the periosteum. The inner meningeal layer is organized into several prominent septa which anchor and protect the regions of the brain: *tentorium cerebelli* supports the occipital lobes of the cerebrum; *falx cerebri* supports and separates the cerebral hemispheres; *diaphragma sellae* forms a roof for the sella turcica and encloses most of the hypophysis; and the *falx cerebelli* which supports and partially separates the cerebellar hemispheres. The meningeal layer also forms a roof over a subdural space that lies between the dura mater and arachnoid. A simple squamous epithelium (mesothelium) lines the free surface of the dura which is exposed to the subdural space.

At the level of the *spinal cord* the dura mater is a single layer of dense collagenous connective tissue, separated from the vertebral periosteum by an epidural space. Both the upper and lower surfaces of the dura are lined with a simple squamous epithelium. Some of the dural tissue is continuous with the epineurium of the spinal nerve roots.

PIA-ARACHNOID LAYER (leptomeninges). Although the arachnoid and pia mater are usually considered as separate membranes, they are derived from a common embryonic structure and may be collectively designated as leptomeninges. During development the leptomeninges are separated into an upper arachnoid and a lower pia layer by a large fluid-filled cavity, the subarachnoid space, and blood vessels. The two layers are partially interconnected by cobweblike strands of tissue, the trabeculae. Cerebrospinal fluid moves between the subarachnoid space and the fourth venticle through three apertures in the roof of the medulla oblongata: a dorsomedian foramen of Magendie and two lateral foramina of Luschka.

Arachnoid. This is a thin, nonvascular layer lying below the subdural space and above the subarachnoid space. The arachnoid is lined with simple squamous epithelium. It is composed of collagen and elastic fibers, fibroblasts, and a few macrophages. Trabeculae extend below the arachnoid and are continuous with the pia mater.

Pia mater. The pia mater contains delicate reticular and collagen fibers, fibroblasts, and some elastic fibers. It also is a thin layer, but unlike the arachnoid it is quite vascular and closely follows the CNS topography. The pia is anchored to the surface of the CNS by processes of astrocytes. Its upper surface is lined by a simple squamous epithelium.

BLOOD AND LYMPHATIC VESSELS OF THE CNS. The vertebral arteries give rise to the posterior and anterior spinal arteries which run the length of the spinal cord. Spinal branches of the vertebral, ascending cervical, intercostal, iliolumbar, and lumbar arteries give rise to small radicular arteries which divide into anterior and posterior branches. The branches run toward the spinal cord, via the roots of the spinal nerves, and eventually form dense plexuses within the pia mater around the periphery of the cord. Vessels from these plexuses extend into the white matter and also some gray matter. At various levels a few large anterior radicular arteries anastomose to form longitudinal vessels near the anterior median fissure of the spinal cord. These branches anastomose with the anterior spinal artery to form a large single vessel along the anterior median fissure. Central arteries arise from the anterior spinal artery, pass into the fissure, and enter the left or right side of the spinal cord. They enter the medial aspect of the anterior gray columns and supply blood to most of the gray matter and some adjacent white matter. The venous pattern is anatomically distinct from that of the arteries. Diffuse plexuses are formed in the pia by venous branches coming from the periphery of the cord and the anterior median fissure. These plexuses are drained by six longitudinal and tortuous veins: one anterior, one posterior, one anterolateral pair, and one posterolateral pair. At the lower levels of the spinal cord these six veins are drained by the intervertebral veins, but at the base of the skull they unite and their common trunks are drained by the vertebral veins.

Arterial blood is carried to the brain by the vertebral arteries and internal carotids. The vertebral arteries fuse to form an unpaired basilar artery. A fusion between branches of the basilar artery and the internal carotids form the posterior portion of the circle of Willis, an anastomosis at the base of the brain. The anterior part of the circle of Willis is completed by an anastomosis between anterior branches of the internal carotid arteries. The circle of Willis also supplies the brain with arterial vessels. Venous blood is drained by branches of cerebral veins which form plexuses in the pia mater. The veins extend through the subarachnoid space and eventually drain into large venous sinuses (dural sinuses). These sinuses, in turn, are drained by the internal jugular veins. Lymphatics are not present in the CNS.

NERVES. Smooth muscles of blood vessels located in the dura, pia, and CNS are innervated by myelinated and unmyelinated fibers of the autonomic nervous system. The meninges also have myelinated afferent fibers innervating sensory receptors.

Blood 7

Blood is a specialized connective tissue containing formed elements (erythrocytes, leucocytes, and platelets) suspended in a fluid plasma. In normal blood the formed elements compose about 46 percent of the total volume, while plasma makes up the remaining 54 percent. *Plasma* is a pale yellow, slightly alkaline (pH 7.40) fluid which provides an isotonic medium for cells and tissues of the body. It functions as a buffer and also transports nutrients (amino acids, carbohydrates, and lipids), wastes (carbon dioxide, urea, etc.), enzymes, hormones, and antibodies. Other functions include its participation in the blood clotting processes and distribution of heat. Of the formed elements, *erythrocytes* transport oxygen and carbon dioxide between the lungs and tissues of the body; *leucocytes* provide a natural defense against inflammatory agents by their phagocytic nature, and production of antibodies and anti-inflammatory substances; *blood platelets* contribute to the blood clotting mechanism.

Blood smears are routinely stained with Romanowsky stains (Giemsa's and Wright's stain), containing acid dyes (eosin), basic dyes (methylene blue, azures A, B, or C), and neutral dyes (eosinates of methylene blue and azures). These dyes color specific organic compounds in the cells by forming electrostatic links with their negatively and positively charged radicals. The Giemsa staining technique is more time-consuming than Wright's, but it consistently produces uniform results and is better for the demonstration of cytoplasmic granules.

Erythrocytes (red blood corpuscles)

These saclike structures carry a respiratory pigment, *hemoglobin*, which transports oxygen and some carbon dioxide. Hemoglobin forms a loose association with oxygen and provides the means whereby carbon dioxide can be carried in the corpuscle; it contributes the base used to convert carbonic acid to a bicarbonate. Erythrocytes normally compose 45 percent of the total blood volume. Although there is considerable developmental overlap during the prenatal period, erythrocytes are successively produced in the yolk sac (4th week), blood vessels (5th week), liver (6th week), spleen, thymus, and lymph nodes (2d to 4th month), and bone marrow (4th month). After birth, they are produced only in bone marrow of the normal individual.

PLATE 1 _____

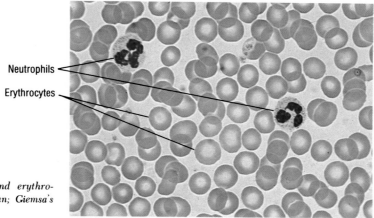

Neutrophils

Erythrocytes

FIGURE 1.
Neutrophilic leucocyte and erythro-
cytes; blood smear; human; Giemsa's
stain; ×1000.

Erythropoietic centers may develop in other organs as a response to certain pathologic conditions. Erythrocytes circulate in the peripheral blood for approximately one hundred and twenty days. At the end of that time the old, usually ruptured, erythrocytes are removed from the blood by phagocytic macrophages in splenic cords and sinusoids of liver and bone marrow. As the erythrocytes are digested by the macrophages, hemoglobin will be degraded into its component parts—globin and heme (an organic compound containing iron). The iron is removed from heme and then is either transported by a blood globulin, transferrin, to the marrow for the synthesis of new hemoglobin or stored in the liver as ferritin. The noniron portion of heme will be converted to bilirubin in the liver and excreted as a bile pigment.

Morphology. The erythrocyte is a small (7.5 μm), biconcave disk with a thin, pale center and a thick, dark rim. It appears round in a surface view, but is dumbbell-shaped in profile. At times normal erythrocytes may be distorted (oval, elongate, crenate, or broken) because of improper laboratory techniques used in preparing the blood smear. The mature erythrocyte lacks a nucleus, and the hemoglobin-filled cytoplasm is surrounded by a thin plasma membrane. The acidophilic hemoglobin stains a pale reddish pink with Giemsa's or Wright's stains. **Plate 1, Fig. 1.**

Leucocytes (white blood cells)

In normal blood these cells compose 1 percent of the total blood volume. Unlike erythrocytes, they are nucleated and lack hemoglobin, and some are actively amoeboid. Of the five types of leucocytes, three (neutrophilic leucocytes, basophilic leucocytes, and eosinophilic leucocytes) are classified as granulocytes because they have specific granules (see Chap. 8) in their cytoplasm. The remaining two types are designated as agranular leucocytes (lymphocytes and monocytes), since they lack specific granules; they may, however, contain nonspecific granules in the cytoplasm (see Chap. 8). Granulocytes have a polymorphonuclear nucleus with two or more connected lobes, and agranular leucocytes have a spherical or kidney-shaped nonlobate nucleus (some monocytes, however, may be lobate). Although leucocyte proportions are relatively constant, they may vary because of allergies, diseases, or unusual stresses. In normal adult blood, leucocytes are present in the following

PLATE 1 *continued*

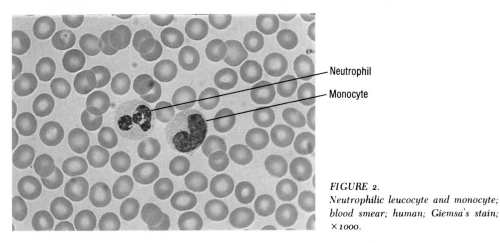

FIGURE 2.
Neutrophilic leucocyte and monocyte;
blood smear; human; Giemsa's stain;
×1000.

approximate proportions: neutrophilic leucocytes, 50 to 80 percent; eosinophilic leucocytes, 1 to 3 percent; basophilic leucocytes, 0 to 1 percent; lymphocytes, 20 to 50 percent.

Leucocytes are produced in the same embryonic hematopoietic centers as erythrocytes (see page 89), but in the adult granulocytes develop only in bone marrow and agranular leucocytes develop in bone marrow and lymphoid organs. Granulocytes circulate briefly in the blood, but eventually most of them enter the extravascular spaces in connective tissues where they become functional. Those remaining in the blood will be removed by the macrophages in the liver and spleen as they die, while the ones in connective tissue will ultimately disintegrate, form pus, or migrate through epithelial surfaces to be eliminated from the body. Agranular leucocytes have a more complex life history (see below).

NEUTROPHILIC LEUCOCYTES (neutrophils, polymorphonuclear neutrophils). These cells constitute approximately 50 to 80 percent of the leucocyte population in blood. Their main function is to phagocytize and digest bacteria or foreign particles which have invaded the body tissues. Destruction and digestion of bacteria are accomplished by the release and activation of hydrolytic enzymes, lysozyme, and phagocytin (an antibacterial basic protein), all of which are present in the cytoplasmic granules.

Morphology. The mature cells are 12 to 15 μm in diameter, approximately twice the size of erythrocytes. The nucleus has three or more lobes connected by thin filaments. The heterochromatin is coarse and stained dark bluish purple; nucleoli are not present. The abundant cytoplasm is light pink and contains many evenly distributed granules. The granules are of two types: numerous tiny specific granules, grayish lavender in color, and a few large nonspecific granules (stained reddish purple). A less mature cell, the neutrophilic band, may appear in circulating blood. It is identified by a U-shaped nucleus, lacking filaments. **Plate 1, Figs. 1 and 2; Plate 2, Figs. 1 and 2; Plate 4, Figs. 1 and 2.**

Female sex chromatin ("drumstick" nuclear appendage). Davidson and Smith (1954) discovered and named a characteristic appendage or extra chromatin lobe in the nucleus of neutrophils found in the peripheral blood of the human female. It occurs in 2.6 percent of the female neutrophils, but has not been found in the male

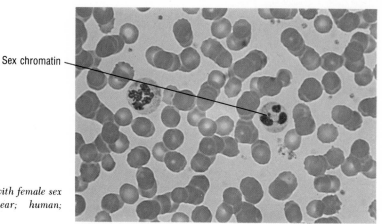

Sex chromatin

FIGURE 3.
Neutrophilic leucocyte with female sex chromatin; blood smear; human; Wright's stain; ×1000.

neutrophils. Neither age of the female nor removal of the gonads have any influence on the occurrence of the structure. It is a well-defined, solid, round head, 1.5 μ in diameter, joined by a single fine chromatin strand to one lobe of the neutrophil nucleus. The male human neutrophil occasionally may show a budding of the nuclear chromatin, but the clubs are much smaller (less than 1.0 μ in diameter) and have pale centers. They are termed "racket" structures and are not considered true sex lobes. **Plate 1, Fig. 3.**

EOSINOPHILIC LEUCOCYTES (eosinophils, polymorphonuclear eosinophils). These cells represent about 1 to 3 percent of the leucocytes in blood. Compared with neutrophils, eosinophils have similar, but reduced, abilities for phagocytizing and destroying bacteria. They are mainly concerned with phagocytosis of antigen-antibody complexes produced during an immune response. The ingested complex, then, may be inactivated, destroyed, or modified to reduce its effect in the body. Also, eosinophils are attracted to sites where histamine and toxic histaminelike substances are released by basophils. Their function is to detoxify and inactivate these substances, thereby controlling the extent of inflammatory reactions.

Morphology. The eosinophil is about the same size as the neutrophil, 12 to 15 μm in diameter. The nucleus has three lobes, one small and two large, connected by nuclear filaments; the small lobe is usually not seen in routine preparations. There is no nucleolus, and the heterochromatin is coarse, clumped, and stained dark bluish purple. The cytoplasm contains large, spherical, eosinophilic (reddish orange) granules of uniform size. Even though the granules fill the cytoplasm, they usually do not cover the nucleus. **Plate 2, Figs. 1 and 2; Plate 4, Fig. 4.**

BASOPHILIC LEUCOCYTES (basophils, polymorphonuclear basophils). The basophils compare favorably with eosinophils in their phagocytic and antibacterial properties but they are less effective in this respect than the neutrophils. Although their granules contain some of the antibacterial substances present in neutrophil granules, they also possess heparin (an anticoagulant) and histamine (a vasoactive amine). If the basophil is stimulated by an antigen or by injury to tissues, it will respond with a degranulation and subsequent release of histamine. The released histamine will initiate an inflammatory reaction by causing vasodilation and increased permeability of blood vessels. Basophils are scarce in blood, representing about 1 percent or less of the leucocytes.

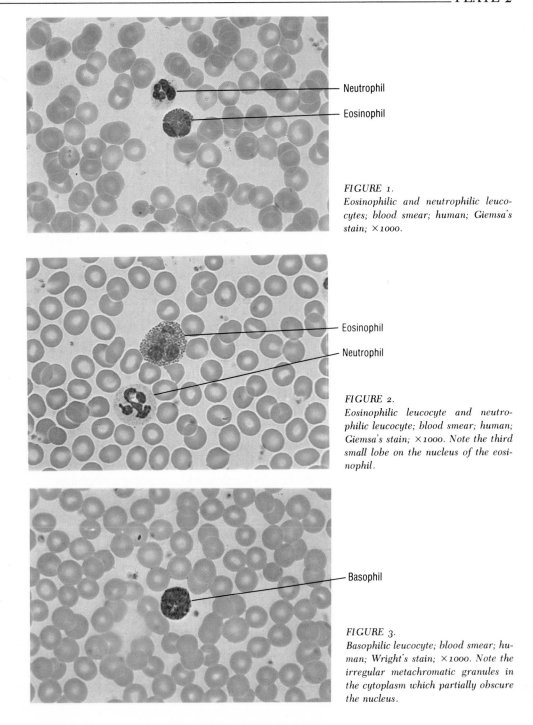

FIGURE 1.
Eosinophilic and neutrophilic leuco-
cytes; blood smear; human; Giemsa's
stain; ×1000.

FIGURE 2.
Eosinophilic leucocyte and neutro-
philic leucocyte; blood smear; human;
Giemsa's stain; ×1000. Note the third
small lobe on the nucleus of the eosi-
nophil.

FIGURE 3.
Basophilic leucocyte; blood smear; hu-
man; Wright's stain; ×1000. Note the
irregular metachromatic granules in
the cytoplasm which partially obscure
the nucleus.

Morphology. Basophils are approximately 12 to 15 μm in diameter, and therefore are in the same size range as neutrophils and eosinophils. The elongate, contorted nucleus has two or three poorly defined lobes, appearing as slight bumps, along its length. Nucleoli are absent and the chromatin is less dense, paler, and more indistinct than the heterochromatin in other granulocytes. Prominent cytoplasmic granules usually obscure the nucleus. These granules are metachromatic (dark blue to purple), variable in numbers, and unevenly distributed. Depending on their state of preservation, the granules may appear spherical and uniform or irregular in size and shape. **Plate 2, Fig. 3.**

LYMPHOCYTES. These cells compose about 20 to 50 percent of the leucocytes in circulating blood, and participate in immune responses. Three sizes of lymphocytes may be present in the blood: small, intermediate, and large. In addition to relative size, the types of lymphocytes are distinguished by the appearance of their chromatin (dark-stained, dense heterochromatin, or light-stained, vesicular euchromatin), and the intensity of the stain of their basophilic cytoplasm. The small lymphocytes are most common, but occasionally intermediate and, more rarely, large ones are present in blood. The large lymphocytes have euchromatin rather than heterochromatin, and their cytoplasm is usually more basophilic than that of the small ones. The intermediate and large lymphocytes may represent antigenically stimulated cells or premitotic phases of unstimulated cells. Although the immune response may be initiated in any part of the body, it usually will continue within the spleen, lymph nodes, or other lymphoid tissues (except the thymus).

There are two types of small lymphocytes: *T cells* (thymus-dependent lymphocytes) and *B cells* (bursa-dependent lymphocytes). Both are derived from multipotential hematopoietic stem cells in the marrow. They cannot be distinguished from each other with the light microscope, but each type has its own unique function and life history.

Immunologically incompetent stem cells originating in bone marrow are carried by the blood to the thymus. Here, they leave the blood, proliferate, and become immunologically competent T cells in the thymic tissues. About 5 percent of these cells reenter the blood as small, long-lived lymphocytes. For many years they recirculate through lymphoid tissues and organs, except the thymus. T cells are the most common (70 to 80 percent) small lymphocytes in circulating blood because of their high rate of recirculation and their long life. As they recirculate, most of the T cells migrate into extravascular regions, but eventually return to the blood via the lymphatic system. When stimulated by antigens, within lymphoid tissues, the T cells differentiate into large lymphocytes (lymphoblasts). These give rise to more T cells with various immunologic functions. The different T cells may stimulate antibody production in B cells, or be capable of destroying antigens directly, without antibody production (cell-mediated immunologic response).

Some investigators believe that B cells differentiate and become competent in bone marrow, while others think that immunological competency occurs in unknown lymphoid structures apart from the marrow. In birds, it is known that immunologically competent B cells are processed in the bursa of Fabricius, a lymphoid diverticulum in the anterior wall of the proctodeum, and released into the blood.

Competent B cells recirculate slowly through lymphoid tissues and organs, except the thymus. Due to their slow rate of recirculation and short life (about 2 weeks), B cells constitute only 20 to 30 percent of the small lymphocytes in blood. Depending on the type of antigen, B cells can be stimulated to produce blood-borne antibodies either independently or by forming close physical associations with macrophages and stimulated T cells. When B cells are stimulated, they may differentiate into large antibody-producing lymphocytes (lymphoblasts) within lymphoid tissues. These highly prolific lymphoblasts may also give rise to antibody-producing plasma cells and more B cells.

Morphology of small lymphocytes. These cells are about 8 μm in diameter, slightly larger than erythrocytes. The large nucleus is spherical or slightly indented. The heterochromatin is dense and coarse, and appears in dark-stained, purple clumps. Nucleoli are present but not evident. The light blue cytoplasm surrounds the nucleus

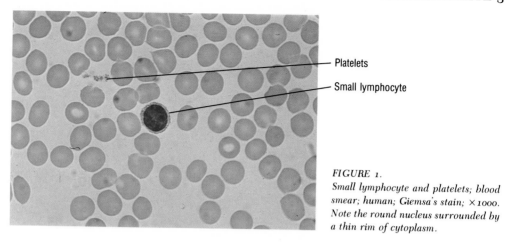

Platelets

Small lymphocyte

FIGURE 1.
Small lymphocyte and platelets; blood
smear; human; Giemsa's stain; ×1000.
Note the round nucleus surrounded by
a thin rim of cytoplasm.

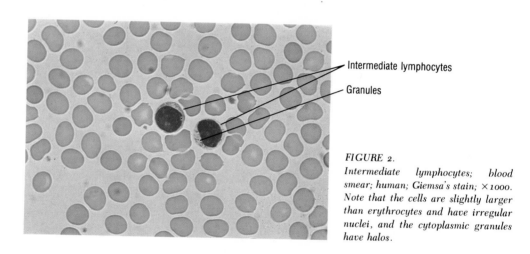

Intermediate lymphocytes

Granules

FIGURE 2.
Intermediate lymphocytes; blood
smear; human; Giemsa's stain; ×1000.
Note that the cells are slightly larger
than erythrocytes and have irregular
nuclei, and the cytoplasmic granules
have halos.

as a thin ring, and may contain some small reddish purple granules. Lymphocytes are fragile and easily distorted during the preparation of a smear, and so the cytoplasm may be frayed or filamentous, or appear in one of many odd forms. **Plate 3, Figs. 1 and 3; Plate 4, Figs. 1 and 2.**

Morphology of intermediate lymphocytes. This type of lymphocyte is about 12 μm, approximately 1½ times larger than the erythrocyte. Compared with a small lymphocyte, the nucleus is well indented or irregular in form. Some heterochromatin has been replaced by euchromatin, and so the nucleus appears less dense than that of a small lymphocyte. The chromatin is reddish purple, and a nucleolus may be observed within the nucleus. The basophilic cytoplasm is relatively more abundant so that it usually forms an ample, unequal ring around the nucleus. At times the cytoplasm contains scattered, irregularly shaped, reddish purple granules, and each granule is surrounded by a clear zone or halo. **Plate 3, Fig. 2; Plate 4, Fig. 2.**

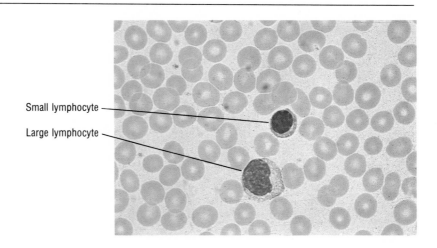

Small lymphocyte

Large lymphocyte

FIGURE 3.
Large and small lymphocytes; blood smear; human; Giemsa's stain; ×1000. The small lymphocyte is distorted, and so the cytoplasm does not appear as a continuous ring around the nucleus. Note that the chromatin in the large lymphocyte is not as dense and dark as the chromatin in the small and intermediate lymphocytes.

Morphology of large lymphocytes. These lymphocytes are about 18 μm in diameter, approximately twice the size of small lymphocytes and about the same size as granular leucocytes. The nucleus may be irregular, indented, or ovoid and contains more euchromatin than heterochromatin. Although some clumps are present, the euchromatin is diffuse and stains light reddish purple; one or two nucleoli may be visible. The basophilic cytoplasm is quite abundant, comprising about one-half of the cell, and may contain granules similar to those described for the intermediate lymphocytes. **Plate 3, Fig. 3.**

MONOCYTES. These are present in circulating blood and constitute from 2 to 10 percent of the leucocytes. They are produced in bone marrow, circulate briefly in blood, and upon reaching extravascular areas, such as spaces in connective tissues, may differentiate into free or fixed macrophages. Monocytes are excellent phagocytic cells and ingest small or large masses of matter (such as bacteria, dead cells, erythrocytes, and tissue debris). They are attracted to sites of inflammation where they may differentiate into macrophages. The macrophages are better phagocytes than monocytes and, in addition, facilitate antibody production by lymphocytes.

Morphology. Monocytes are the largest leucocytes in normal blood, varying in size from 12 to 25 μm. The nucleus may be oval, kidney-shaped, or lobate. If lobes are present, they are superimposed and give the nucleus a convoluted appearance. The chromatin, unlike that of lymphocytes, is less dense, and has pale reddish blue, netlike strands rather than clumps. Nucleoli are present, but are usually not visible. The cytoplasm forms better than one-half of the cell and may have one or more short, blunt pseudopods. It stains dull grayish blue and usually contains vacuoles, granules, and phagocytized particles. Occasionally a few large reddish purple granules will be scattered among the numerous tiny gray ones. **Plate 1, Fig. 2; Plate 4, Figs. 1, 2, and 3.**

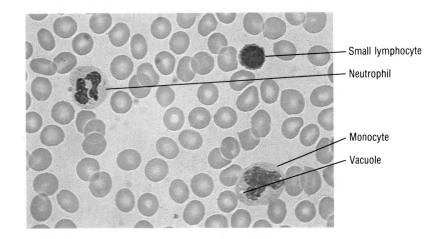

Small lymphocyte

Neutrophil

Monocyte

Vacuole

FIGURE 1.
Monocyte, small lymphocyte and neutrophilic leucocyte; blood smear; human; Giemsa's stain; ×1000. Note the vacuolated cytoplasm in the monocyte.

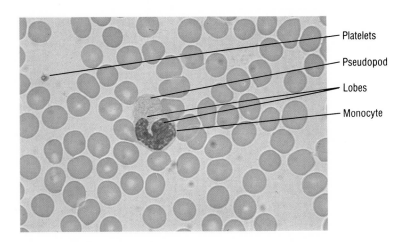

Small lymphocyte

Intermediate lymphocyte

Neutrophil

Monocyte

FIGURE 2.
Monocyte, small lymphocyte, intermediate lymphocyte, and neutrophil; blood smear; human; Giemsa's stain; ×1000.

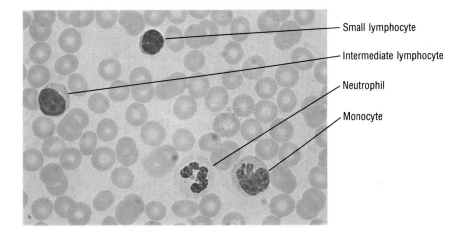

Platelets

Pseudopod

Lobes

Monocyte

FIGURE 3.
Monocyte and platelets; blood smear; human; Giemsa's stain; ×1000. In the monocyte, note the folded lobes in the nucleus, granular cytoplasm, and pseudopods.

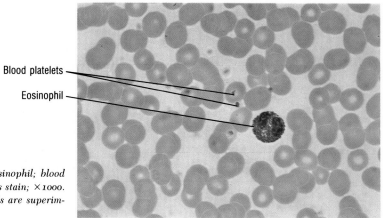

Blood platelets

Eosinophil

FIGURE 4.
Blood platelets and eosinophil; blood
smear; human; Wright's stain; ×1000.
Note that some platelets are superim-
posed on erythrocytes.

Blood platelets

These structures are derived from the cytoplasm of megakaryocytes located in the bone marrow. They have a life-span of about 10 days and are removed by macrophages lining the sinusoids of the liver and bone marrow. When activated, platelets release a substance, *thromboplastin*, which plays a role in fibrin fiber formation in blood clots. Platelets improve a clot by becoming enmeshed between the fibers and anastomosing to form a continuous, viscous mass. They are also responsible for the later shrinkage and retraction of the clot. It is possible that clot shrinkage is due to the activity of a contractile protein, thrombostenin, present in activated platelets. When the platelet is activated, this protein may be synthesized from components similar to actin and myosin filaments in muscle.

Morphology. Platelets are small, approximately 3 μm, round or oval disks, but may appear stellate with many cytoplasmic extensions. The central part of the platelet is the granulomere, containing small reddish purple granules. The peripheral part of the platelet, that surrounding the granulomere, is the nongranulated, pale blue hyalomere. These two regions of the platelet may not be readily visible in some preparations. **Plate 4, Fig. 4.**

Hematopoietic Tissue 8

Blood cells develop in hematopoietic tissues which are present in the yolk sac, blood vessels, liver, spleen, and bone marrow of the embryo. In the normal adult the most important hematopoietic tissue is bone marrow. Although hematopoiesis occurs primarily in extravascular regions, some blood-forming activity may be found within the vascular system. According to the monophyletic theory of hematopoiesis, which is followed by this atlas, hematopoietic tissue of the marrow contains a single type of multipotential hematopoietic stem cell which is derived from mesenchymal cells. These stem cells are precursors of erythrocytes, granular leucocytes (neutrophils, eosinophils, and basophils), monocytes, lymphocytes, and megakaryocytes. Some hematologists, however, favor the concept of several types of stem cells as precursors of blood cells (polyphyletic theory).

Multipotential hematopoietic stem cells are morphologically undefined because they are undistinguished, slowly reproducing cells, and are a very small proportion of the blood cell population. Their presence in marrow and lymphoid tissues has been established by indirect evidence. Their progeny, undistinguished stem cells with less developmental potential and greater reproductive rates, differentiate into blast cells as a response to hormones and other possible environmental factors.

Blast cells are the immediate precursors to the various lineages of blood cells. Unlike the stem cells from which they were derived, blast cells are more numerous, are morphologically distinct, and may be recognized in a marrow smear (except monoblasts). Depending on the particular lineage of blood cells, blast cells may be designated as *myeloblasts*, for granulocytopoiesis; *proerythroblasts*, for erythropoiesis; *lymphoblasts*, for lymphocytopoiesis; *promonocytes* (not blast cells), for monocytopoiesis; and *megakaryoblasts*, for megakaryocyte development.

In a study of this type one will encounter many cells which are difficult to identify for one or more of the following reasons: distortion, cell degeneration, transitional stages of maturation, or poorly stained cells. It is important, therefore, to scan several fields with an oil immersion lens, to get a "feel for the smear," and then to concentrate on locating the best specimens according to their description.

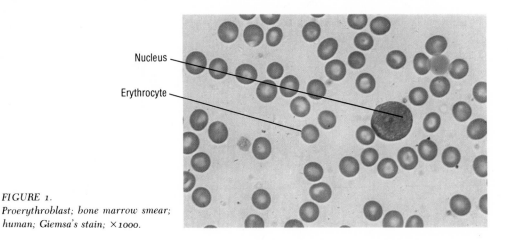

Nucleus ————

Erythrocyte ————

FIGURE 1.
Proerythroblast; bone marrow smear;
human; Giemsa's stain; ×1000.

Erythropoiesis

Multipotential hematopoietic stem cells give rise to less primitive cells which are influenced by a renal-produced hormone, erythropoietin, to differentiate into proerythroblasts. These latter cells are the immediate precursors of the maturation stages in the erythrocyte lineage. The chronological order of these stages are *proerythroblasts, basophilic erythroblasts, polychromatophil erythroblasts, normoblasts, reticulocytes,* and *erythrocytes.* During maturation, hemoglobin synthesis begins in the basophilic erythroblast, increasing in concentration until a maximum is reached in the normoblast. Ribosomes, on the other hand, will decrease throughout maturation, becoming scarce in the reticulocyte. Hemoglobin is acidophilic and stains red with the Romanowski blood stains, while the basophilic ribosomes stain blue. The cytoplasmic color of a cell, then, depends on the proportions of red-stained hemoglobin and blue-stained ribosomes. Young cells with low hemoglobin concentrations may stain blue, grayish blue, or gray, but as the hemoglobin increases in concentration, the more mature cells stain pinkish blue to pink. During maturation, the nucleus becomes smaller and heterochromatin replaces euchromatin.

PROERYTHROBLASTS (rubriblast). These cells are derived from stem cells in the marrow. They are capable of proliferating and giving rise to basophilic erythroblasts. They represent about 1 percent of the blood cells in marrow.

Morphology. The cells are round and large, approximately three times the diameter of erythrocytes (about 20 to 30 μm). A large, pale, oval or round nucleus is surrounded by a thin ring of dark bluish violet cytoplasm. The pale reddish blue chromatin is granular or netlike, and one or two pale nucleoli are present. **Plate 1, Fig. 1.**

BASOPHILIC ERYTHROBLASTS (prorubricyte). These are the progeny of proliferating proerythroblasts and, like them, can reproduce. As the basophilic erythroblasts mature and differentiate, they give rise to polychromatophil erythroblasts. Although hemoglobin synthesis begins with the basophilic erythroblasts, the hemoglobin is masked by the basophilic ribosomes. The cytoplasm is dark blue but is usually less

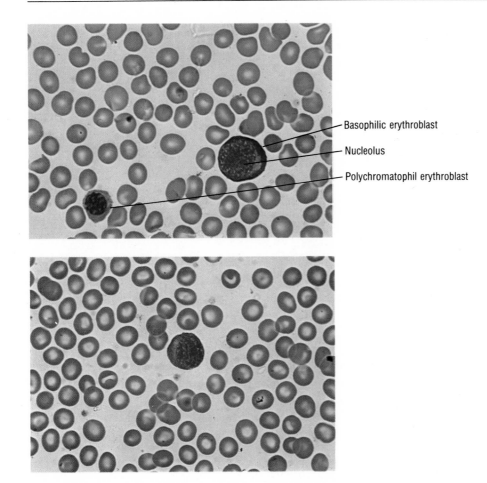

— Basophilic erythroblast

— Nucleolus

— Polychromatophil erythroblast

FIGURE 2.
Basophilic erythroblast (early); bone
marrow smear; human; Giemsa's stain;
×1000.

FIGURE 3.
Basophilic erythroblast (late); bone
marrow smear; human; Giemsa's stain;
×1000. Note that the nucleus is some-
what spotted.

intensely stained than that of the proerythroblasts. Basophilic erythroblasts make up about 1 to 4 percent of the marrow blood cells.

Morphology. The round cells are approximately twice the diameter of erythrocytes, about 15 to 20 μm. The relatively large, round nucleus is surrounded by a prominent ring of cytoplasm stained medium to dark bluish violet. The dark reddish purple chromatin strands are condensed and slightly clumped, so that the nucleus appears spotted. This spotting is an important morphological characteristic for these and later maturation stages in the erythropoietic series. One or more poorly defined nucleoli may be present. **Plate 1, Figs. 2 and 3.**

POLYCHROMATOPHIL ERYTHROBLASTS (rubricyte). These cells are derived from basophilic erythroblasts and are quite prolific. They are precursors to the next stage of maturation, the normoblasts. As the polychromatophil erythroblasts mature, they decrease in size, the cytoplasm fills with hemoglobin, the nucleus becomes smaller with condensed chromatin, and nuclear spotting is prominent. These cells constitute about 5 to 10 percent of the blood cells in marrow.

Morphology. Although the size may vary (12 to 15 μm in diameter), the cells are about 1½ times larger than erythrocytes. Depending on the concentration of

PLATE 2 _____

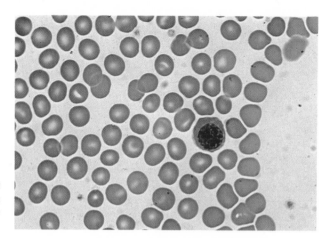

FIGURE 1.
Polychromatophil erythroblast; bone marrow smear; human; Giemsa's stain; ×1000. Note the prominent spotted nucleus.

hemoglobin, the cytoplasm stains grayish blue, gray, or pinkish blue. The nucleus is small and round, and spotted with densely clumped chromatin that stains dark purplish blue. Nucleoli are usually hidden by the chromatin. **Plate 2, Fig. 1.**

NORMOBLASTS (metarubricyte). These cells, unlike the polychromatophil erythroblasts from which they were derived, do not proliferate and contain high concentrations of hemoglobin in their cytoplasm. As normoblasts transform into reticulocytes, the nucleus becomes nonfunctional and pycnotic, and is lost from the cytoplasm. The nucleus may appear in the smear as a small, dark, oval body with shreds of cytoplasm clinging to it. Normoblasts are quite abundant, composing about 10 to 20 percent of the marrow cells.

Morphology. The normoblasts are slightly larger than erythrocytes; usually the diameter is about 1¼ times greater, or approximately 8 to 10 μm. The small nucleus may be pycnotic, with the chromatin appearing as deeply stained purplish black clumps or as a solid mass. The cytoplasm may be pinkish blue or pink. **Plate 2, Figs. 2 and 3.**

RETICULOCYTES (polychromatophilic erythrocytes). Reticulocytes are the end products of normoblast maturation. They transform into erythrocytes by a continued loss of ribosomes and cytoplasmic basophilia. Reticulocytes, as they are produced in the marrow, may be held in reserve or released into the blood. They represent about 1 percent of the circulating erythrocytes.

Morphology. Reticulocytes are about the size as normoblasts (8 to 10 μm), but slightly larger than erythrocytes. They are enucleate and stain pinkish blue, still showing a slight degree of basophilia. When the cells are stained with a supravital stain, such as brilliant cresyl blue, the remaining ribosomes appear as a fine blue network in the cytoplasm. **Plate 2, Figs. 3 and 4.**

ERYTHROCYTES. Mature erythrocytes are derived from reticulocytes. As the reticulocytes lose their ribosomes, they leave a concentration (about 33 percent) of hemoglobin within a matrix of organic and inorganic compounds.

Morphology. Erythrocytes are enucleate, biconcave disks which are thick at the periphery and thin in the center. They are approximately 7.5 μm in diameter and stain reddish pink (see Chap. 7). **Plate 2, Fig. 3.**

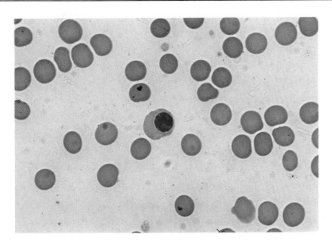

FIGURE 2.
Normoblast; bone marrow smear; human; Giemsa's stain; ×1000. Note the dense, almost homogeneous nucleus.

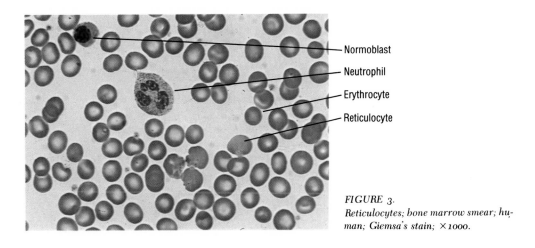

Normoblast

Neutrophil

Erythrocyte

Reticulocyte

FIGURE 3.
Reticulocytes; bone marrow smear; human; Giemsa's stain; ×1000.

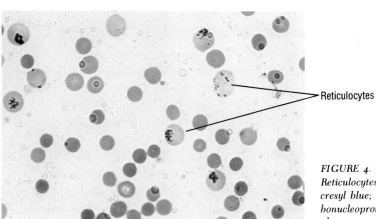

Reticulocytes

FIGURE 4.
Reticulocytes; blood smear; human; cresyl blue; ×1000. Note the blue ribonucleoprotein network in the cytoplasm.

Multipotential hematopoietic stem cells give rise to less primitive daughter cells which proliferate and differentiate into myeloblasts. The myeloblasts are precursor cells, specific for a particular lineage of granulocytic leucocytes—neutrophils, basophils, or eosinophils. The differentiation of myeloblasts is influenced by a hormone, *leukopoietin*, probably comparable to erythropoietin. The stages of maturation for any specific granulocyte lineage are given in the following chronological order: *myeloblasts, promyelocytes, myelocytes, metamyelocytes, bands,* and *segmented mature granulocytes* (leucocytes). Only the myelocytes and later stages can be readily identified as belonging to a particular lineage because the cytoplasm contains many *specific granules*. Depending on the granulocyte lineage (neutrophil, eosinophil, or basophil), these granules may be one of three types: *neutrophilic granules* are small and irregular, and stain blue-gray or light purple or are colorless; *eosinophilic granules* are large, uniform, and round, and stain reddish orange; *basophilic granules* are large and irregular, and stain dark blue or reddish purple.

All granulocytes mature in a similar manner. During the early stages of maturation, the young cells are large and have a large, oval, pale-stained euchromatin-filled nucleus; the cytoplasm gradually fills with large azurophilic *primary granules* (lysosomes). As the cells mature, they become smaller. The nucleus becomes smaller and segmented, and fills with dense clumps of dark-stained heterochromatin. Specific or secondary granules (see above), containing mainly bacteriocidal substances, are produced and these eventually outnumber the primary granules. Both types of granules persist in mature granulocytes, but their ratios depend on the type of cell.

MYELOBLASTS. These cells are derived from the progeny of the multipotential hematopoietic stem cells. The myeloblasts proliferate, differentiate, and mature, eventually giving rise to promyelocytes. They are the earliest cells to be recognized in the granulocytopoietic lineage and represent about 0.3 to 0.5 percent of the blood marrow cells.

Morphology. Myeloblasts are relatively large cells (15 to 21 μm in diameter), about 2½ times the diameter of erythrocytes. A large, pale reddish blue nucleus occupies about two-thirds of the cell, and two or more pale nucleoli are usually visible. The nucleus can be oval but is usually irregular. The cytoplasm lack granules and is stained an uneven medium to light blue color. **Plate 3, Fig. 1.**

PROMYELOCYTES (progranulocytes). These cells are derived from myeloblasts, and they in turn multiply and differentiate to become myelocytes. A few primary granules are produced in the cytoplasm of early promyelocytes; they increase in number as the cell matures. Approximately 1 to 8 percent of the blood marrow cells are promyelocytes.

Morphology. The cells may be as small as myeloblasts, but usually they are larger (18 to 30 μm in diameter), approximately four times the diameter of erythrocytes. The large, oval (or slightly indented) nucleus is surrounded by a medium-blue-stained cytoplasm containing some scattered, large, irregular, azurophilic (reddish purple) primary granules. Pale blue nucleoli are present but may be hidden by the condensed, coarse, reddish blue clumps of chromatin. **Plate 3, Fig. 2.**

MYELOCYTES. The myelocytes develop from promyelocytes and are precursors to metamyelocytes. In addition to the primary granules, which are already present, new specific or secondary granules are produced that almost fill the cytoplasm (see above. Young myelocytes, of course, have fewer specific granules than older cells.

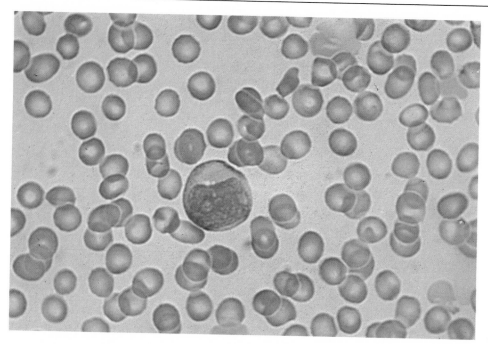

FIGURE 1.
Myeloblast; bone marrow smear; human; Giemsa's stain; ×1000.

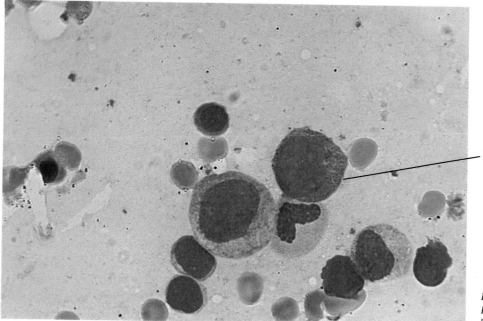

Promyelocyte

FIGURE 2.
Promyelocytes; bone marrow smear; human; Giemsa's stain; ×1000.

Myelocytes constitute the following approximate proportions in bone marrow: neutrophilic myelocytes, 5 to 19 percent; eosinophilic myelocytes, 0.5 to 3 percent; basophilic myelocytes, 0 to 0.5 percent.

Morphology. The cells vary in size, depending on the particular granulocyte lineage, but are much smaller than promyelocytes. They are about twice the diameter of erythrocytes (12 to 15 μm). The nucleus is oval or flattened on one side and may be more prominently indented than the nucleus of a promyelocyte. The chromatin is organized into dark reddish purple clumps; nucleoli may be present or absent. The cytoplasm is filled with specific granules of one of three types: neutrophil, eosinophil, or basophil (refer to page 104). **Plate 4, Fig. 1; Plate 5, Fig. 1; Plate 6, Fig. 1.**

METAMYELOCYTES (juveniles). These cells are the progeny of myelocytes and compose approximately 13 to 32 percent of the blood cells in marrow. Unlike myelocytes, metamyelocytes do not proliferate or produce more granules. As they mature, they transform into the next developmental stage, the band. Both meta-myelocytes and bands may occasionally be present in blood, especially as a response to a systemic bacterial infection.

Morphology. Metamyelocytes are only slightly smaller than myelocytes, so they are also about twice the diameter of erythrocytes (12 to 15 μm). The nucleus is deeply indented on one side so that it appears bent or kidney-shaped. The chromatin is coarse and densely clumped, and stains dark purple. Specific granules, either neutrophil, eosinophil, or basophil (see page 104), fill the cytoplasm and usually hide the primary granules (refer to page 104). **Plate 4, Fig. 2; Plate 5, Fig. 2; Plate 6, Fig. 2.**

BANDS The metamyelocytes transform into bands, which eventually become the mature, segmented, granulocytic leucocytes. Bands are quite numerous in bone marrow, composing about 10 to 40 percent of the blood cells, but some may also circulate in blood.

Morphology. Bands are about the same size or slightly smaller than metamyelocytes. The cytoplasm is well packed with specific granules; either neutrophil, eosinophil, or basophil (see page 104). The nucleus is so deeply indented that it forms a U-shaped structure, and the arms of the U are parallel for most of their length. In late bands, the ends of the arms may be constricted into lobes. The nucleus is filled with very coarse clumps of chromatin; which stain dark purplish blue. Nucleoli are absent. **Plate 4, Fig. 3; Plate 5, Fig. 3; Plate 6, Fig. 3..**

SEGMENTED GRANULOCYTES (polymorphonuclear leucocytes). These cells are derived from the bands and represent the end products of granulocytopoiesis. With these late stages of maturation, the nucleus becomes segmented (except basophilic leucocytes) with several lobes connected by thin filaments. Granulocytes are present in bone marrow in the following approximate proportions: eosinophils, 0.5 to 4 percent; neutrophils, 7 to 30 percent; basophils, 0 to 0.7 percent.

Morphology. The cells are about the same size as bands (12 to 15 μm in diameter). The nucleus may have two or more lobes (except basophils) connected by thin filaments. It is filled with very dense clumps of chromatin which stain dark purplish blue. Nucleoli are absent. The cytoplasm is slightly acidophilic for neutrophilic leucocytes and somewhat basophilic for eosinophilic and basophilic leucocytes. Specific granules—neutrophil, eosinophil, or basophil (see page 104)—fill the cytoplasm and obscure the primary granules, which are also present. See Chap. 7 for examples of segmented leucocytes.

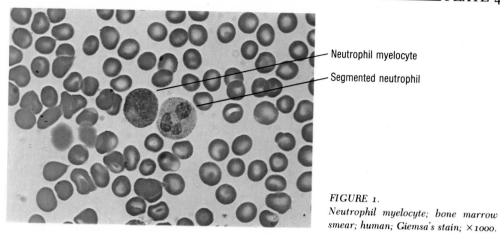

Neutrophil myelocyte

Segmented neutrophil

FIGURE 1.
Neutrophil myelocyte; bone marrow smear; human; Giemsa's stain; ×1000.

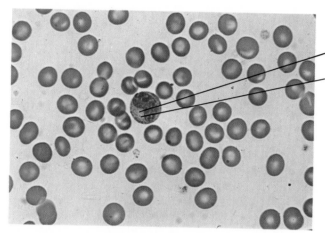

Secondary granules

Primary granules

FIGURE 2.
Neutrophil metamyelocyte; bone marrow smear; human; Giemsa's stain; ×1000. Note the deeply indented nucleus, the large primary azurophilic granules, and the tiny, pale secondary granules.

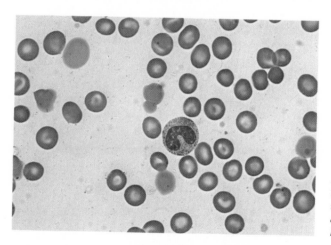

FIGURE 3.
Neutrophil band; bone marrow smear; human; Giemsa's stain; ×1000. Note the parallel arms of the U-shaped nucleus which is characteristic for the bands.

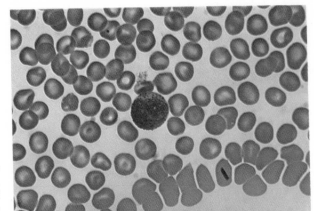

FIGURE 1.
Eosinophil myelocyte; bone marrow smear; human; Giemsa's stain; ×1000. Note both the primary azurophilic and specific eosinophilic granules in the cytoplasm.

Eosinophil metamyelocyte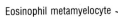

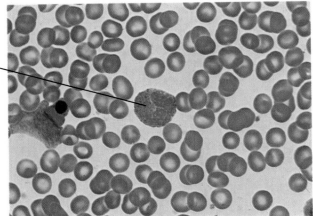

FIGURE 2.
Eosinophil metamyelocyte; bone marrow smear; Giemsa's stain; human; ×1000. Note the deeply indented nucleus.

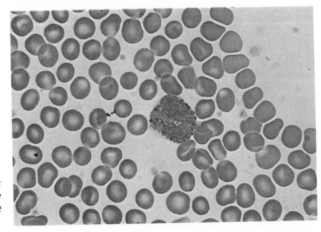

FIGURE 3.
Eosinophil band; bone marrow smear; human; Giemsa's stain; ×1000. Note that one arm of the nucleus is somewhat lobate.

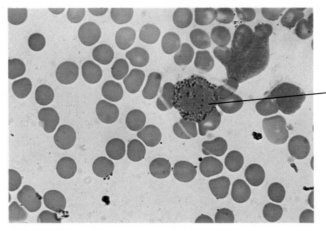

Basophil myelocyte

FIGURE 1.
Basophil myelocyte; bone marrow smear; human, Giemsa's stain; ×1000. Note the large, irregular, specific basophilic granules.

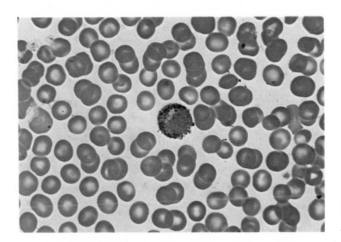

FIGURE 2.
Basophil metamyelocyte; bone marrow smear; human; Giemsa's stain; ×1000.

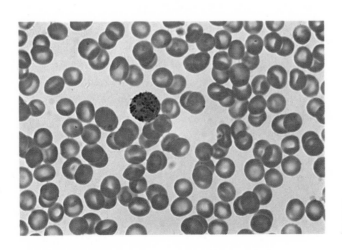

FIGURE 3.
Basophil band; bone marrow smear; human; Giemsa's stain; ×1000.

PLATE 7 _____

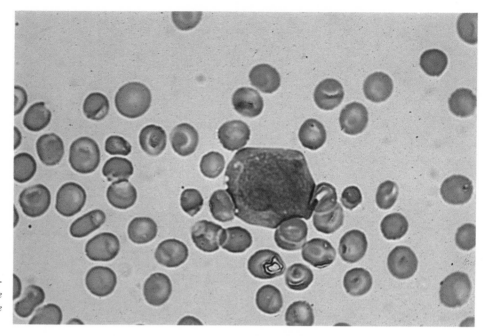

FIGURE 1.
Promonocyte; bone marrow smear; human; Giemsa's stain; ×1000. Note the irregular nucleus which almost fills the cytoplasm.

Monocytopoiesis

The earliest recognizable stages of maturation in the monocyte lineage are the promonocytes. They originate from undistinguished precursor cells (monoblasts) in the marrow. Here, promonocytes differentiate into monocytes, which represent about 0.5 to 5 percent of the marrow blood cells. The monocytes are then released into the blood. After a short period of circulation, they may enter extravascular areas and may differentiate to become free or fixed macrophages (histiocytes).

Promonocyte morphology. The cells resemble monocytes, but usually are larger (up to 30 μm in diameter) and have an immature nucleus. The large, irregularly shaped nucleus almost fills the entire cytoplasm, and may have one or more deep indentations. The chromatin is a delicate network of pale reddish blue strands in which two or more nucleoli are visible. The grayish blue cytoplasm may be vacuolated and have tiny reddish purple primary granules scattered through it; pseudopods may be present. **Plate 7, Fig. 1.**

Monocyte morphology. These cells are smaller than the promonocytes, but are variable in size (12 to 25 μm in diameter). The irregularly shaped nucleus fills about two-thirds of the cytoplasm. The chromatin network is moderately coarse and stains reddish blue; nucleoli usually are not visible. The cytoplasm is grayish blue and may have pseudopods, vacuoles, azurophilic granules, and phagocytized particles (see Chap. 7).

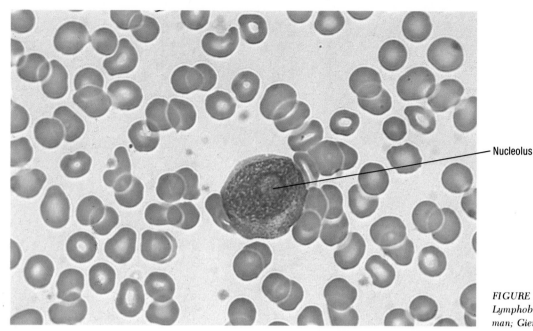

— Nucleolus

FIGURE 2.
Lymphoblast; bone marrow smear; human; Giemsa's stain; ×1000.

Lymphocytopoiesis

Lymphoblasts are the precursors of lymphocytes and plasma cells. They represent the earliest stages of lymphocytopoiesis to be recognized in a marrow smear. Lymphoblasts may be derived from the progeny of the multipotential hematopoietic stem cells, or from small lymphocytes participating in an immune response (refer to Chap. 7). Lymphoblasts are probably the same as large circulating lymphocytes, but are much larger and rarely or never circulate in blood.

Lymphoblast morphology. The cells are very large, about 18 to 30 μm in diameter, and may be oval or irregular in shape. The large, oval, pale nucleus fills most of the cytoplasm. The delicate network of chromatin stains reddish purple, and one or more irregularly shaped nucleoli may be visible. The cytoplasm stains medium to dark blue and usually lacks the reddish purple granules sometimes present in lymphocytes. **Plate 7, Fig. 2.**

Lymphocyte morphology. The lymphocytes (small, intermediate, and large) are smaller than the lymphoblasts and have clumps of darker-stained chromatin. The cytoplasm is less basophilic than that of the lymphoblast, and may have some scattered reddish purple granules. These cells constitute about 3 to 17 percent of the blood cells in marrow (see Chap. 7).

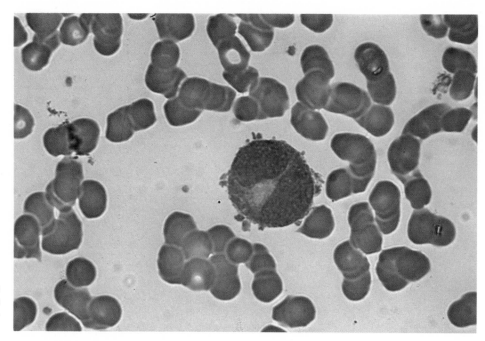

FIGURE 1.
Megakaryoblast; bone marrow smear; human; Giemsa's stain; ×1000. Note the two nuclei and pseudopodlike projections.

Megakaryocyte development

Multipotential hematopoietic stem cells give rise to large megakaryoblasts within the marrow. These in turn mature to become the larger megakaryocytes. During maturation the oval, diploid nucleus becomes polyploid and lobate, the cells increase in size, and the cytoplasm becomes granular and less basophilic. Blood platelets are parceled and usually separated from the peripheral cytoplasm of the megakaryocytes.

Megakaryoblast morphology. These are relatively large mononuclear or binuclear cells, about 20 μm in diameter. The large, oval nucleus (or nuclei) is indented and contains reddish purple, granular chromatin. The cytoplasm is moderately basophilic and agranular, and may have pseudopodlike projections. **Plate 8, Fig. 1.**

Megakaryocyte morphology. These are the largest cells in bone marrow, approximately 100 μm in diameter, and are quite visible even with low-power magnification. The large, irregular, lobate nucleus is filled with dark-stained chromatin organized into a network of coarse strands or clumps. The cytoplasm is somewhat basophilic and stains pinkish blue. If the cell is not producing blood platelets, then reddish-stained granules may be scattered throughout the cytoplasm. If platelets are being produced, they will appear as prominent granular bodies, either throughout the cytoplasm or at its periphery. **Plate 8, Fig. 2.**

Other cell types present in hematopoietic tissues

Other cell types, such as fat cells, reticular cells, plasma cells, and macrophages, may be present in bone marrow along with the hematopoietic cells.

RETICULAR CELLS (reticulum cells). These are cells which, along with reticular fibers, form a delicate network supporting hematopoietic cells. They represent about 0.1 to 2 percent of the marrow cells. In a smear they may appear as distorted cells,

PLATE 8 *continued*

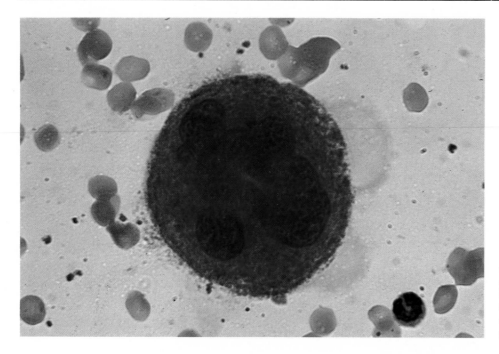

FIGURE 2.
Megakaryocyte; bone marrow smear; human; Giemsa's stain; ×1000. Note the multilobed nucleus and granular cytoplasm. The cell is inactive and not producing blood platelets.

PLATE 9

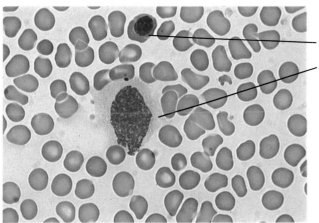

— Polychromatophil erythroblast

— Reticular cell

FIGURE 1.
Reticular cell; bone marrow smear; human; Giemsa's stain; ×1000.

with ruptured nuclear membranes and frayed cytoplasmic margins. This appearance is common because these large, fragile cells have been torn from the reticular network. It is also quite common to find a reticular cell nucleus surrounded by only a few strands of cytoplasm.

Morphology. In bone marrow smears, the intact cell is quite large, about 20 to 40 μm in diameter (approximately five times the diameter of the erythrocytes). The cells have a large, pale, nucleus which stains reddish pink and is surrounded by an agranular, almost colorless basophilic cytoplasm. The chromatin appears as a reticulum of granules and delicate strands. Several large, pale nucleoli are usually visible. In tissues other than bone marrow, reticular cells are relatively large, and stellate or fusiform. They have a large, oval, vesicular, pale nucleus surrounded by sparse, pale-stained cytoplasm. (see Chap. 3). **Plate 9, Fig. 1.**

Macrophage
Pseudopods

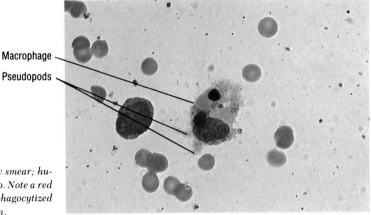

FIGURE 2.
Macrophage; bone marrow smear; human; Giemsa's stain; ×1000. Note a red blood cell and other phagocytized structures in the cytoplasm.

Eosinophil metamyelocyte
Plasma cell
Vacuole

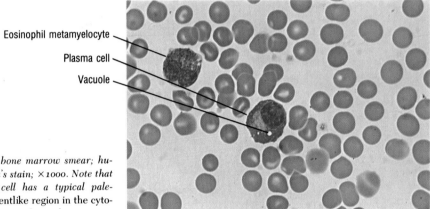

FIGURE 3.
Plasma cell; bone marrow smear; human; Giemsa's stain; ×1000. Note that the plasma cell has a typical pale-stained, cresentlike region in the cytoplasm adjacent to the nucleus.

MACROPHAGES. These cells may be free and amoeboid or fixed and attached to the reticular network supporting the hematopoietic tissues. The latter type of macrophages are designated as histiocytes. Both types of macrophages may be derived from monocytes and are quite phagocytic. They compose about 0.1 to 3 percent of the marrow cells. Macrophages, in addition to being excellent scavengers, may also contribute to the immunological mechanism by altering antigens, thereby stimulating a stronger antibody response by lymphocytes (see Chaps. 3 and 7).

Morphology. Macrophages are large cells, about 15 to 30 μm in diameter, and may appear round, oval, or irregularly shaped. In a smear, the free macrophages usually have pseudopods, while the histiocytes have torn or fragmented margins. The abundant cytoplasm is light bluish gray and usually contains phagocytized particles. The relatively small, oval or round nucleus is usually indented and is filled with coarse, dark reddish purple chromatin strands. **Plate 9, Fig. 2.**

PLASMA CELLS. These cells are present in hematopoietic tissues and can be found in especially large numbers during an immune response. If B lymphocytes (B cells) are antigenically stimulated, then they may differentiate into lymphoblasts which, in turn, give rise to plasma cells. Plasma cells are important sources for blood-borne antibodies, the immunoglobulins.

Morphology. The cells are relatively large, covering a wide range of sizes (8 to 20 μm in diameter). They are oval or round and are among the most deeply stained basophilic cells in a marrow smear because of their high concentration of ribosomes. The small, round, eccentric nucleus contains massive clumps of coarse, purplish blue chromatin, sometimes arranged in a spokelike manner. In the dark bluish violet cytoplasm next to the nucleus, there is a pale crescentlike region containing the Golgi apparatus and centrioles. The cytoplasm may also contain vacuoles, and the margins of the cell may be somewhat ragged (see Chap. 3). **Plate 9, Fig. 3.**

Cardiovascular System 9

The cardiovascular system functions to circulate, distribute, and move blood through the tissues of the body. The muscular, pumping heart exerts pressure on the blood which circulates through blood vessels in the body and eventually returns to the heart. *Arteries* direct blood away from the heart; the blood may be richly oxygenated (systemic arteries) or poorly oxygenated (pulmonary arteries). All *veins* carry blood toward the heart; the blood may be richly oxygenated (pulmonary veins) or poorly oxygenated (systemic veins). *Capillaries* connect the arterial and venous sides of the circulatory system and will allow for an exchange of nutrients, gases, and fluids between the blood and tissues of the body.

The histology of the cardiovascular structures described in this chapter are indicated below. They are given in their anatomical order, going from the heart to the capillaries and then back to the heart.

The major circulatory pathways are indicated by solid lines on the diagram; others are shown by dotted lines. The *arteriovenous* pathways are characteristic of skin on the extremities; the *arteriole-sinusoid-venule* pathways are found in the spleen and bone marrow; and the *venule-sinusoid-venule* pathways are present in the pituitary and liver.

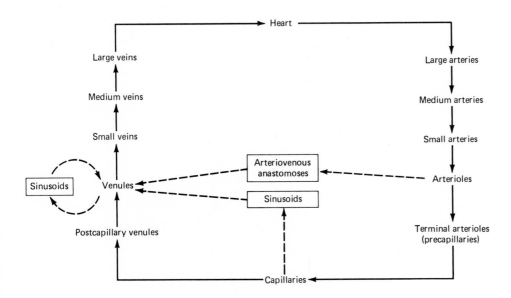

Heart

The heart is a four-chambered double pump (two atria and two ventricles). A pulmonary pump on the right side sends oxygen-poor blood to the lungs for oxygenation, and a systemic pump on the left side sends oxygen-rich blood into the general circulation.

A dense collagenous connective tissue framework of fibrous rings separates the atria from the ventricles. It also supports the cardiac valves (bicuspid and tricuspid) and the roots of major cardiac vessels, and provides attachments for cardiac muscles. An interventricular extension of the framework separates the ventricles. The walls of the heart are composed of three distinct layers: an outer *epicardium*, a middle *myocardium*, and an inner *endocardium*. The walls are thicker in the ventricles than the atria, and the left ventricular wall is thicker than the right one.

EPICARDIUM (visceral pericardium). This is the most superficial layer of the heart and forms the innermost wall of the pericardial sac. It is continuous with the outer wall (parietal pericardium) of the sac. The epicardium is a thin layer of loose connective tissue containing collagen and some elastic fibers. It also contains nerves, blood and lymphatic vessels, and adipose tissue. The epicardium is covered by a simple squamous epithelium, the mesothelium. **Plate 1, Fig. 1.**

MYOCARDIUM. This layer forms the musculature of the heart and is more massive than either the endocardium or epicardium. It is composed of cardiac muscle (see Chap. 5), which is under the control of the autonomic nervous system and the impulse conducting system (see below). Like other layers of the heart wall, the myocardium has an extensive supply of blood and lymphatic vessels. Cardiac fibers are organized into sheets and fasciculi by connective tissue composed of collagen, elastic, and reticular fibers. These sheets and fascicles form prominent spiral muscles in the ventricles, and so during a ventricular systole they "wring" blood out of the cavities. The ventricular myocardium forms ridges, *trabeculae carneae*, and conelike *papillary muscles* which are attached to cardiac valves by thin tendons, the *chordae tendineae*. These latter structures are composed of dense collagenous connective tissues and covered with endocardium. They prevent the eversion of cardiac valves into the atria during a ventricular systole. **Plate 1, Figs. 1** and **2.**

ENDOCARDIUM. This is a relatively thin layer of tissue lining the cardiac chambers. It is continuous with the major blood vessels entering and leaving the heart and is folded to form the valves of the heart. These are the atrioventricular valves, the bicuspid and tricuspid valves which separate the atria from the ventricles, and the semilunar valves within the aorta and pulmonary trunk. The endocardium is composed of three distinct layers.

1 *Endothelium*. This is a simple squamous epithelium lining the cavities of the heart.

2 *Subendothelium*. This is a thin, delicate layer of collagen fibers just below the endothelium. In the lower regions, the subendothelium is a relatively dense tissue containing elastic and collagen fibers and some smooth muscle.

3 *Subendocardium*. This layer binds the endocardium to the myocardium. It is composed of loose connective tissue containing fat cells, fibers of the impulse-conducting system (see below), autonomic nerve fibers, coronary blood vessels, lymphatic vessels, and sensory nerves.

See **Plate 1, Fig. 2; Plate 2, Fig. 1.**

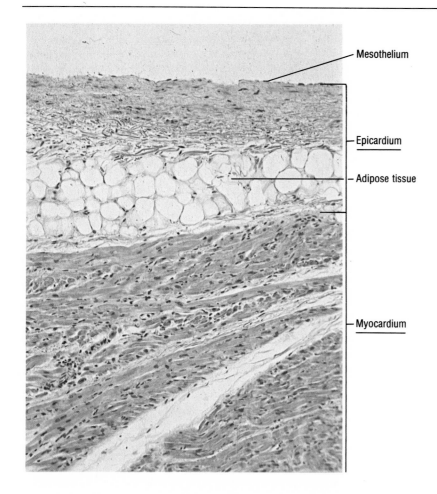

Mesothelium

Epicardium

Adipose tissue

Myocardium

FIGURE 1.
Epicardium of the ventricle; human heart; H&E; ×100.

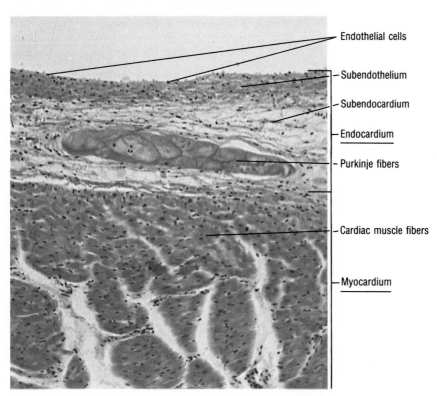

Endothelial cells

Subendothelium

Subendocardium

Endocardium

Purkinje fibers

Cardiac muscle fibers

Myocardium

FIGURE 2.
Myocardium and endocardium of the ventricle; bovine heart; H&E; ×100.

Endothelium

Subendothelium

Subendocardium

Purkinje fibers

Cardiac muscle fibers

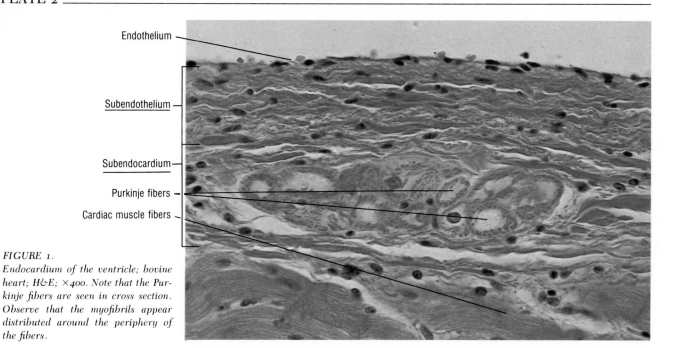

FIGURE 1.
Endocardium of the ventricle; bovine heart; H&E; ×400. Note that the Purkinje fibers are seen in cross section. Observe that the myofibrils appear distributed around the periphery of the fibers.

Impulse conducting system (ICS). The ICS is a modified cardiac tissue which transmits bioelectric impulses and is important in coordinating the heart beat. An impulse originates in a mass of ICS tissue, the *sinoatrial node* (SA node) or pacemaker, at the junction of the superior vena cava and wall of the right atrium. The atria then contract as the impulse spreads out over nonspecialized cardiac fibers. Eventually the impulse reaches a second node of ICS tissue, the *atrioventricular node* (AV node), located in the wall of the interatrial septum, adjacent to the right atrial cavity, above the opening of the coronary sinus. From the AV node the impulse is transmitted into the interventricular septum, via the *atrioventricular bundle* (bundle of His). This bundle, also composed of ICS tissue, divides into two major fasciculi within the interventricular septum. Each fasciculus then subdivides into many smaller branches, the *Purkinje fibers*, which continue into the subendocardium (see above) and are continuous with muscle fibers in the ventricular myocardium. These fibers conduct the impulse to cardiac muscle in the ventricles. **Plate 1, Fig. 2; Plate 2, Figs. 1** and **2.**

PURKINJE FIBERS. Although these fibers are located in the ventricular myocardium, they are best seen in the subendocardium as complex plexuses of tissue. They resemble cardiac fibers, but are larger and have fewer cross-striated myofibrils within an abundant pale-stained sarcoplasm. The glycogen-filled sarcoplasm contains one or two centrally positioned oval nuclei and peripheral myofibrils. **Plate 2, Figs. 1** and **2.**

In humans, the conductile tissues of the nodes and atrioventricular bundle resemble myocardial muscle. The nodal fibers, however, show greater differences when compared with cardiac muscle than do the fibers of the atrioventricular bundle; they are smaller, fusiform, darker stained, have less sarcoplasm, more cross striations, and are embedded within a dense connective tissue.

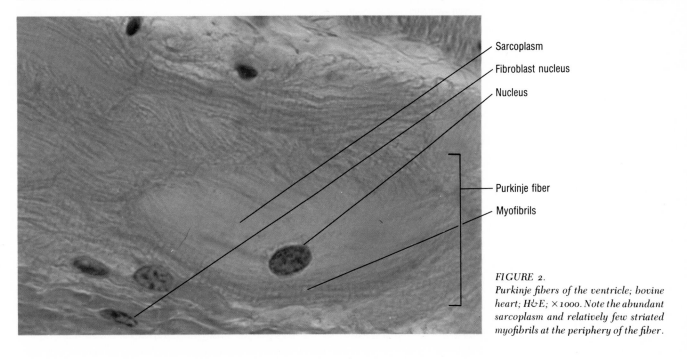

Sarcoplasm

Fibroblast nucleus

Nucleus

Purkinje fiber

Myofibrils

FIGURE 2.
Purkinje fibers of the ventricle; bovine
heart; H&E; ×1000. Note the abundant
sarcoplasm and relatively few striated
myofibrils at the periphery of the fiber.

BLOOD AND LYMPHATIC VESSELS. Coronary arteries carry oxygen-rich blood to the epicardium. Branches of these vessels form extensive capillary networks in the myocardium and subendocardium. They supply blood to cardiac muscle and tissues of the ICS. Venous blood is drained from the capillaries by venules and then by cardiac veins in the epicardium. These veins, in turn, drain into the coronary sinus and then into the right atrium.

Lymphatic vessels are present in all regions of the wall of the heart, but are more abundant in the myocardium.

NERVES. Preganglionic parasympathetic fibers (supplied by the vagus nerve), postganglionic sympathetic and parasympathetic fibers, and visceral sensory fibers are abundant around blood vessels, the ICS, and cardiac tissues. The telodendrons of the axons are bare fibers lying adjacent to the cells of these tissues. Ganglion cells of the parasympathetic division of the autonomic system will also be found in the ICS and cardiac tissues.

Blood vessels

VASCULAR SYSTEM. Except for some specialized vessels (see below), the walls of the larger blood vessels are composed of three coats or tunicae of tissue: (1 the *tunica intima* is adjacent to the lumen and its tissue elements are arranged longitudinally; (2) the *tunica media* is just peripheral to the intima and composed of circumferentially arranged tissue; (3) the *tunica adventitia* is the outermost coat and its longitudinally arranged tissues may blend with connective tissues of adjacent structures.

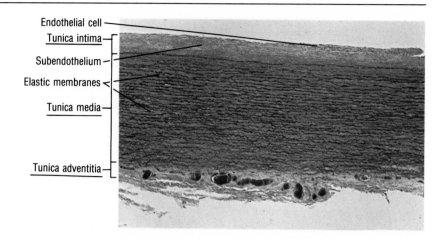

Endothelial cell
Tunica intima
Subendothelium
Elastic membranes
Tunica media
Tunica adventitia

FIGURE 1.
Large artery; human aorta; Verhoeff's elastic stain with eosin; ×40. Note the vasa vasorum in the tunica adventitia.

When tracing either an artery or vein distally from the heart, the diameter becomes smaller and the tunicae are reduced by a loss of tissue. These are gradual changes, and an abrupt transition from one type of vessel to another is usually not evident. To begin a study of the vascular system, one should first scan a section of any organ, looking for well-stained cross sections of vessels (longitudinal sections are more difficult to analyze). At comparable levels, veins are generally distinguished from arteries in the following ways:

1 Veins have a larger diameter and a wider lumen relative to their thin walls.

2 The walls are irregular and usually collapsed.

3 Tunicae usually are not as sharply defined as in the arteries.

4 Muscle and elastic fibers are more scarce and scattered through an abundant fibrous connective tissue.

5 Valves formed by the tunica intima extend into the lumina of small and medium-sized veins. They are cuplike flaps of elastic tissue covered by an endothelium, and function to keep blood moving unidirectionally.

6 An internal elastic membrane (see below) is absent, except for a certain few veins.

In general, arteries and to a lesser degree veins may be classified as small, medium, or large. Although most vessels may be classified by their size and morphology of tunicae, some diseased, aged, or specialized vessels (see below) are difficult to classify.

Large arteries (elastic arteries). These are easily identified as large vessels with a prominent tunica media filled with fenestrated elastic membranes. These conducting arteries are important in sustaining blood pressure as the blood leaves the heart. Examples are the aorta and pulmonary arteries. **Plate 3, Fig. 1.**
TUNICA INTIMA. An endothelium (simple squamous epithelium) lies on a relatively thick subendothelial layer of elastic and collagen fibers containing a few smooth muscle cells. The nuclei of the endothelial cells bulge into the lumen of the vessel; the cytoplasm is indistinct.
TUNICA MEDIA. This is the widest tunica, composed of 45 to 70 concentric fenestrated membranes of elastic tissue. The membranes are separated by collagen fibers, fibroblasts, and some smooth muscle cells, all of which are embedded in a

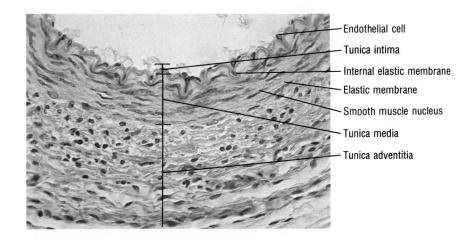

FIGURE 2.
Small artery; human; H&E; ×400. Note that the external elastic membrane is not present in this specimen.

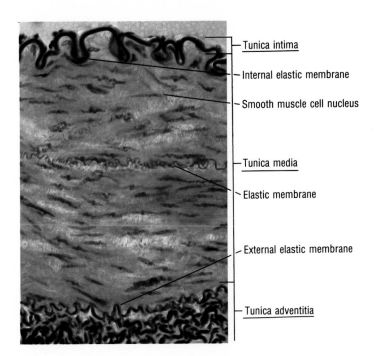

FIGURE 3.
Medium artery; rabbit; Weigert's elastic stain with eosin; ×400. Note that this artery is larger than the one in Plate 3, Fig. 2; therefore an external elastic membrane is present. The preparation shows light regions which are artifacts.

glycoprotein ground substance. Near the heart, the bases of the aorta and pulmonary arteries contain some cardiac muscle fibers.

TUNICA ADVENTITIA. This tunica of moderately dense, irregular connective tissue is slightly thinner than the tunica intima and contains longitudinal spirals of collagen and elastic fibers. It also has small blood vessels (vasa vasorum), lymphatics, and nerve fibers. At the periphery of the artery the tunica adventitia merges with loose connective tissue of adjacent organs.

Medium to small arteries (muscular arteries). These vessels are quite numerous. An example is any artery from 0.5 to 10 mm in diameter with a well-developed tunica media of smooth muscle. These are distributing arteries which can control the flow of blood to a specific organ. **Plate 3, Figs. 2** and **3.**

PLATE 4 _____

Smooth muscle tissue
Smooth muscle cell nucleus
Internal elastic membrane
Tunica adventitia
Tunica intima
Endothelium
Venule
Tunica media
Loose connective tissue

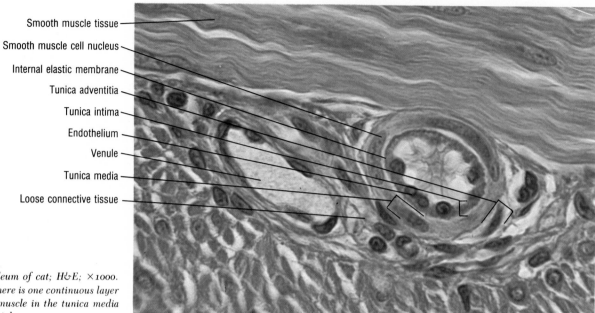

FIGURE 1.
Arteriole; ileum of cat; H&E; ×1000.
Note that there is one continuous layer
of smooth muscle in the tunica media
of the arteriole.

TUNICA INTIMA. The endothelium (simple squamous epithelium) lies on a fenestrated layer of a dense network of elastic fibers, the *internal elastic membrane*, which appears as a thick, homogeneous, scalloped structure. The scalloped condition is the result of collapse or muscular contraction of the vessel as it is prepared for sectioning. The internal elastic membrane usually appears refractile and bright pink with an H& E stain. A subendothelium of collagen, elastic, and reticular fibers, and occasionally some smooth muscle, is present in the largest vessels of this type. It is located between the endothelium and internal elastic membrane.

TUNICA MEDIA. The 4 to 40 closely packed layers of concentric smooth muscle fibers is the most prominent feature of this tunica. The muscle layers are slightly separated by a glycoprotein matrix containing collagen, elastic, and reticular fibers. Some fenestrated elastic membranes may be found in the largest muscular arteries.

TUNICA ADVENTITIA. This tunica is variable in size; it may be thicker, the same size as, or thinner than the media. In the medium-sized arteries an *external elastic membrane* lies just peripheral to the media. It usually appears as a relatively thick, homogeneous structure, similar to but not as prominent as the internal elastic membrane (see above). The adventitia is composed of loose connective tissue containing fibroblasts and collagen and elastic fibers. Vasa vasorum, small nerve fibers, and adipose tissue are present in the outer less dense region of the adventitia.

Arterioles. These vessels range in size from about 30 to 300 μm in diameter. They have one to three continuous layers of smooth muscle surrounding the endothelium and possess three tunicae. **Plate 4, Fig. 1.**

TUNICA INTIMA. The endothelium (simple squamous epithelium) is flat, but nuclei of the endothelial cells bulge into the lumen. The endothelium lies on an internal elastic membrane, but unlike the condition in the larger arteries, the membrane is nonfenestrated (see above). A subendothelial layer is lacking.

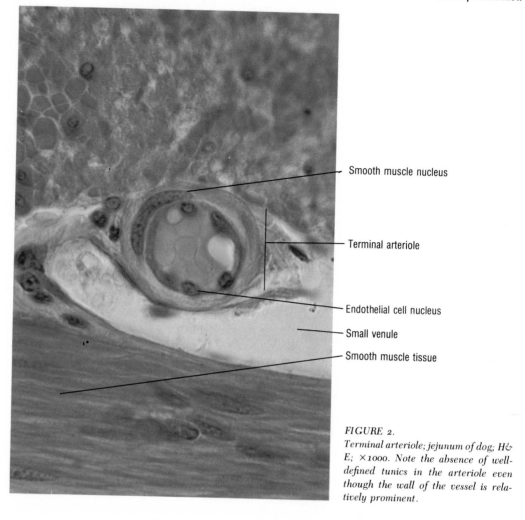

Smooth muscle nucleus

Terminal arteriole

Endothelial cell nucleus

Small venule

Smooth muscle tissue

FIGURE 2.
Terminal arteriole; jejunum of dog; H&
E; ×1000. Note the absence of well-
defined tunics in the arteriole even
though the wall of the vessel is rela-
tively prominent.

TUNICA MEDIA. One to three complete layers of concentrically or spirally arranged smooth muscle tissue is present within a bed of fibroelastic tissue. The cells are tightly packed, with only small amounts of connective tissue appearing between them.

TUNICA ADVENTITIA. This is a thin layer of loose connective tissue. It is composed of collagen and elastic fibers, fibroblasts, and some nerve fibers. Like the small muscular arteries, an external elastic membrane is lacking.

Terminal arterioles (precapillaries). These vessels carry blood from the smallest arterioles to the capillaries. They are about 10 to 30 μm in diameter, and have no well-defined tunicae. A few smooth muscle cells, collagen and elastic fibers, and fibroblasts form an incomplete, discontinuous, poorly organized layer around the endothelium. The histology resembles that of small venules (see below), but the diameter of these vessels is much smaller. **Plate 4, Fig. 2; Plate 5, Figs. 2 and 3.**

Capillaries. These are the smallest vessels in the vascular system, approximately 3 to 10 μm in diameter. They are thin cellular tubes supported only by a network of delicate reticular fibers. In cross section a capillary appears as a tube formed by 1

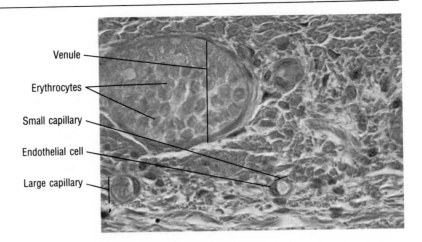

Venule —
Erythrocytes —
Small capillary —
Endothelial cell —
Large capillary —

FIGURE 1.
Capillaries; respiratory mucosa of rhesus monkey; H&E; ×1000.

to 3 longitudinally arranged squamous endothelial cells. The cells may be evident only by their nuclei bulging into the lumen of the capillary, since the cytoplasm usually appears as a thin line. *Pericytes* (Rouget cells in earlier literature) may be found sitting on the capillary wall and scattered along its length. They are stellate cells of unknown function. The nucleus is distinguished from fibroblast nuclei by being darker and not as flattened.

Capillaries are semipermeable vessels whereby water, gases, salts, foods, and other substances may pass through cell junctions, across the cytoplasm via micropinocytotic vesicles, or through cytoplasmic pores. Because capillaries are selectively permeable, they form effective barriers, keeping certain substances from passing between the blood and tissues. An example of this is the blood-brain barrier. There are two main types of capillaries; they are classified according to endothelial ultrastructures which cannot be detected with the light microscope:

1 *Fenestrated capillaries.* The endothelial cells have tiny pores in their thin cytoplasm and are important in the movement of fluids through the capillary walls. These capillaries are present in endocrine glands, the choroid plexus, and the renal glomerulus.

2 *Continuous capillaries.* The endothelial cells in these capillaries lack pores, but they have micropinocytotic vesicles in the cytoplasm which function to transport substances across the cell. These capillaries are found in muscle, the central nervous system, and the lungs. **Plate 5, Figs. 1 and 3.**

Postcapillary venules. These vessels drain the capillaries and are about 10 to 50 μm in diameter. The flat endothelium is surrounded only by reticular and collagen fibers and fibroblasts. Although these vessels are about the same size as terminal arterioles, they may be distinguished by their complete lack of smooth muscle tissue. The postcapillary venules, like the capillaries, selectively allow substances to pass between the blood and tissues. This activity occurs mainly at cell junctions and is most dramatic with injury, inflammation, or temperature changes. **Plate 5, Figs. 2 and 3.**

Venules. The venules may be distinguished from the postcapillary venules by their larger size—they are approximately 50 to 200 μm in diameter—and the presence of smooth muscle within their walls. The smaller venules have an incomplete layer of smooth muscle cells, scattered within a fibroelastic bed of connective tissue, partially surrounding the endothelium. The larger venules have a continuous one to two

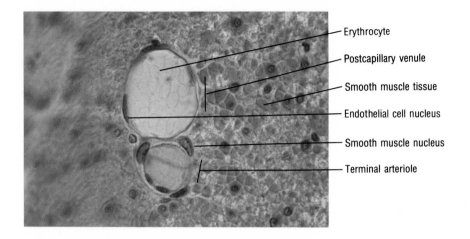

- Erythrocyte
- Postcapillary venule
- Smooth muscle tissue
- Endothelial cell nucleus
- Smooth muscle nucleus
- Terminal arteriole

FIGURE 2.
Postcapillary venule; jejunum of dog; H&E; ×1000. Note the relatively large size (therefore it is not a capillary) and the thin walls, which lack smooth muscle.

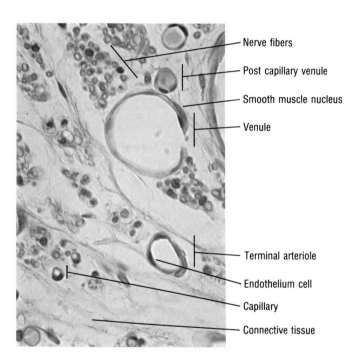

- Nerve fibers
- Post capillary venule
- Smooth muscle nucleus
- Venule
- Terminal arteriole
- Endothelium cell
- Capillary
- Connective tissue

FIGURE 3.
Venule; pulp of human tooth; H&E; ×1000. Note the large size of the venule with thin walls containing scattered smooth muscle cells. Tunicae are absent.

layers of smooth muscle surrounding the endothelium, and three tunicae. The larger venules may be distinguished from arterioles of the same size since they lack an internal elastic membrane; the walls are very thin relative to the large lumen; the walls are usually irregular or collapsed; and the smooth muscle cells are more widely separated by collagen and elastic fibers. **Plate 4, Fig. 1. Plate 5, Figs. 1 and 3.**
TUNICA INTIMA. The endothelium (simple squamous epithelium) is relatively thin, and an internal elastic membrane is lacking.
TUNICA MEDIA. The tunica appears as one to two layers of circumferentially arranged smooth muscle cells scattered through a fibroelastic layer.
TUNICA ADVENTITIA. This is a thin layer of collagen fibers, some elastic fibers, fibroblasts, and nerve fibers.

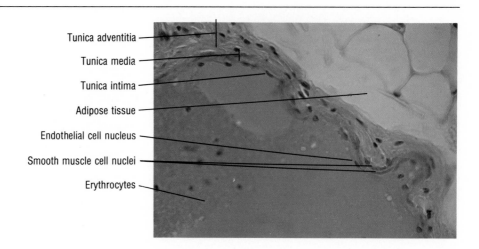

Tunica adventitia —
Tunica media —
Tunica intima —
Adipose tissue —
Endothelial cell nucleus —
Smooth muscle cell nuclei —
Erythrocytes —

FIGURE 1.
Medium vein; jejunum of dog; H&E;
×400. Note that muscle bundles are
present in the tunica media and sepa-
rated by fibroelastic tissue.

Small and medium veins. These vessels are approximately between 200 μm and 9 mm in diameter. The small veins resemble the larger venules (see above), but their walls contain smooth muscle which is organized into bundles. Except for the major veins and their branches, these vessels represent most of the anatomically named veins in the body; an example would be veins located close to or within an organ. **Plate 6, Fig. 1.**

TUNICA MEDIA. This thin tunica has small scattered bundles of circumferentially internal elastic membrane is lacking. Larger veins of this type, however, may have a thin subendothelium of fibroblasts and elastic fibers.
TUNICA MEDIA. This thin tunic has small scattered bundles of circumferentially oriented muscle which form a coat peripheral to the endothelium. The bundles are somewhat separated by collagen and elastic fibers. The small veins have one to two layers of smooth muscle, and the medium-sized veins have three or more layers.
TUNICA ADVENTITIA. The loose connective tissue of this layer blends imperceptibly with the tissue of the media. It is wider than the media, containing longitudinal collagen and elastic fibers and some smooth muscle.

Large veins. These veins are approximately 9 mm or more in diameter. Their walls are composed of predominately loose connective tissue, but smooth muscle bundles are present. Examples of large veins would be the inferior vena cava and pulmonary and hepatic portal veins. **Plate 6, Fig. 2.**
TUNICA INTIMA. The endothelium (simple squamous epithelium) lies on a usually well-developed subendothelium composed of collagen and elastic fibers, fibroblasts, and some longitudinal smooth muscle. In some vessels a delicate, somewhat fragmented, internal elastic membrane may be present.
TUNICA MEDIA. This tunica is poorly developed or may be lacking. If present, it is a thin layer composed of loose connective tissue with scattered bundles of smooth muscle.
TUNICA ADVENTITIA. This tunica constitutes the major portion of the wall and is thicker than the intima and media combined. The loose connective tissue of the adventitia blends with the connective tissue of the media and contains many bundles of longitudinal smooth muscle, collagen and elastic fibers, vasa vasorum, lymphatic vessels, and nerves.

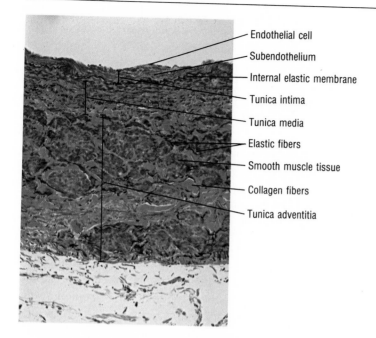

- Endothelial cell
- Subendothelium
- Internal elastic membrane
- Tunica intima
- Tunica media
- Elastic fibers
- Smooth muscle tissue
- Collagen fibers
- Tunica adventitia

FIGURE 2.
Large vein; human vena cava; Verhoeff's elastic tissue and eosin stains; ×100. Note the many large bundles of smooth muscle in the tunica adventitia.

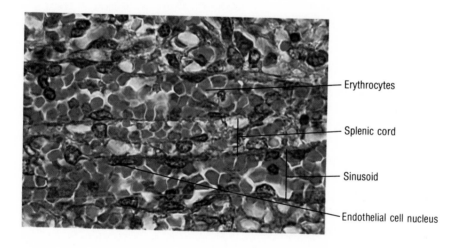

- Erythrocytes
- Splenic cord
- Sinusoid
- Endothelial cell nucleus

FIGURE 3.
Sinusoids; human spleen; Masson's trichrome stain; ×1000.

Sinusoids. These are similar in structure to capillaries. They have a thin wall of simple squamous epithelium supported by reticular fibers. They differ by having a larger diameter (approximately 10 to 35 μm); they are irregular rather than cylindrical in cross section; and the epithelium may be continuous or discontinuous. Also, sinusoids lie close to the parenchyma of organs rather than being separated by connective tissue. The cells lining the sinusoids may be one or more of three possible types: nonphagocytic endothelium, slightly phagocytic reticular cells, or highly phagocytic fixed macrophages. The cells lining sinusoids of the spleen, hypophysis, and adrenal glands are nonphagocytic endothelium. They are fusiform cells with small, oval, dense, dark-stained nuclei. In the liver, the sinusoids are lined by fixed macrophages (Kupffer cells) and endothelium. The macrophages are considered as part of the reticuloendothelial or macrophage system (see Chap. 3). They are fusiform or stellate in shape and have a moderately large, dark-stained, oval nucleus. **Plate 6, Fig. 3.**

Arteriovenous anastomoses. This is a special vascular shunt usually connecting arterioles directly to venules. It is present in the skin of extremities and mucosa of the gastrointestinal tract. With a contraction or relaxation of the smooth muscles in its wall, the shunt directs blood to capillaries (when it is closed) or to venules (when it is open). This regulation of blood flow through tissues is necessary for physiological processes which have fluctuating demands for blood volume, for example, temperature regulation and digestion. The shunt is usually a short, twisted vessel which appears somewhat like an arteriole. It has a prominent tunica media with modified smooth muscle cells, which forms a sphincter muscle.

TUNICA INTIMA. The endothelium (simple squamous epithelium) lies directly on the tunica media.

TUNICA MEDIA. The smooth muscle cells are several layers in thickness and form a sphincter muscle around the vessel. The muscle cells are short and thick, appearing somewhat like stratified cuboidal epithelium.

TUNICA ADVENTITIA. This is a thin layer of loose connective tissue containing many fibers of vasomotor nerves of the autonomic nervous system.

Specialized vessels. Although there is a general histologic format for the vascular system, it must be realized that many vessels do not fit into the format because they are diseased or aged, or belong to a specialized category. Some of these specialized vessels (cerebral veins, for example) may lack some tunicae; others (superior vena cava) have longitudinal smooth muscle where there is normally circumferential muscle. Still other specializations exist.

BLOOD AND LYMPHATIC VESSELS WITHIN BLOOD VESSELS. The walls of the larger arteries and veins, usually greater than 1.0 mm, are supplied by small blood vessels, the *vasa vasorum*. These vessels extend through the adventitia, carrying blood to and draining blood from capillary networks within the tunica adventitia in large arteries or tunica media in large veins. Small lymphatic vessels are present within the tunica adventitia of the larger blood vessels.

NERVES IN BLOOD VESSELS. There are abundant unmyelinated postganglionic axons of sympathetic neurons present within the outer tunicae of blood vessels. These are vasomotor neurons which innervate smooth muscle cells within the media. Myelinated fibers of visceral sensory neurons may also be present within the walls of the vessels. A limited distribution of parasympathetic nerves is present in some vessels.

Lymphoid Tissues, Lymphoid Organs, and Lymphatic Vessels 10

All lymphoid tissues and organs have heavy concentrations of lymphocytes trapped within the interspaces of a fibrous mesh of reticular tissue, or a cytoreticulum (see below). These structures may appear as a simple *diffuse lymphoid tissue;* a more highly organized *tonsil* or *nodule;* or as complex *lymphoid organs* (thymus, spleen, and lymph nodes).

Diffuse lymphoid tissue

This tissue is abundant in the loose connective tissue of the lamina propria of the respiratory system and alimentary canal, as well as in various regions of lymphoid organs. It appears as a relatively dense, stippled cellular mass of lymphocytes of various sizes concentrated in the interspaces of reticular tissue. Although large and medium-sized lymphocytes are present, small lymphocytes are most abundant. The boundaries of diffuse lymphoid tissue are indistinct, as lymphocytes blend with loose connective tissue at the periphery. Reticular cells (see Chap. 3) may be distinguished from lymphocytes by their large, pale, oval nucleus. Their fusiform or branched cytoplasm stains lightly, and usually is not visible. These cells may produce fibers or be somewhat phagocytic. Other cell types which may be present are macrophages, monocytes, and plasma cells (see Chaps. 3 and 8 for their morphology). Diffuse lymphoid tissue responds to antigens entering the body by the production of lymphocytes. **Plate 1, Figs. 1** and **2.**

Lymphoid nodule

LYMPHOID NODULES (primary nodules). These structures are composed of cell types similar to those in diffuse lymphoid tissue. They usually appear as a very dense spherical mass of lymphocytes, sharply set off from a surrounding bed of diffuse lymphoid tissue. Lymphoid nodules occur in tonsils, lymph nodes, spleen, and the lamina propria of the alimentary canal and respiratory system. They may be present as *solitary* nodules or *aggregates* of nodules. Aggregates are prominent as *Peyer's patches* in the lamina propria of the ileum, just opposite to the attachment of the mesentery. They are large oval-shaped structures which may extend through the muscularis mucosae and into the submucosa. The aggregates are composed of several oval lymphoid nodules, the bases of which may be fused. **Plate 2, Figs. 1** and **2.**

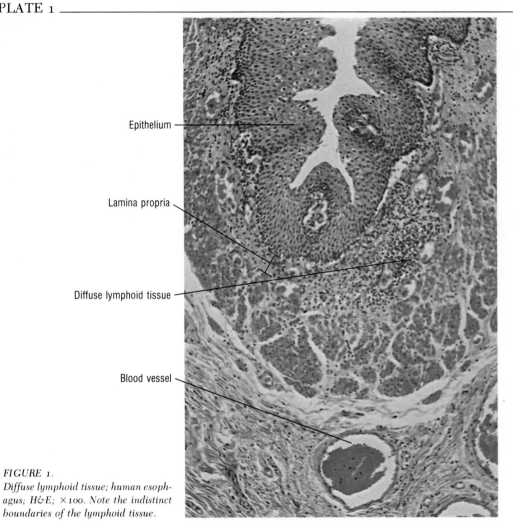

Epithelium

Lamina propria

Diffuse lymphoid tissue

Blood vessel

FIGURE 1.
Diffuse lymphoid tissue; human esoph-
agus; H&E; ×100. Note the indistinct
boundaries of the lymphoid tissue.

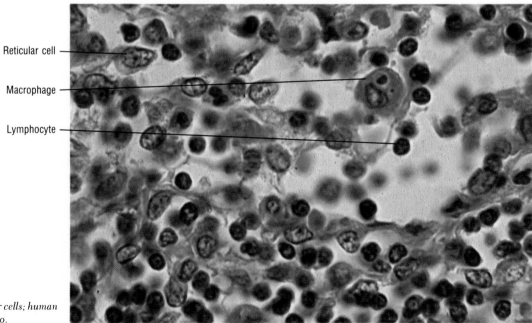

Reticular cell

Macrophage

Lymphocyte

FIGURE 2.
Macrophage and reticular cells; human
lymph node; H&E; ×1000.

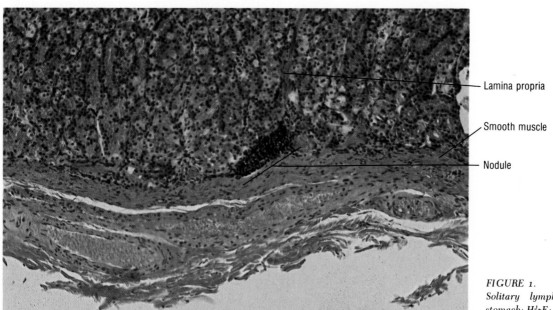

Lamina propria

Smooth muscle

Nodule

FIGURE 1.
Solitary lymphoid nodule; human stomach; H&E; ×100. Note the distinct borders of the solitary nodule.

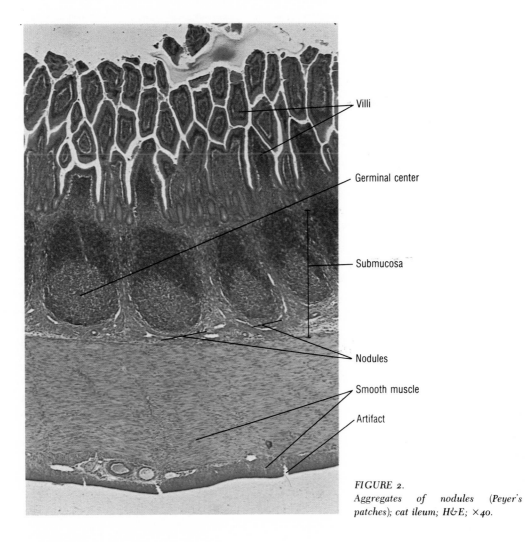

Villi

Germinal center

Submucosa

Nodules

Smooth muscle

Artifact

FIGURE 2.
Aggregates of nodules (Peyer's patches); cat ileum; H&E; ×40.

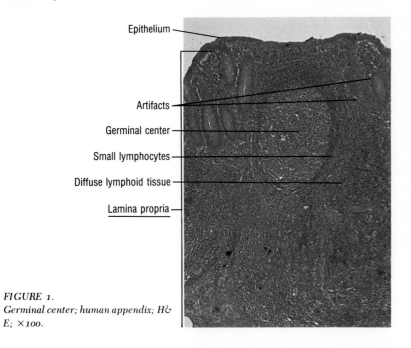

Epithelium

Artifacts

Germinal center

Small lymphocytes

Diffuse lymphoid tissue

Lamina propria

FIGURE 1.
Germinal center; human appendix; H&
E; ×100.

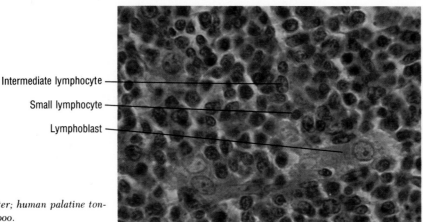

Intermediate lymphocyte

Small lymphocyte

Lymphoblast

FIGURE 2.
Germinal center; human palatine ton-
sil; H&E; ×1000.

GERMINAL CENTERS (secondary nodules). These are prominent, pale, ovoid areas of lymphoid tissue, completely or partially surrounded by a dark ring of concentrated small lymphocytes and separated from diffuse lymphoid tissue. The germinal center contains a high concentration of large-sized lymphocytes (lymphoblasts) and medium-sized lymphocytes, but macrophages and reticular and plasma cells are also present (see Chaps. 3, 7, and 8). A germinal center is indicative of lymphocytosis and corresponding antibody production during a primary and secondary immune response. Some investigators believe that the germinal centers have no association with primary nodules and do not represent transitional stages derived from these structures; others, however, hold the opposite view. Unlike other lymphoid organs, the thymus lacks germinal centers. **Plate 2, Fig. 2; Plate 3, Figs. 1 and 2.**

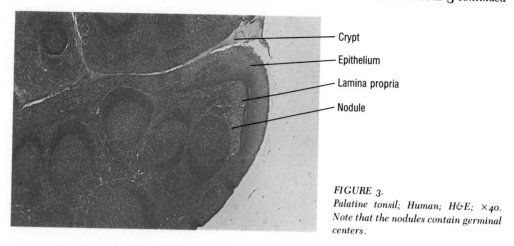

— Crypt
— Epithelium
— Lamina propria
— Nodule

FIGURE 3.
Palatine tonsil; Human; H&E; ×40.
Note that the nodules contain germinal centers.

Tonsils

Tonsils are relatively complex lymphoid structures surrounding the entrance to the throat. They are located on the root of the tongue and at the junction of the nasopharynx and oropharynx. There are three types of tonsils: *lingual, pharyngeal,* and *palatine.* Although they vary in anatomical position (see Chap. 13), their structures are somewhat similar. A tonsil is an organized mass of diffuse lymphoid tissue and nodules (usually containing germinal centers) within the lamina propria of the oral mucous membrane. It is separated from surrounding connective tissue by a fibrous capsule and is lined on its oral surface with epithelium. The capsule is composed of collagen fibers and has thin septa, carrying vessels and nerves, extending into the interior of the tonsil. The *palatine* and *lingual* tonsils have deeply branched or unbranched crypts. These crypts extend into the tonsil and are lined with stratified squamous epithelium. The *pharyngeal* tonsils (adenoids) have only deep folds rather than crypts. They are lined with pseudostratified columnar ciliated epithelium containing goblet cells. The epithelium of all tonsils is characteristically heavily infiltrated with lymphocytes migrating from underlying lymphoid tissues. The crypts may be filled with debris, leucocytes, desquamated cells, and bacteria.

Tonsils lack lymphatic sinuses, but do have plexuses of peripheral lymphatic capillaries which drain lymph into efferent lymphatic vessels (see below). **Plate 3, Fig. 3.**

Lymph nodes and lymphatic vessels

As lymph is drained from the tissues of the body and carried by lymphatic vessels toward the heart, it is filtered through lymph nodes. The nodes remove toxic and foreign substances, produce antibodies, and release lymphocytes into the lymph.

LYMPH NODE. A lymph node is a small (up to 30 mm in diameter), oval or round lymphoid organ connected to a system of lymphatic vessels. A node has an indented region, the hilus, through which vessels and nerves enter and leave the structure.

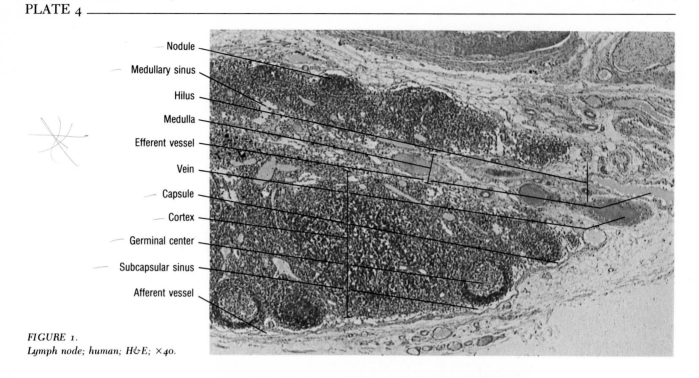

Nodule
Medullary sinus
Hilus
Medulla
Efferent vessel
Vein
Capsule
Cortex
Germinal center
Subcapsular sinus
Afferent vessel

FIGURE 1.
Lymph node; human; H&E; ×40.

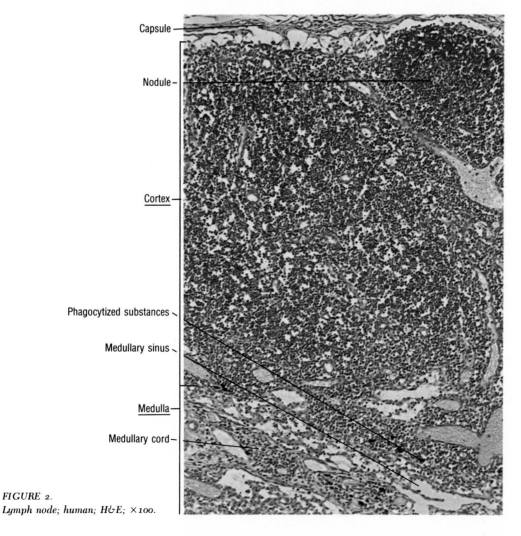

Capsule

Nodule

Cortex

Phagocytized substances

Medullary sinus

Medulla

Medullary cord

FIGURE 2.
Lymph node; human; H&E; ×100.

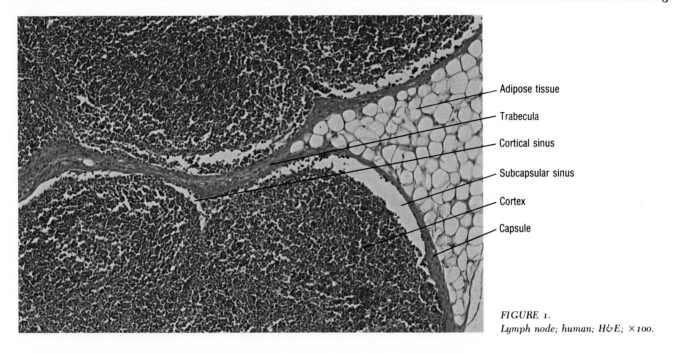

— Adipose tissue

— Trabecula

— Cortical sinus

— Subcapsular sinus

— Cortex

— Capsule

FIGURE 1.
Lymph node; human; H&E; ×100.

The node is surrounded by a dense, irregular collagenous connective tissue *capsule* containing some smooth muscle. The capsule has many branched trabeculae which organize the lymphoid tissue into an outer *cortex* of incomplete compartments and an inner noncompartmentalized *medulla*. The outer cortex is composed of dense lymphoid tissue containing nodules, with or without germinal centers (see above), while the medulla is a loose network of anastomosing cords of lymphoid tissue. **Plate 4, Figs. 1 and 2.**

Lymph enters a node through afferent lymphatic vessels located within the capsule, percolates through sinuses toward the medulla, and then leaves the node via efferent vessels. The afferent vessels are drained by *subcapsular sinuses*. These sinuses are drained by *cortical sinuses*, located between the trabeculae and cortical tissue. The cortical sinuses, in turn, are drained by *medullary sinuses*, located between the trabeculae and medullary cords. These latter sinuses are then drained by efferent vessels at the hilus of the node. The thin-walled sinuses are composed of reticular fibers which are continuous with the fibers of the parenchyma. The sinuses are irregular in size, highly branched, and crisscrossed with reticular fibers. Although some histologists believe that an incomplete layer of reticular cells line the sinuses and accompany the intraluminal fibers, others think that the sinuses and fibers are lined by macrophages and stellate or flattened endothelial cells. While all of these cells have varying degrees of phagocytic abilities and could filter lymph by phagocytizing foreign substances, the macrophages are the most effective phagocytes. **Plate 4, Figs. 1 and 2; Plate 5, Figs. 1 and 2.**

Arteries and veins have approximately the same pathway through a lymph node. Arteries enter the hilus, are distributed to the medullary cords via the trabeculae, and then continue into the cortex. The arteries give rise to capillary plexuses, both in the medulla and around the cortical nodules. Some vascular branches also enter the capsule. Vasomotor nerve fibers accompany the blood vessels.

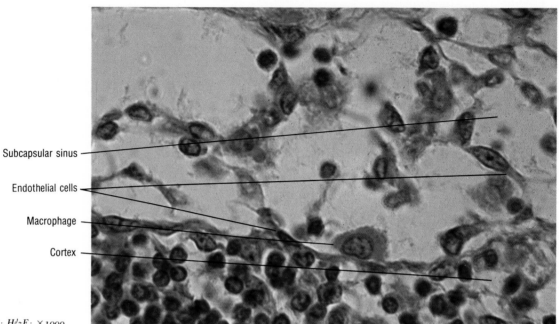

Subcapsular sinus —

Endothelial cells —

Macrophage —

Cortex —

FIGURE 2.
Lymph node; human; H&E; ×1000.

LYMPHATIC VESSELS. Tiny *lymphatic capillaries* drain lymph from the body tissues. They converge to form larger *collecting vessels* as the lymph is drained centrally and toward the heart. Eventually, large *lymphatic ducts* drain the collecting vessels and conduct the lymph to the right brachiocephalic vein and junction of the left jugular and subclavian veins near the heart.

Lymphatic capillaries. These are the smallest of the lymphatic vessels. Although they resemble vascular capillaries, they are larger in diameter (up to 100 μm) and usually irregular in shape; they are lined by a flattened endothelium but lack pericytes. The endothelium is surrounded by a delicate layer of collagen and reticular fibers. **Plate 6, Fig. 1.**

Collecting vessels. The vessels of this type are about 100 to 1000 μm in diameter. They have valves and resemble veins of comparable size, but their walls are extremely thin relative to the large lumen. The walls of the *larger collecting* vessels (300 μm and larger) are organized into three superimposed layers, or tunicae, similar to the condition found in blood vessels, but the demarcation between the tunicae is ill defined. The inner layer is the *tunica intima*, composed of an endothelium lying on a thin layer of elastic fibers; the middle layer is the *tunica media*, composed of one or two layers of smooth muscle cells; the outer *tunica adventitia* contains a network of collagen and elastic fibers, and some scattered smooth muscle. The adventitital tissue is continuous with surrounding connective tissue. The valves are a pair of folds of the tunica intima which extend into the lumen. They are designed to ensure a unidirectional lymph flow.

The walls of the *smaller collecting vessels* are not organized into separate layers. They are lined by an endothelium lying on a thin bed of reticular and collagen fibers with some scattered smooth muscle cells. **Plate 6, Fig. 2.**

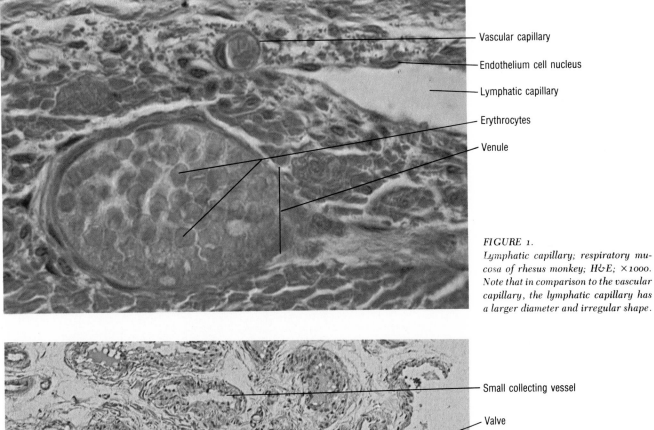

Vascular capillary

Endothelium cell nucleus

Lymphatic capillary

Erythrocytes

Venule

FIGURE 1.
*Lymphatic capillary; respiratory mu-
cosa of rhesus monkey; H&E; ×1000.
Note that in comparison to the vascular
capillary, the lymphatic capillary has
a larger diameter and irregular shape.*

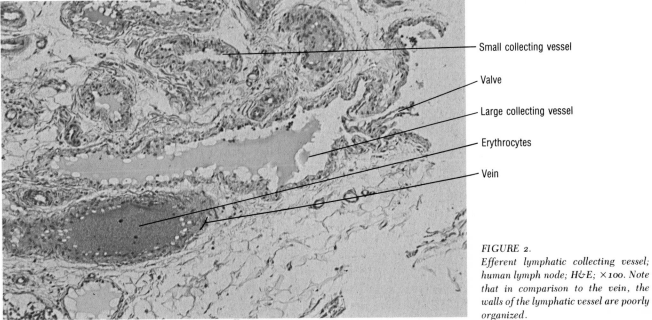

Small collecting vessel

Valve

Large collecting vessel

Erythrocytes

Vein

FIGURE 2.
*Efferent lymphatic collecting vessel;
human lymph node; H&E; ×100. Note
that in comparison to the vein, the
walls of the lymphatic vessel are poorly
organized.*

Lymphatic ducts. These are the largest vessels of the lymphatic system, usually
several millimeters in diameter. Their walls are thin relative to the size of the lumen,
valves are present, and the wall of the vessel is composed of an inner *tunica intima*,
middle *tunica media*, and an outer *tunica adventitia*. The lymphatic ducts differ
from veins of similar size because the three tunicae are very poorly defined and the
tunica media contains a prominent layer of smooth muscle tissue.

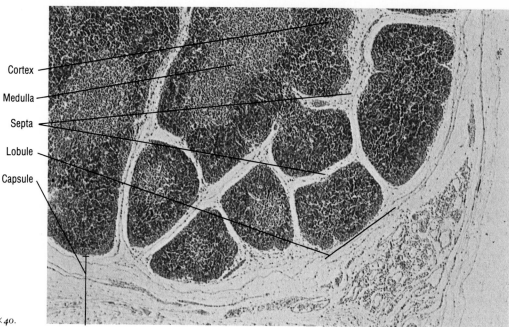

Cortex

Medulla

Septa

Lobule

Capsule

FIGURE 1.
Thymus; human fetus; H&E; ×40.

Thymus

The thymus is located within the anterior mediastinum dorsal to the sternum in the upper thorax, and extends into the neck. It is largest during prepuberty, it starts to regress at puberty, and will be mainly replaced by adipose tissue in middle age. It is composed of two long lobes, united by connective tissue. Each lobe is surrounded by a capsule of fibroelastic tissue. Septa extend from the capsule to subdivide each lobe into many incomplete rectangular lobules. Each lobule is composed of a peripheral *cortex* which is dense with lymphocytes and which surrounds a less dense, lightly stained central *medulla*. The inner region on each lobule lacks a septum, so the medullary portions are continuous with each other. **Plate 7, Fig. 1.**

CORTEX. This is a cytoreticulum (only a meshwork of cells), composed of reticuloepithelial cells in which are located great numbers of small, medium, and large lymphocytes. Although the cells of the cytoreticulum resemble reticular cells, they do not produce fibers, are derived from entoderm rather than mesenchyme, and have desmosomes which are characteristic of epithelial cells. These are large, stellate, acidophilic cells with a large, pale nucleus and a prominent nucleolus. Usually only the nucleus is visible. Other cells, such as macrophages, fat cells, mast cells, and plasma cells, may also be present in the cortex. **Plate 7, Fig. 1.**

MEDULLA. This innermost region of both the lobes and lobules is composed of elements similar to those of the cortex (see above). Since lymphocytes are not as numerous here as in the cortex, more of the cytoreticulum is visible and the entire medulla appears less dense and paler. Cells in the cytoreticulum appear more like epithelial cells in the medulla than the cortex because they may occur in clumps and are either cuboidal, columnar, or polygonal. Lymphocytes in the medullary tissue

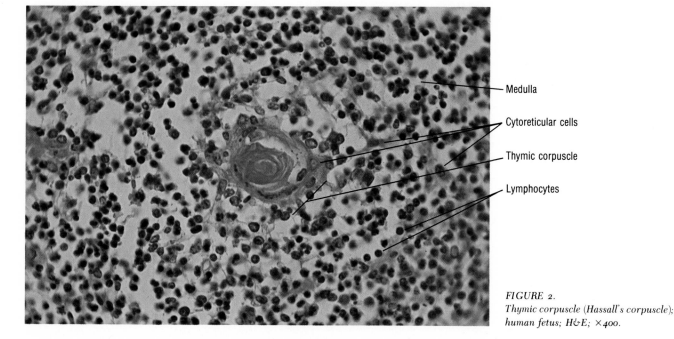

- Medulla
- Cytoreticular cells
- Thymic corpuscle
- Lymphocytes

FIGURE 2.
Thymic corpuscle (Hassall's corpuscle);
human fetus; H&E; ×400.

are usually in transit; they migrate from the cortex through the medulla and leave the thymus via medullary veins. **Plate 7, Figs. 1 and 2.**

Thymic corpuscles (Hassall's corpuscles). These are prominent, dark pink, spherical structures located within the medulla. They are composed of layered, degenerate reticuloepithelial cells and vary in size from 15 to 200 μm in diameter. The cells in the interior of the corpuscle may be keratinized, calcified, or disintegrated, so that the center may appear pale or hollow. The corpuscles are present in the fetal thymus and increase in numbers and size as cells from the cytoreticulum are added to its periphery. Although development of the corpuscles continues throughout the life of the individual, their function is unknown. **Plate 7, Fig. 2.**

BLOOD AND LYMPHATIC VESSELS. Arterial branches from the internal thoracic and inferior thyroid arteries enter the capsule and are carried within the interlobular septa. These vessels extend to the corticomedullary junction where they give rise to arterioles ensheathed with reticuloepithelial cells. From this junction, branches mainly supply capillary beds in the cortex and capsule, but some go to the medulla. Capillaries are thick-walled, having a prominent basement membrane and an incomplete layer of reticuloepithelial cells surrounding an endothelium. This unique arrangement constitutes a *blood-thymus barrier* and is common to the cortex rather than the medulla. The barrier is effective in preventing the movement of macromolecules from the blood to cortical tissues, and therefore lymphocytes in this region are not exposed to antigens. Capillaries in the cortical and medullary regions are drained by postcapillary venules at the corticomedullary junction. Lymphocytes enter the bloodstream at the corticomedullary junction by migrating from thymic tissue through the venule walls. The venules then form larger veins in the interlobular septa. These veins drain into major veins which carry blood to the left brachiocephalic, internal thoracic, and inferior thyroid veins.

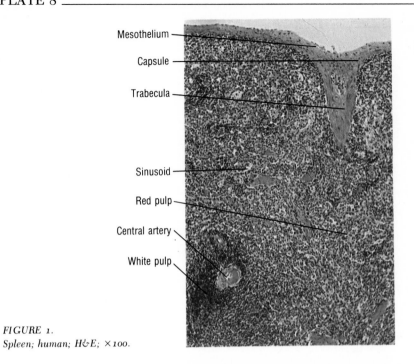

Mesothelium

Capsule

Trabecula

Sinusoid

Red pulp

Central artery

White pulp

FIGURE 1.
Spleen; human; H&E; ×100.

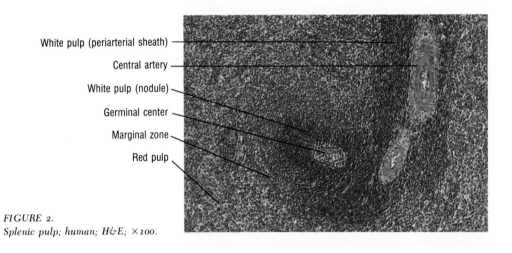

White pulp (periarterial sheath)

Central artery

White pulp (nodule)

Germinal center

Marginal zone

Red pulp

FIGURE 2.
Splenic pulp; human; H&E; ×100.

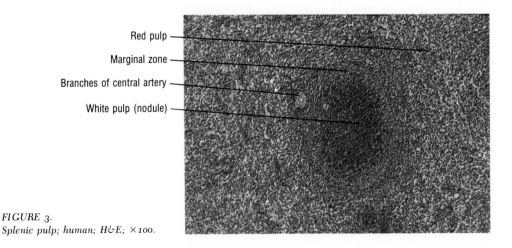

Red pulp

Marginal zone

Branches of central artery

White pulp (nodule)

FIGURE 3.
Splenic pulp; human; H&E; ×100.

Lymphatic vessels of the efferent type are present in the interlobular septa. They drain lymph toward the hilus and eventually into the tracheobronchial and brachiocephalic lymph nodes. Afferent lymphatic vessels and sinuses are not present in the thymus.

NERVES. Vasomotor nerve fibers of the sympathetic and parasympathetic divisions of the autonomic nervous system are present in the capsule, but only sympathetic fibers accompany the blood vessels.

Spleen

The spleen is an ovoid, vascular organ which is about 12 cm long and lies between the stomach and diaphragm. It contains lymphatic and hematopoietic tissues. Of its various functions of blood storage, hematopoiesis, and antibody production, the most important is the removal of foreign matter and nonfunctional blood cells from the plasma. The spleen has a long medial fissure, the *hilus*, which receives arteries, veins, lymphatics, and nerve branches at various points along its length.

CAPSULE. The spleen is surrounded by a capsule of dense, irregular collagenous connective tissue containing some elastic fibers and smooth muscle. A mesothelium, the *peritoneum*, covers the surface of the capsule. A network of *trabeculae* extends from the capsule to the interior of the spleen, subdividing the splenic pulp (see below) into small interconnecting compartments. The capsule and trabeculae carry blood vessels, lymphatic vessels, and nerves. **Plate 8, Fig. 1.**

SPLENIC PULP. This is the parenchyma of the spleen and it has three histologic regions: (1) *red pulp*, which is quite vascular and has many stored red blood corpuscles; (2) *white pulp*, which is typical lymphoid tissue containing nodules; (3) the *marginal zone*, which separates the red and white pulp and has some characteristics of both regions. **Plate 8, Figs. 1, 2, and 3; Plate 9, Figs. 1 and 2.**

Red pulp. This tissue has large (10 to 45 μm diameter), branching *sinusoids* separating thin plates of parenchyma, the *splenic cords* (Billroth cords). The sinusoidal wall has loosely joined fusiform endothelial cells sitting on a fenestrated basement membrane. This arrangement in the sinusoidal wall facilitates passage of blood cells between sinusoids and cords. The splenic cords are composed of a network of reticular tissue which is continuous with the marginal zone. Spaces in the reticular network contain blood plasma, many erythrocytes, leucocytes, plasma cells, macrophages, and hematopoietic cells. Reticular cells and particularly macrophages phagocytize foreign matter, nonfunctional erythrocytes, leucocytes, and cell debris from the blood. **Plate 8, Figs. 1 and 2; Plate 9, Figs. 1 and 2.**

White pulp. This is a dense sheath of lymphatic tissue which surrounds central arteries in the parenchyma. The sheath itself is surrounded by red pulp. The white pulp is composed of reticular tissue forming a loose mesh containing small, medium, and large lymphocytes, plasma cells, and macrophages (see Chaps. 7 and 8). Where solitary lymphatic nodules, with or without germinal centers, are present in the sheath, they displace the central artery or its branches to an eccentric position. **Plate 8, Figs, 1, 2, and 3; Plate 9, Fig. 2.**

Marginal zone. This tissue is peripheral to the white pulp and resembles it, except that it is less dense and more vascular. It is a transitional area from the white to the red pulp. **Plate 8, Figs. 2 and 3; Plate 9, Fig. 2.**

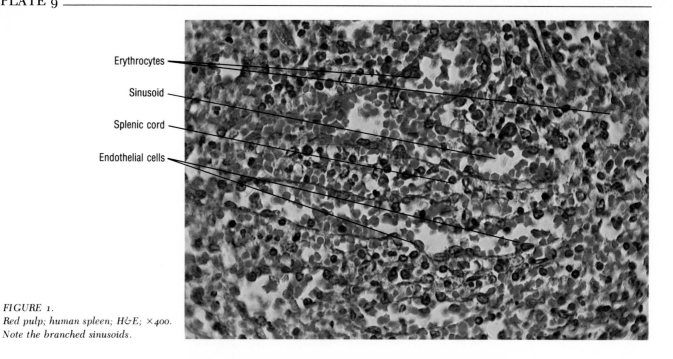

Erythrocytes

Sinusoid

Splenic cord

Endothelial cells

FIGURE 1.
Red pulp; human spleen; H&E; ×400.
Note the branched sinusoids.

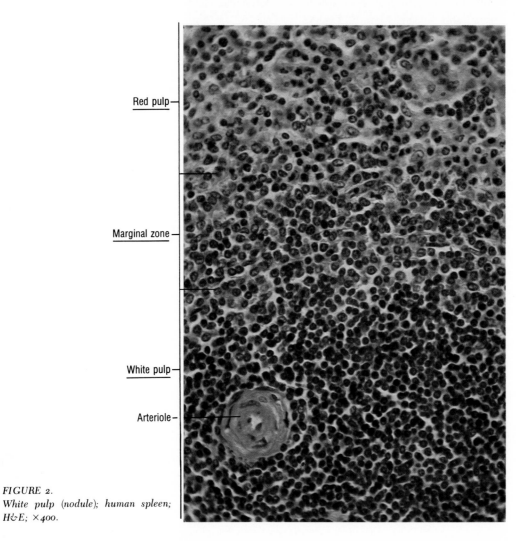

Red pulp

Marginal zone

White pulp

Arteriole

FIGURE 2.
White pulp (nodule); human spleen;
H&E; ×400.

BLOOD AND LYMPHATIC VESSELS. The vascular pattern of the spleen is quite complex. Table 1 is a schematic representation of that pattern, with special emphasis given to the type and location of blood vessels.

Lymphatic vessels are lacking in the splenic pulp because of the easy exchange of tissue fluids between the sinusoids and the cords; only prominent vessels are present in the trabeculae and capsule. The capsule is drained by large lymphatic vessels which leave the spleen at the hilus.

NERVES. Unmyelinated sympathetic nerve fibers accompany blood vessels in the spleen.

TABLE 1
Circulatory pattern in the spleen

Location	Name of vessel	Type of vessel
Hilus	Splenic artery	Muscular artery.
Trabeculae	Trabecular artery	Muscular artery.
White pulp	Central artery	Small muscular artery to arterioles. Adventitia is filled with lymphoid tissue.
Red pulp	Penicillus	This has several straight branches which form a tuft of vessels. Each vessel is divided into three segments (see box).
	Pulp arteriole	Small arteriole; one layer of smooth muscle; internal elastic membrane is lacking; one to two layers of lymphoid tissue in a thin adventitia; tall endothelium.
Red pulp	Sheathed arteriole (ellipsoid) (sheathed capillary)	Terminal arteriole; tall endothelium surrounded by a dense ellipsoid sheath of reticular tissue and macrophages, the Schweigger-Seidel sheath. The sheath is poorly developed in humans.
	Terminal arterial capillaries	Capillaries.
Red pulp	Open / Closed → Splenic cords	There are three theories on how blood circulates through this part of the pattern. (1) Open circulation; blood leaves the vascular system, percolating through the cords to the sinuses. (2) Closed circulation; blood remains within the vascular system. (3) Both open and closed types of circulation are functional at the same time.
Red pulp	Venous sinusoids (sinuses)	
Red pulp	Pulp veins	Venules to small veins.
Trabeculae	Trabecular veins	Small to medium-sized veins.
Hilus	Splenic vein	Medium-sized to large veins.

Integument 11

The integument is a superficial covering of the body surface and is composed of skin, nails, hair, and glands. Among its numerous functions, the integument is adapted to prevent desiccation and provide physical protection to underlying tissues. It exerts a regulatory influence on the homeostatic functions of the body through thermo-regulation, maintenance of water balance, and excretion of metabolic waste sub-stances. Also, the integument contains sensory receptors which provide the body with information about the environment.

Skin

The skin covers the surface of the body and is approximately 0.5 to 5.0 mm in thickness. This thickness varies directly with friction and pressure exerted on the skin. Skin is composed of two layers: an outer *epidermis* of ectodermal origin, and an underlying *dermis*, derived from mesoderm. The boundary between the two layers is irregular, except for the skin of the scrotum and ear. In some regions the dermis may be firmly attached to underlying bone by a fusion of the dermis with the periosteum, but in most regions it is loosely attached to underlying muscles by a loose connective tissue, the *subcutaneous layer* (hypodermis or superficial fascia). **Plate 1, Fig. 1.**

EPIDERMIS. This outer layer of stratified squamous keratinized epithelium is resistant to physical and chemical stresses. In areas such as the soles and palms, where friction and pressure is most intense, five distinct superimposed layers are present in the epidermis. In areas with less physical stresses (skin of chest, scalp, etc.), there are fewer than five layers. In going from the lower to the upper surface of the epidermis, the five layers are designated as the *stratum germinativum, stratum spinosum, stratum granulosum, stratum lucidum,* and *stratum corneum.* The lucidum and granulosum layers may be absent in some skin (scalp). **Plate 1, Figs. 1, 2,** and **3.**

The stratum germinativum is regenerative, and as cells are produced by this layer, they migrate up through the overlying strata. During their migration they undergo morphologic and physiologic changes, becoming flattened, dead, dry,

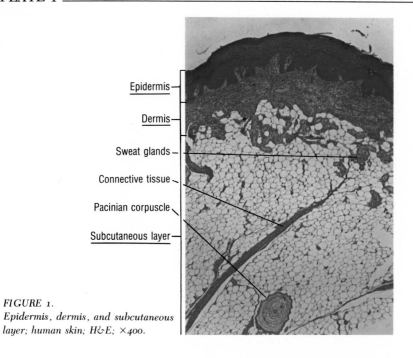

Epidermis —

Dermis —

Sweat glands —

Connective tissue —

Pacinian corpuscle —

Subcutaneous layer —

FIGURE 1.
Epidermis, dermis, and subcutaneous
layer; human skin; H&E; ×400.

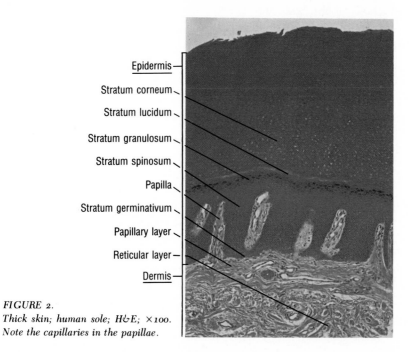

Epidermis —

Stratum corneum —

Stratum lucidum —

Stratum granulosum —

Stratum spinosum —

Papilla —

Stratum germinativum —

Papillary layer —

Reticular layer —

Dermis —

FIGURE 2.
Thick skin; human sole; H&E; ×100.
Note the capillaries in the papillae.

keratinized flakes. As these cells are desquamated at the surface, they are replaced by later generations of keratinized cells. The epidermis is avascular but is supplied with fluids from capillary plexuses in the dermis.

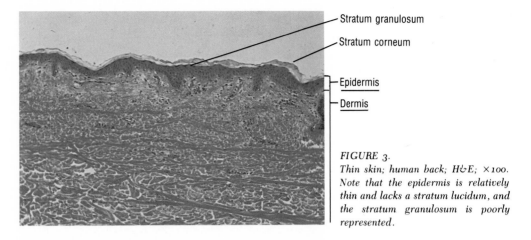

FIGURE 3.
*Thin skin; human back; H&E; ×100.
Note that the epidermis is relatively
thin and lacks a stratum lucidum, and
the stratum granulosum is poorly
represented.*

_____ PLATE 2

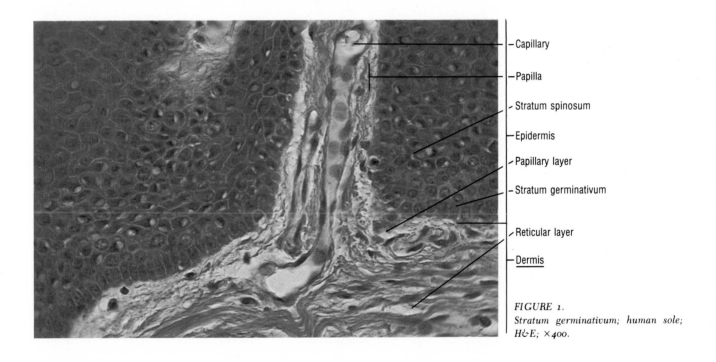

FIGURE 1.
*Stratum germinativum; human sole;
H&E; ×400.*

Stratum germinativum. This is the lowermost layer of cells. It lies on a thin basement membrane and conforms to the ridges and grooves of the dermis. The cells may be either cuboidal or low columnar, and each cell has a large, oval nucleus surrounded by sparse, deeply stained, basophilic cytoplasm. Randomly oriented fibrous bundles, *tonofibrils*, are present in the cytoplasm and contribute to the later keratinization of the cells. The tonofibrils converge on *desmosomes*, which are points of attachment between adjacent cells. **Plate 2, Fig. 1.**

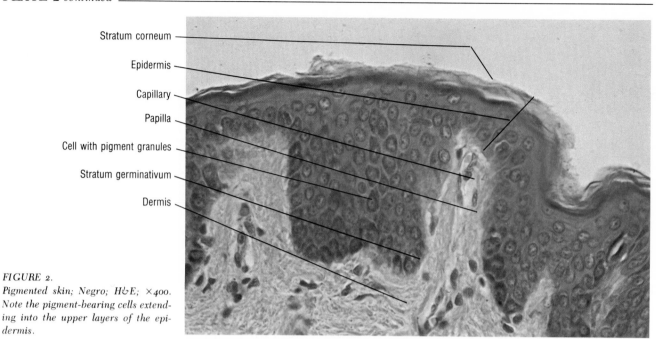

Stratum corneum —

Epidermis —

Capillary —

Papilla —

Cell with pigment granules —

Stratum germinativum —

Dermis —

FIGURE 2.
Pigmented skin; Negro; H&E; ×400.
Note the pigment-bearing cells extend-
ing into the upper layers of the epi-
dermis.

In addition to the generative cells in the stratum germinativum, *melanocytes*, or pigment-producing cells, are also present. Melanocytes represent about 10 to 25 percent of the cells in this layer; they do not undergo keratinization and lack tonofibrils and desmosomes. Melanocytes may extend into the dermis and the upper layers of the epidermis. Since they transfer their dark brown pigment to the adjacent epidermal cells, they are difficult to identify in H&E–stained preparations. In a section of epidermis they may appear as shrunken, branched, poorly stained cells, isolated from adjacent stained cells by a clear zone. During development of the embryo, melanocytes originate from neural crest tissue. They migrate to the stratum germinativum and synthesize melanin, which is the pigment responsible for dark skin colors. Melanin is incorporated into tiny (about 0.3 μm), oval, concentrically lamellated, cytoplasmic organelles, the *melanosomes* or *pigment granules*. The melanosomes are transferred to adjacent cells in the stratum germinativum, but will disappear as the epithelial cells migrate to the surface. In dark-skinned people melanosomes are present in the upper layers of the epidermis. The melanosomes disappear at the lower stratum spinosum layer in light-skinned people. **Plate 2, Fig. 2.**

Stratum spinosum. This is a relatively thick layer of slightly flattened, polyhedral cells lying above the stratum germinativum. Their large nuclei may be rounded or flattened with a prominent nucleolus, and the cytoplasm is slightly basophilic. The cells have a spiny appearance due to the wide intercellular spaces exposing cytoplasmic processes and desmosomes. The desmosomes bind adjacent cells by joining their processes. Tonofibrils form fibrous bundles in the cytoplasm, insert on the desmosomes, and are more easily seen than those in the cells of the stratum germinativum. **Plate 1, Fig. 2; Plate 2, Fig. 1; Plate 3, Figs. 1 and 2.**

Stratum granulosum. In thick skin (palms and soles) the stratum granulosum may have up to five layers of tissue, but in thin skin (chest) these layers may be absent

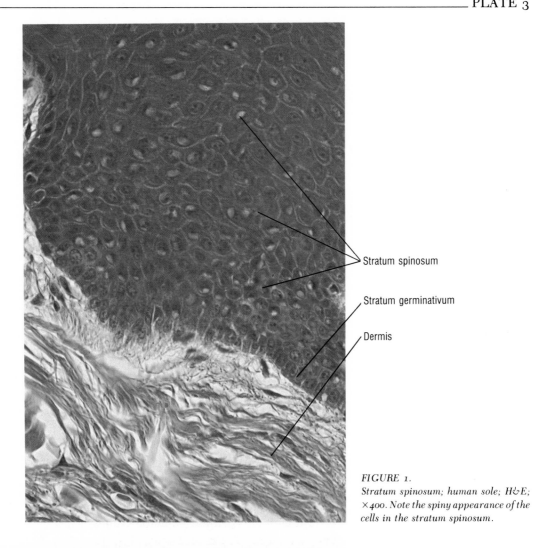

Stratum spinosum

Stratum germinativum

Dermis

FIGURE 1.
Stratum spinosum; human sole; H&E;
×400. Note the spiny appearance of the
cells in the stratum spinosum.

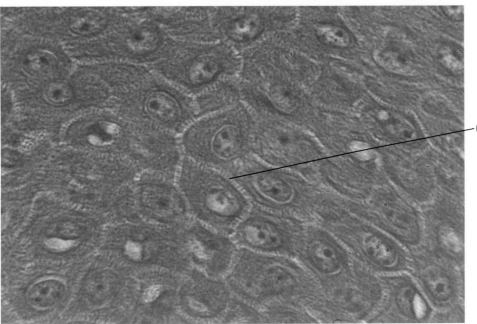

Cytoplasmic processes

FIGURE 2.
Stratum spinosum; human sole; H&E;
×1000. Note the wide intercellular
spaces and the cytoplasmic processes
(bridges) which are joined by desmo-
somes.

PLATE 4 ⎯⎯⎯⎯⎯⎯⎯⎯⎯⎯⎯⎯⎯⎯⎯⎯⎯⎯⎯⎯⎯⎯⎯⎯⎯⎯⎯⎯⎯⎯

Stratum corneum —

Stratum lucidum —

Stratum granulosum —

Stratum spinosum —

Papilla —

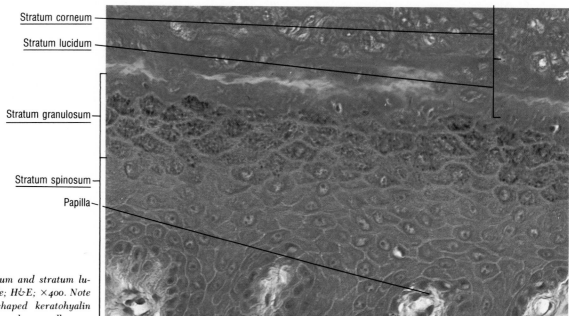

FIGURE 1.
Stratum granulosum and stratum lu-cidum; human sole; H&E; ×400. Note the irregularly shaped keratohyalin granules in the granulosum cells.

or poorly represented. The cells are more squamous and usually larger than those of the underlying stratum spinosum. The degenerating nucleus may be ovoid or flat and stains lightly, and the cytoplasm is filled with large (1 to 5 μm), irregularly shaped, basophilic *keratohyalin granules*. Although these granules are conspicuous in many keratinized tissues and are incorporated into keratin during the keratinization process, they are not present in all keratinized tissues, for example, hair and nails. The cellular interspaces are obliterated as tiny membrane-coating granules (a second type of granule also synthesized in the cytoplasm) are released to thicken the plasma membranes. **Plate 1, Fig. 2; Plate 4, Fig. 1.**

Stratum lucidum. This tissue lies above the stratum granulosum. It is about three to five cell layers in thickness, somewhat refractile, and stains poorly with H&E because the cells are dying and becoming keratinized. Since the nucleus, cell organelles, and plasma membranes are indistinct, the several layers of flat cells may appear as one consolidated homogeneous mass. Keratohyalin granules are not visible because they form *keratin*, a dense, amorphous matrix in which tonofibrils are embedded. The keratin is of the "soft type" because the fibrous proteins contain low levels of sulfur. Some integumentary structures (nails) may not achieve keratinization in this man-ner since they lack the stratum granulosum (see above). **Plate 1, Fig. 2; Plate 4, Fig. 1.**

Stratum corneum. This is the outermost keratinized layer of the epidermis. The number of cell layers varies from a few in thin skin to many in thick skin. The extremely flattened cells appear as thin, elongate, poorly stained, anucleate structures with thickened plasma membranes. Although the cytoplasm is replaced with fibrous

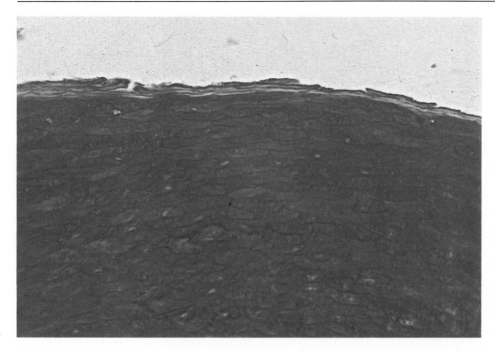

FIGURE 2.
*Stratum corneum; human sole; H&E;
×400. Note that the cells are anucleate
and become extremely flattened at the
surface.*

keratin, it appears homogeneous with the light microscope. These tightly packed, dead cells migrate to the surface, where they are desquamated as individuals or as sheets of cells, the *stratum disjunctum*. **Plate 1, Fig. 2; Plate 4, Figs. 1 and 2.**

DERMIS (corium). The dermis is a layer of fibroelastic tissue lying below the epidermis and continuous with the deeper subcutaneous layer. It varies between 0.3 and 4 mm in thickness. Since the dermis imparts the characteristics of strength, durability, and pliability to the skin, it normally is thicker in areas receiving maximal mechanical stresses. It is thicker in the palms and soles than the skin of the back. The dermis is organized into an upper, moderately dense *papillary layer*, which lies below the epidermis, and a lower, more dense *reticular layer*, which is continuous with the subcutaneous layer. The boundary between the two dermal layers is not distinct since there is some intergradation of tissues. **Plate 1, Figs. 1 and 2; Plate 2, Figs. 1 and 2; Plate 5, Figs. 1 and 2.**

Papillary layer (pars papillaris). This upper layer of the dermis is composed of a loose network of thin collagen, elastic, and reticular fibers. The ground substance is moderately abundant, containing many fibroblasts, some macrophages, mast cells, melanocytes (absent in palms and soles), and a few lymphocytes. In the skin of the soles and palms, where physical stresses are greatest, the papillary layer may be organized into tall and sometimes branched *dermal papillae*. These papillae form a complex interlocking system with ridges and grooves of the epidermis. In other areas, the face for example, the papillary layer forms only low, irregular hillocks. Although the papillae have an excellent vascular and lymphatic supply, only certain

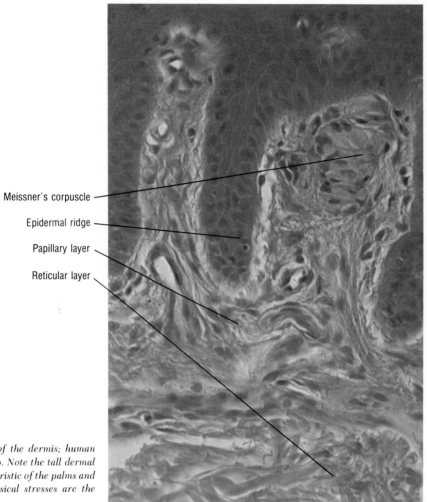

Meissner's corpuscle

Epidermal ridge

Papillary layer

Reticular layer

FIGURE 1.
Papillary layer of the dermis; human sole; H&E; ×400. Note the tall dermal papilla, characteristic of the palms and soles where physical stresses are the greatest.

ones have sensory receptors for touch, *Meissner's corpuscles*. The papillary layer lies below a thin basement membrane, which is usually indistinguishable in H&E–stained sections; it separates the epidermis and dermis. **Plate 1, Fig. 2; Plate 5, Fig. 1.**

Reticular layer (pars reticularis). This is the lower layer of the dermis, it is composed of dense, irregular collagenous connective tissue. The coarse collagen fibers are mainly parallel to the surface of the skin. A network of elastic fibers is also present and interspersed with the collagen fiber bundles. The reticular layer has fewer cell types than the papillary layer; the predominant cells are fibroblasts and macrophages. Sweat glands, hair follicles, sebaceous glands, and pressure receptors (pacinian corpuscles) are present in this layer. Smooth muscle fibers are located in the reticular layer of the scrotum, penis, labia majora, and nipples. They also are associated with hair follicles as the *arrector pili muscles*. In facial skin, the striated muscles of expression insert into the lower region of the reticular layer. **Plate 1, Fig. 2; Plate 2, Fig. 1; Plate 5, Figs. 1 and 2.**

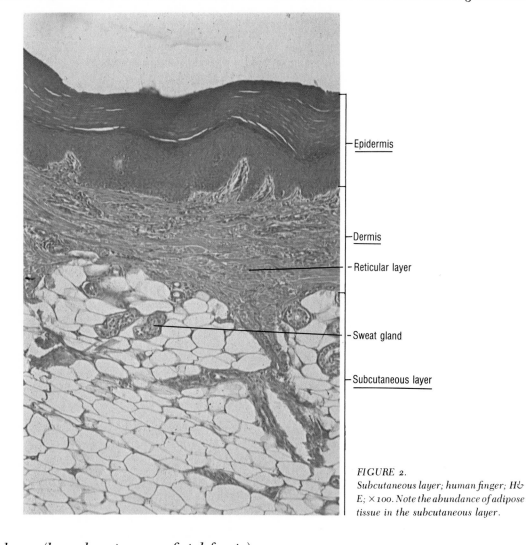

- Epidermis

- Dermis

- Reticular layer

- Sweat gland

- Subcutaneous layer

FIGURE 2.
Subcutaneous layer; human finger; H&
E; ×100. Note the abundance of adipose
tissue in the subcutaneous layer.

Subcutaneous layer (hypodermis, superficial fascia)

The subcutaneous layer is usually studied with the skin, but is not a part of it. It is composed of loose connective tissue, is usually thicker than the dermis, and extends from the reticular layer of the dermis to the underlying deep fasciae of muscles. The mobility of the skin varies indirectly with the amount of collagen and elastic fibers present in the subcutaneous layer. In most regions, excluding the scrotum, penis, and eyelids, the subcutaneous layer contains some scattered adipose tissue. Prominent sheets of adipose tissue, the *panniculus adiposus*, are located in the deeper regions of the subcutaneous layer and occur on the abdomen, for example. Large blood vessels, pressure sensory receptors (Pacinian corpuscles), nerves, and lymphatics may be found in this layer. Also, parts of hair follicles, sweat glands, and smooth or striated muscle tissue may be present. **Plate 1, Fig. 1; Plate 5, Fig. 2.**

The human nail is an integumentary structure derived entirely from the epidermis. It is a rectangular and curved *nail plate* of fused stratum corneum cells attached to a stratum germinativum, the *nail bed*. The proximal portion of the nail plate is the unexposed *root;* distally it is the exposed *body*. A fold of skin, the *nail wall*, covers the root and lateral margins of the body. The space between the nail wall and plate is the *nail groove*. **Plate 6, Figs. 1 and 2.**

NAIL BED. This is a stratum germinativum lying under the nail plate. The proximal portion of the nail bed, the *nail matrix*, is also the thickest. As the nail grows, matrix cells give rise to root cells by proliferation, differentiation, and keratinization. This process allows the nail to grow distally about 2 mm a month. The deepest layer of matrix cells are columnar with a large nucleus surrounded by an abundant basophilic cytoplasm. They give rise to upper layers of polyhedral cells with a pale basophilic cytoplasm filled with tonofibrils. These polyhedral matrix cells then differentiate into flattened, keratinized, fused root cells. During nail growth the cells do not pass through the granulosum or lucidum stages, which characterize keratinization in certain regions of the skin. **Plate 6, Figs. 1 and 2.**

The portion of the nail bed lying directly under the nail body does not contribute to the growth of the nail. It anchors the nail but still allows the body to slide distally as growth occurs at the root. In this region the stratum germinativum is composed of a few layers of polyhedral cells lying over a basal layer of cuboidal cells. The nail bed is fastened to the dermis by an interlocking system of longitudinal ridges and grooves. The system is best seen in cross section as tall dermal papillae extend up into the epidermis of the nail bed. The dermis itself is anchored directly to the perisoteum. **Plate 6, Figs. 1 and 2.**

NAIL. The root and body of the nail are composed of many layers of fused and keratinized squamous cells which do not undergo desquamation. The plasma membranes are indistinguishable since they are fused; thus the nail appears as a translucent, homogeneous structure which stains poorly with H&E. **Plate 6, Figs. 1 and 2.**

EPONYCHIUM (cuticle). This is a thin layer of keratinized stratum corneum of the nail wall covering the proximal surface of the nail body. **Plate 6, Fig. 1.**

HYPONYCHIUM. This is the thickened stratum corneum of the skin, lying directly under the distal free edge of the nail. The hyponychium represents the junction where the stratum germinativum of the nail bed and skin are continuous. **Plate 6, Fig. 2.**

LUNULA. The lunula is a white, opaque, crescent-shaped structure on the proximal surface of the nail body near the nail wall. Its appearance is due to the presence of the underlying thickened nail matrix.

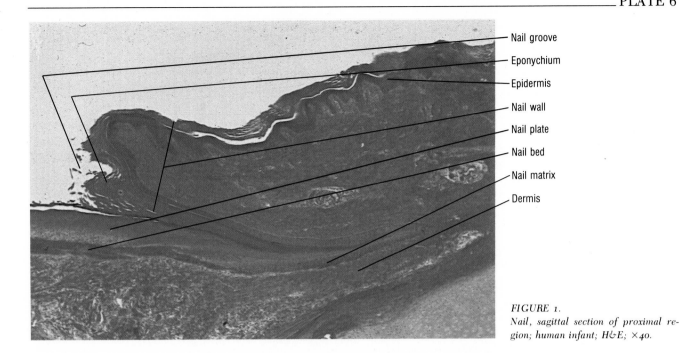

Nail groove

Eponychium

Epidermis

Nail wall

Nail plate

Nail bed

Nail matrix

Dermis

FIGURE 1.
Nail, sagittal section of proximal region; human infant; H&E; ×40.

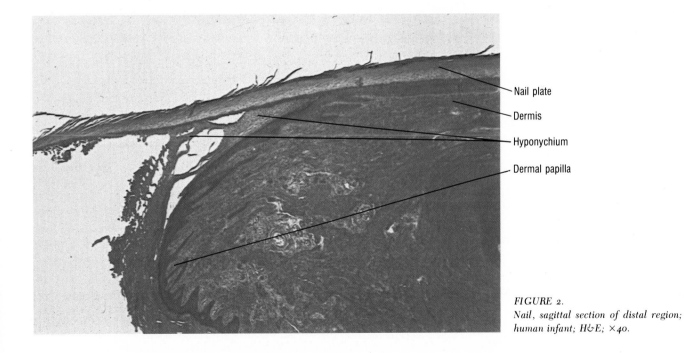

Nail plate

Dermis

Hyponychium

Dermal papilla

FIGURE 2.
Nail, sagittal section of distal region; human infant; H&E; ×40.

A hair is an epidermal thread produced by the activity of a *hair follicle*. These follicles are located over most of the skin; exceptions are the palms and soles. A hair follicle is a tubular extension of the epidermis into the dermis and subcutaneous layers. It is surrounded by a connective tissue sheath of the dermis and is closely associated with sebaceous glands and arrector pili muscles (see below). The follicle terminates as an enlarged epithelial bulk of generative matrix cells. The matrix cells give rise to the hair and contribute to its growth. As the hair grows, it pushes up through the follicle and extends from the surface of the skin. Matrix cells also form the inner sheath root of the hair follicle (see below). The lower region of the bulb is indented with connective tissue, nerves, and blood vessels. This tissue fills the center of the bulb as the *dermal papilla*. The metabolic activities and differentiation of both the hair and sheath are influenced by the dermal papillae. **Plate 7, Figs. 1 and 2.**

HAIR. A hair has a root and a shaft. The shaft is the fully keratinized upper portion extending from the surface of the skin. The root is contained within the follicle below the surface of the skin, and is continuous with the deeper matrix cells. It is only partially keratinized at its lower levels. The hair is composed of three concentric layers which differentiate from the matrix cells: *medulla, cortex,* and *cuticle*.

Medulla. This is a central longitudinal core of a few lightly packed, cuboidal, vacuolated or keratinized cells partially separated by air spaces. The medulla does not extend to the tip of the hair and is absent in fine hairs. **Plate 7, Fig. 1; Plate 8, Figs. 1 and 2.**

Cortex. This is a peripheral layer of cells surrounding the medulla, and constitutes most of the hair mass. It is composed of dense, compact layers of pigmented squamous keratinzed cells. **Plate 7, Fig. 1; Plate 8, Figs. 1, 2, and 3.**

Cuticle. This is a single layer of enucleated squamous keratinized cells lying on the surface of the hair. The cells overlap each other and have free serrated edges. The edges are directed upward and interlock with the downward-directed edges of the cells lining the follicle. **Plate 7, Figs. 1 and 2; Plate 8, Figs. 1 and 3.**

HAIR FOLLICLE. The follicle is composed of an outer and inner root sheath of epidermal origin and is surrounded by a connective tissue sheath of the dermis.

Inner root sheath. This sheath is peripheral to the hair and organized into three sublayers of tissue: *cuticle, Huxley's layer,* and *Henle's layer*. Like the hair, these layers are also derived from matrix cells. As the cells grow toward the surface of the skin, they are desquamated at the level of the sebaceous glands. During this time they undergo stages of keratinization, and so at the uppermost level they desquamate as keratinized tissues. Keratin in these cells, unlike that of hair and nail cells, is of the "soft type" and contains small amounts of sulfur in its fibrous proteins. **Plate 7, Figs. 1 and 2; Plate 8; Figs. 1, 2, and 3.**

CUTICLE. At the upper levels of the follicle this layer is composed of keratinized squamous cells. The cells are organized as downward-directed scales which interlock with the upturned scales of the hair cuticle. **Plate 7, Fig. 1; Plate 8, Figs. 1 and 3.**

HUXLEY'S LAYER. This layer is peripheral to the cuticle and composed of several layers of cells. At the lower levels of the follicle the cells are transparent and polygonal, but at higher levels they become flattened, and filled with tonofibrils and trichohyalin granules (similar to keratohyalin). Near the sebaceous glands they are fully keratinized cells. **Plate 7, Fig. 1; Plate 8, Fig. 3.**

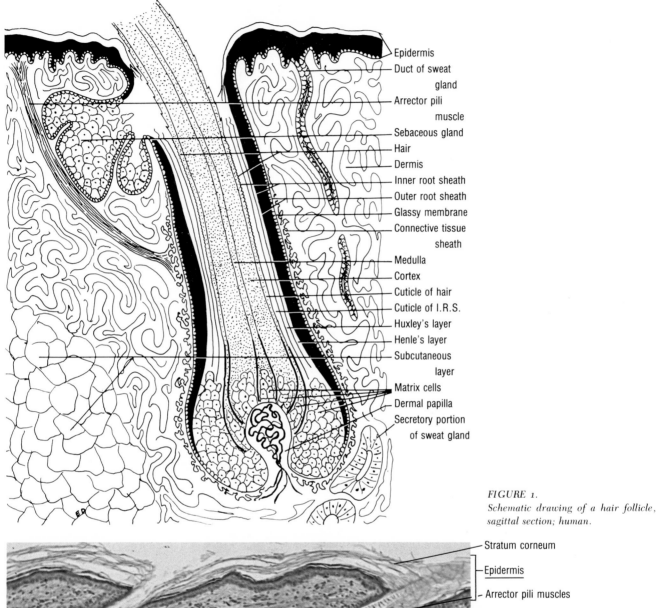

Epidermis
Duct of sweat
gland
Arrector pili
muscle
Sebaceous gland
Hair
Dermis
Inner root sheath
Outer root sheath
Glassy membrane
Connective tissue
sheath
Medulla
Cortex
Cuticle of hair
Cuticle of I.R.S.
Huxley's layer
Henle's layer
Subcutaneous
layer
Matrix cells
Dermal papilla
Secretory portion
of sweat gland

FIGURE 1.
Schematic drawing of a hair follicle,
sagittal section; human.

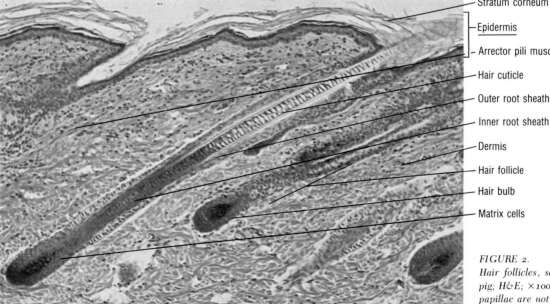

Stratum corneum
Epidermis
Arrector pili muscles
Hair cuticle
Outer root sheath
Inner root sheath
Dermis
Hair follicle
Hair bulb
Matrix cells

FIGURE 2.
Hair follicles, sagittal section; guinea
pig; H&E; ×100. Note that the dermal
papillae are not showing in these sec-
tions of the follicles.

HENLE'S LAYER. Just peripheral to Huxley's layer, and at the lower levels, Henle's layer is composed of a single layer of cuboidal cells. They undergo the same stages of keratinization as the Huxley layer, but the process occurs deeper so the flattened cells with trichohyalin granules and the fully keratinized cells are located deeper in the sheath. **Plate 7, Fig. 1; Plate 8, Fig. 3.**

Outer root sheath. This sheath is peripheral to the inner root sheath and extends from the sebaceous glands down to the bottom of the hair follicle. It is composed of stratified nonkeratinized epithelial tissue which is continuous with and comparable to the stratum spinosum and stratum germinativum layers of the skin. At the level of the dermal papilla these layers are reduced to a single layer of cells, and these eventually mix with matrix cells. Just below the sebaceous glands the tissue of the outer root sheath, lying peripheral to Henle's layer, is composed of spiny-looking cells with cytoplasmic processes filled with tonofibrils. Peripheral to the spiny cell layer, and representing the outer region of the outer root sheath, is a single layer of low columnar cells lying on a basement membrane, the *glassy membrane* (see below). **Plate 7, Figs. 1 and 2; Plate 8, Figs. 1, 2, and 3.**

Connective tissue sheath. This sheath is composed of fibroelastic tissue of the dermis. It surrounds the outer root sheath and is limited to the lower portion of the follicle. The connective tissue sheath forms, in conjunction with the basal lamina of epidermal cells in the outer root sheath, a prominent, homogeneous *glassy membrane* (see above). This structure separates the epidermal and dermal tissues of the follicle, and also separates matrix cells from the dermal papilla. **Plate 7, Fig. 1; Plate 8, Figs. 1, 2, and 3.**

Arrector pili muscles. These are strands of smooth muscle cells associated with hair follicles, except those in eyelashes. Arrector pili muscles originate in the pars papillaris of the dermis and split into several branches, each of which inserts onto the connective tissue sheaths of separate follicles. The branches may pass close to sebaceous glands, and so when the muscles contract they elevate the hair and squeeze an oily sebum into the follicle. **Plate 7, Figs. 1 and 2; Plate 9, Fig. 1.**

Glands

Sebaceous, sweat, and mammary glands are integumentary glands derived from the epidermis. Mammary glands are considered in Chap. 15.

SEBACEOUS GLANDS. Sebaceous glands are of the holocrine type (see Chap. 2); that is, the glandular cells become a part of the secretion. These glands, which produce an oily sebum, are located in all areas of the skin except the sole and palms. They are simple alveolar or branched simple alveolar glands which lie in the dermis and are surrounded by a thin layer of connective tissue. The glands open into a relatively short, wide excretory duct which may open directly into a hair follicle or onto the surface of the skin. The duct is lined by a stratified squamous epithelium and is continuous with the external root sheath of the hair follicle, or the stratum germinativum of the skin. Close to the sebaceous gland, the excretory duct is reduced to a simple cuboidal layer of epithelium which is continuous with the generative cells of the gland. Small, cuboidal, basophilic generative cells are located at the periphery of the gland. They give rise to daughter cells which eventually migrate to the interior. During this migration the cells grow in size and become polygonal, and lipid droplets fill the cytoplasm. Deep within the interior of the gland the cells show signs of deterioration; the nucleus is shrunken or absent, and the cytoplasm appears fragmented. Sebum is produced from the disintegrating cells as a mixture of cell

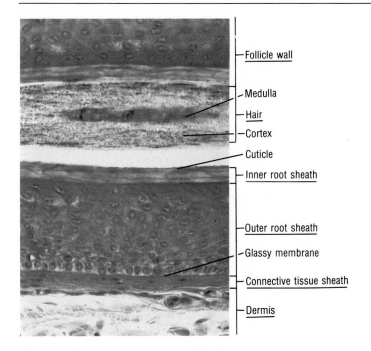

Follicle wall

Medulla

Hair

Cortex

Cuticle

Inner root sheath

Outer root sheath

Glassy membrane

Connective tissue sheath

Dermis

FIGURE 1.
Hair follicle, sagittal section; human scalp; H&E; ×400. Note that the layers of the inner root sheath are keratinized at this level and somewhat indistinct. Note pigment in the cortex of the hair, serrated edges on the cuticle layers, and spiny cells in the outer root sheath.

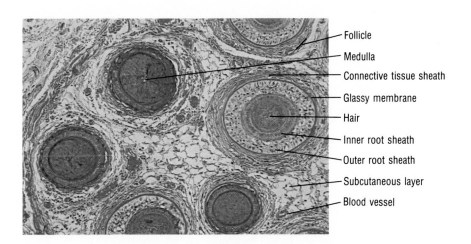

Follicle

Medulla

Connective tissue sheath

Glassy membrane

Hair

Inner root sheath

Outer root sheath

Subcutaneous layer

Blood vessel

FIGURE 2.
Hair follicles, transverse section; human scalp; H&E; ×100. Note that these follicles appear differently because they lie at different levels in the scalp.

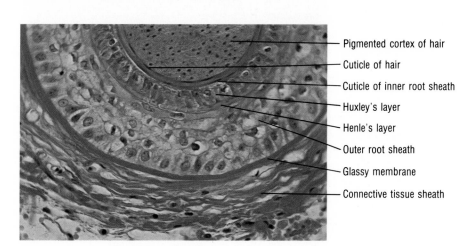

Pigmented cortex of hair

Cuticle of hair

Cuticle of inner root sheath

Huxley's layer

Henle's layer

Outer root sheath

Glassy membrane

Connective tissue sheath

FIGURE 3.
Hair follicle, transverse section; human scalp; H&E; ×400. Note that trichohyalin granules can be seen in the cells of Huxley's layer. Note the keratinized cells of Henle's layer.

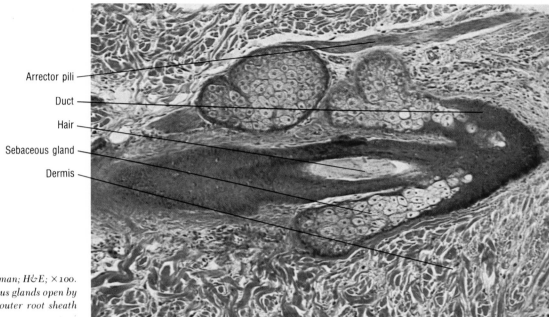

Arrector pili —

Duct —

Hair —

Sebaceous gland —

Dermis —

FIGURE 1.
Sebaceous glands; human; H&E; ×100.
Note that the sebaceous glands open by
short ducts into the outer root sheath
of the hair follicle.

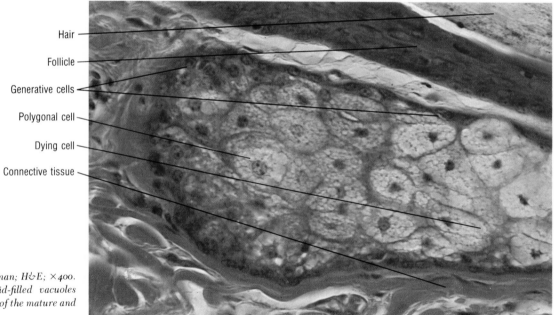

Hair —

Follicle —

Generative cells —

Polygonal cell —

Dying cell —

Connective tissue —

FIGURE 2.
Sebaceous gland; human; H&E; ×400.
Note the large, lipid-filled vacuoles
within the cytoplasm of the mature and
dying cells.

debris and lipids. It is conveyed through the excretory ducts into the upper levels of hair follicles or directly onto the skin surface (meibomian glands in eyelids and the mucocutaneous junction of the lips). Sebum is a lubricant for hair and the skin, and may also be slightly bacteriostatic. **Plate 7, Fig. 1; Plate 9, Figs. 1 and 2.**

SWEAT GLANDS. There are two types of sweat glands: the small, ordinary *eccrine* (*merocrine*) glands, measuring about 0.3 mm in diameter, and the larger *odoriferous* (*apocrine*) glands, which are approximately 3 to 5 mm in diameter. For many years

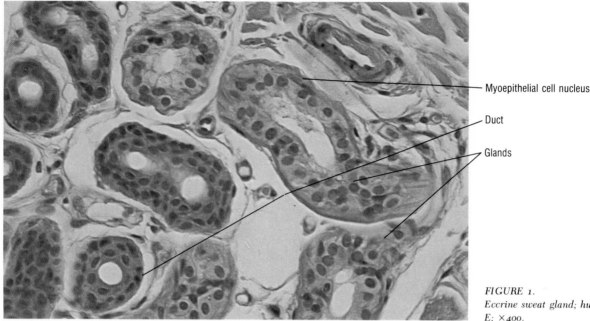

Myoepithelial cell nucleus

Duct

Glands

FIGURE 1.
Eccrine sweat gland; human sole; H&
E; ×400.

the odoriferous glands were believed to produce *apocrine secretions* as the apical cytoplasm of the secretory cells pinch off to become part of the secretion. Recent investigations indicate that both the odoriferous glands and the eccrine glands produce *merocrine secretions* which do not contain apical cytoplasm of the secretory cells. The apocrine sweat gland terminology persists, however, and is used by most authors. Both types of glands have a secretory portion located either in the dermis or subcutaneous layer of the skin. Each type of gland has an excretory duct to transport secretions either to the surface of the skin or into hair follicles. The glands function to eliminate metabolic waste substances and to regulate body temperature by the elimination and evaporation of sweat.

Eccrine sweat glands. These are more numerous than the odoriferous glands. They are not connected to hair follicles, and are distributed over the entire skin, except for the lips, glans penis, clitoris, labia minora, nipples, and nail beds. They are most numerous in the skin of the palms and soles. The gland is a simple, coiled, tubular structure which secretes an aqueous fluid, *sweat*, derived from blood plasma. In addition to other organic and inorganic compounds, sweat contains sodium chloride, potassium ions, cholesterin, urea, and lactic acid. **Plate 7, Fig. 1; Plate 10, Figs. 1 and 2; Plate 11, Fig. 1.**

SECRETORY END PIECE. This is a coiled, unbranched tubule, with a narrow lumen, lying in the dermis or subcutaneous layer. Three cell types are present in the tubule wall: *myoepithelial cells, clear secretory cells,* and *dark secretory cells.* A thin basement membrane is present.

  Myoepithelial cells. These are fusiform cells which have an elongate nucleus lying within an acidophilic cytoplasm containing myofilaments. The cells are scattered around the periphery of the tubule and rest on a thin basement membrane. They are wedged between the bases of secretory cells (see below), and aid in the secretion of sweat as they contract. **Plate 10, Fig. 1.**

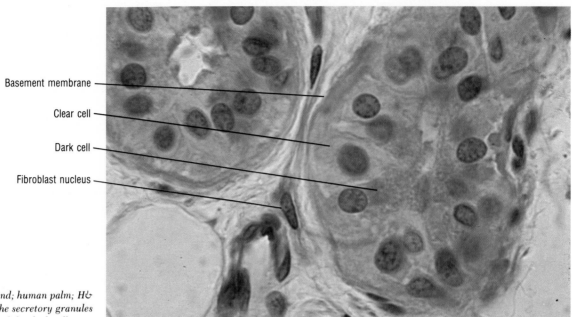

Basement membrane

Clear cell

Dark cell

Fibroblast nucleus

FIGURE 2.
Eccrine sweat gland; human palm; H&
E; ×1000. Note the secretory granules
in the cytoplasm of the dark cell.

Clear secretory cells. These are large, pyramidal cells with their broad bases lying either on a basement membrane or on myoepithelial cells. The pale acidophilic cytoplasm may contain glycogen particles. A prominent, round nucleus is located in the center of the cell. These cells secrete a watery sweat into the lumen of the gland via intercellular canaliculi which are formed by the plasma membranes of adjacent cells. **Plate 10, Fig. 2.**

Dark secretory cells. Unlike the clear secretory cells (see above), these cells are small and pyramidal, with their broad bases lying next to the lumen. They are fewer in number than the clear cells, and their basophilic cytoplasm may be filled with secretory granules of glycoproteins. They have a large, round nucleus in the center of the cytoplasm. These cells may contribute to the mucoid component of sweat, which coats the surface of the duct epithelium. **Plate 10, Fig. 2.**

EXCRETORY DUCT. The duct forms about one-half of the eccrine gland. It is relatively straight in the dermis and subcutaneous layers, but as it enters the epidermis, between dermal papillae, it becomes extremely coiled. In the dermis the duct has a small, round lumen, usually lined by an eosinophilic layer of mucoid material. Myoepithelial cells are absent at its periphery, and the walls are composed of two layers of cuboidal epithelium. The lumen of the duct is a narrow cleft in the epidermis, and its walls are formed of epidermal cells. **Plate 11, Fig. 1.**

Odoriferous sweat glands (apocrine sweat glands). These large glands are found in the skin of the axilla, external auditory canal (ceruminous glands), eyelids (ciliary glands of Moll), mammary areola, scrotum, labia majora, perineum, and circumanal

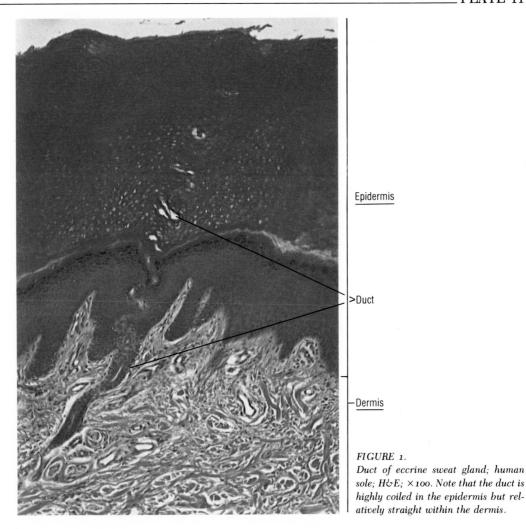

Epidermis

>Duct

Dermis

FIGURE 1.
Duct of eccrine sweat gland; human sole; H&E; ×100. Note that the duct is highly coiled in the epidermis but relatively straight within the dermis.

region. They are simple, branched, tubular glands which are larger and less coiled than the eccrine glands. The secretory portion of a gland lies in the dermis of the subcutaneous layer, and its straight duct usually opens into a hair follicle. Unlike eccrine glands, these glands produce a thick, pigmented (usually light tan) secretion containing lipids and proteins. As skin bacteria decompose these organic compounds, distinctive body odors are produced. **Plate 11, Fig. 2.**

SECRETORY END PIECE. The wide secretory tubules have only one type of glandular cell. The cells may be low cuboidal or low columnar, depending on the functional state of the gland. The more active low columnar cells have an acidophilic cytoplasm filled with vacuoles of glycoprotein and golden brown lipofuscin granules. A large, round nucleus with a prominent nucleolus is located in the lower part of the cytoplasm. Myoepithelial cells are similar to those present in the eccrine sweat glands (see above), but tend to be more numerous and larger. **Plate 11, Fig. 2.**

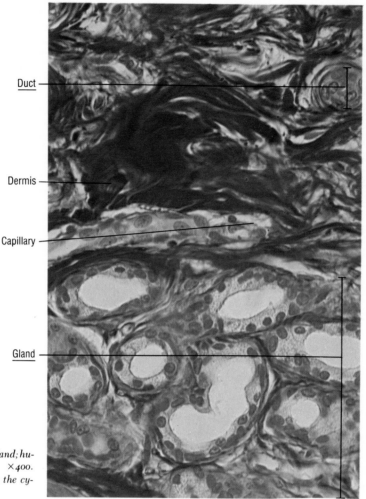

Duct

Dermis

Capillary

Gland

FIGURE 2.
Odoriferous (apocrine) sweat gland; hu-
man scrotum; Mallory-azan; ×400.
Note the secretory granules in the cy-
toplasm of the glandular cells.

EXCRETORY DUCT. The histology of the ducts is similar to that of the eccrine glands (see above), except they are not highly coiled and usually empty into hair follicles. **Plate 11, Fig. 2.**

BLOOD AND LYMPHATIC VESSELS OF THE INTEGUMENT. Branches of large arteries in the subcutaneous layer of the integument anastomose to form prominent plexuses just below the dermis. These plexuses send branches into the lower subcutaneous layer to supply fat lobules, hair follicles, sweat glands, and sebaceous glands with arterial blood. Many branches also extend into the dermis where they terminate as subpapillary plexuses between the papillary and reticular layers. Dermal papillae and integumentary structures (hair follicles, nails, sweat glands, and sebaceous glands) lying in the more superficial regions of the dermis are supplied by vessels from these subpapillary plexuses. The drainage pattern for venous and lymphatic vessels is arranged much in the same manner as the arterial pattern, except lymphatic vessels do not form subpapillary plexuses and do not drain hair follicles or integumentary glands.

NERVES. Both myelinated and nonmyelinated nerves are present as networks lying in the subcutaneous layer, in the subepidermal region, and between the papillary and reticular layers. These networks contain somatic and visceral afferent nerves carrying impulses from sensory receptors. Efferent nerves of the autonomic nervous system, which innervate blood vessels, arrector pili muscles, and sweat glands are also present in the nerve networks.

Digestive System 12

The major function of the digestive system is to prepare food for utilization by the body. The process involves a physical mastication, enzymatic digestion, and absorption of the digested food into the circulatory system for distribution throughout the body. For convenience, the digestive system may be divided into three major divisions: the *oral cavity*, the *digestive tube*, and the *digestive glands*.

Oral cavity

The oral or buccal cavity is the uppermost region of the digestive system. Food and water enter the digestive tube through the buccal cavity; here the food is masticated and mixed with saliva. The oral cavity is organized into two chambers: the *vestibule* and *oral cavity proper*. The vestibule is a pouch which separates *teeth* and *gums* from *lips* and *cheeks;* it is continuous with the oral cavity proper. The latter is bordered anteriorly and laterally by the teeth and gums and posteriorly by the palatoglossal folds and oropharynx (see Chap. 13). The *hard* and *soft palate* form the roof of the oral cavity, while the anterior region of the tongue forms the floor. The oral cavity is lined by an *oral mucosa* (a mucous membrane) which also covers the tongue and continues as a lining of the digestive tube. The oral mucosa forms a crescentic fold, the frenulum linguae, which anchors the ventral surface of the tongue to the floor of the mouth. The oral mucosa is continuous with the skin at the free edge of the lips, and the boundary between the two is the mucocutaneous junction. The oral mucosa is composed of an epithelium lying over a fibrous lamina propria. It is modified in various areas of the oral cavity, according to different functions. In regions that are not subjected to great pressure and friction (the cheeks), the oral mucosa lies on a movable bed of loose connective tissue, the submucosa. In other areas, where food is crushed against parts of the oral cavity, a submucosa is lacking and the oral mucosa is thick and nonmovable. In these regions the mucosa is fused to the periosteum of underlying bone. Its epithelium is stratified, squamous, and keratinized in regions where wear and tear is maximum. Ducts of mucous, serous, and seromucous *salivary glands* open onto the surface of the oral mucosa in specific regions of the oral cavity (see below).

Papillae –

Lamina propria –

Oral mucosa –

Adipose tissue –

Submucosa –

Labial glands –

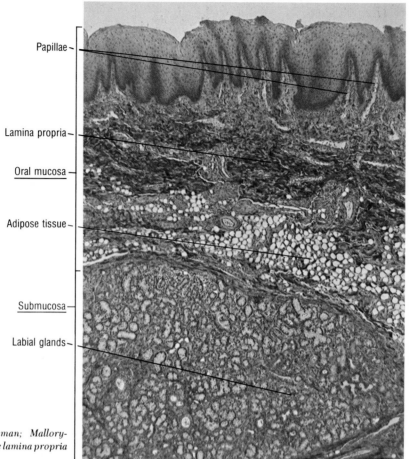

FIGURE 1.
Oral mucosa; lip; human; Mallory-azan; ×40. Note that the lamina propria is quite thick.

LIPS. These are fleshy folds which surround the opening to the mouth. They are lined on their exterior surface by skin which contains hair follicles, sebaceous glands, and eccrine sweat glands. The interior surface is lined by the *oral mucosa*. The core of the lip is composed of fibroelastic connective tissue in which is embedded the orbicularis oris, a skeletal muscle of facial expression, blood and lymphatic vessels, and nerves. Sensory nerve endings are also present in the oral mucosa and dermis. The oral mucosa has a thick stratified squamous nonkeratinized epithelium lying over a thick lamina propria. The latter is composed of moderately dense connective tissue with tall papillae extending up into the epithelium. A thin *submucosa* of loose connective tissue lies between the lamina propria and orbicularis oris muscle. It contains many mixed labial and salivary glands whose ducts open into the vestibule. Compared with other areas of the skin, the mucocutaneous junction of the lip is translucent because the stratum lucidum is exceptionally thick and the stratum cornium is thin. This portion of the lip, then, appears red because the color of blood in the highly vascularized papillae show through the translucent epidermis. The mucocutaneous junction lacks hair follicles, sebaceous glands, and sweat glands. **Plate 1, Fig. 1.**

CHEEK (bucca). This lateral wall of the vestibule forms much of the side of the face and is continuous with the lips. The general histologic organization is much like that of the lips (see above), except that the skeletal muscle is the buccinator muscle, the lamina propria has more elastic fibers, the submucosa contains more adipose tissue, and the mixed glands are designated as buccal glands.

PALATE. The palate forms a horizontal partition between the nasal and oral cavities. The anterior region, the *hard palate*, is composed of the palatine processes of the maxillae and the horizontal processes of the palatine bones. The posterior region is the soft, fleshy *soft palate*. The hard palate provides a strong, hard surface which is utilized by the tongue during mastication, mixing, and swallowing of foods. The soft palate functions to close the nasopharynx from the oropharynx as food or water is swallowed. Both the hard and soft palate are lined by the oral mucosa on their oral surfaces, and a respiratory mucosa on their respiratory surfaces.

Hard palate. The oral mucosa is lined by a stratified squamous keratinized epithelium. The lamina propria is a dense, fibrous layer which indents the epithelium with tall papillae. The lower portion of the lamina propria is continuous with the periosteum of the palatal bone. On the roof of the mouth the oral mucosa forms a midline raphe or ridge which extends the length of the hard palate. The lamina propria contains small mucous glands near the posterior end of the hard palate. The nasal surface of the hard palate is lined with a respiratory mucosa containing pseudostratified columnar ciliated epithelium (see Chap. 13).

Soft palate. This is a movable flap of soft tissue which extends posteriorly from the hard palate and hangs down into the oropharynx. The soft palate has a posteriorly located conical projection, the uvula. The lateral regions of the soft palate are attached to the tongue by the palatoglossal arches and to the oropharynx by the palatopharyngeal arches. The soft palate is composed of an internal layer of fibrous connective tissue, the palatine aponeurosis, which provides structural support for the soft palate. The aponeurosis also is a base on which palatal skeletal muscles can be anchored, e.g., the tensor veli palatini. Blood vessels, nerves and lymphoid tissues are also present within this internal layer of tissue. The soft palate is lined by an oral mucosa on its inferior surface and a respiratory mucosa on its superior surface. The thin lamina propria of the oral mucosa has tall papillae of moderately dense connective tissue which project up into a stratified squamous nonkeratinized epithelium. A thick submucosal layer containing adipose tissue and many mucous glands is present, but is separated from the lamina propria by a dense network of fibroelastic fibers. The respiratory mucosa is similar to the oral mucosa at the posterior end of the soft palate, where the two are continuous over the free edge. At the anterior end of the soft palate the respiratory mucosa has a pseudostratified columnar ciliated epithelium, lacks a submucosa, and has small, scattered mixed glands in the lamina propria. **Plate 1, Fig. 2.**

SALIVARY GLANDS. Many small mixed or mucous salivary glands are present in the oral mucosa, lining portions of the oral cavity, vestibule, and some regions of the lips. They produce saliva which continuously wets the surfaces of these structures. In addition to these small glands, there are three pairs of large salivary glands which produce copious amounts of saliva as an aid to the digestive processes. These are the *parotid, submandibular,* and *sublingual* glands. All three are merocrine-type glands. They are compound branched tubular or tubuloalveolar glands, and each opens into

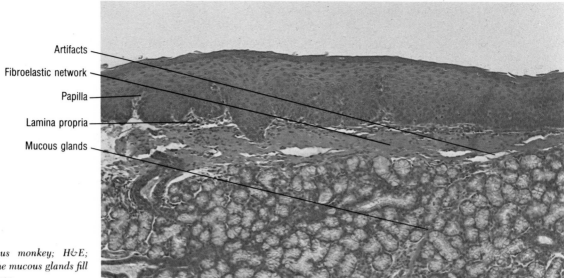

Artifacts

Fibroelastic network

Papilla

Lamina propria

Mucous glands

FIGURE 2.
Soft palate; rhesus monkey; H&E;
×100. Note that the mucous glands fill
the submucosal layer.

the oral cavity by prominent excretory ducts. The ducts are epithelial tubes which are surrounded by a basal lamina and embedded within connective tissue of the gland; myoepithelial cells are located between the basal lamina and epithelium of the lower ducts. As the excretory ducts extend from the oral cavity to the salivary glands, they form three different segments. According to their size, location, and epithelial lining these segments are the *excretory duct proper*, the *secretory duct*, and the *intercalated duct*. The *excretory duct proper* extends from the oral cavity to the salivary gland and is present in the interlobular connective tissue of the gland. Near the oral cavity the duct is a large tube of stratified squamous epithelium, but near or within the gland it becomes smaller and is composed of pseudostratified or simple columnar epithelium containing a few scattered goblet cells. The *secretory duct* (striated duct) is of a smaller diameter than the excretory duct and is located within the intralobular tissues. It is composed of a simple columnar epithelium, but the cells are unique because they have basal striations. The striations are due to a vertical orientation of mitochondria and basal folding of the plasma membrane. The cytoplasm of these cells is strongly acidophilic. It is believed that cells of this type are instrumental in modifying the composition of saliva by an active transport of fluids and ions. The *intercalated duct* is the smallest of the three ducts and is also intralobular. They are long, thin, branched tubules attached directly to the secretory end piece of the gland. The duct is composed of a simple low cuboidal or squamous epithelium lying on a basal lamina. Elongate myoepithelial cells, *basket cells*, are randomly distributed between the epithelium and basal lamina. These cells move saliva along the duct by their contractile properties.

Parotid gland. This is the largest of the three major salivary glands. It is located just below the ear, covering the posterior portion of the mandibular ramus. The excretory duct (Stenson's duct) crosses the masseter muscle and enters the vestibule opposite the second molar. The parotid is a *serous gland* surrounded by a capsule of dense fibroelastic connective tissue. Its glandular parenchyma is divided into lobes and lobules by septa extending from the capsule. The secretory end pieces are elongated alveoli lying in a delicate stroma of reticular tissue. The alveolar epithelium is

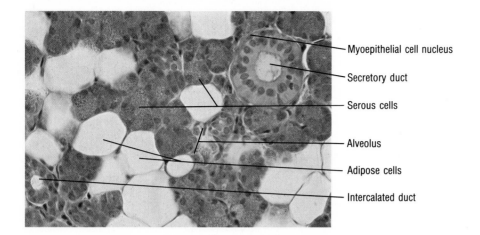

— Myoepithelial cell nucleus

— Secretory duct

— Serous cells

— Alveolus

— Adipose cells

— Intercalated duct

FIGURE 1.
Parotid gland; human; H&E; ×400.
Note the faint basal striations on the
secretory duct cells. Granules fill the
basophilic cytoplasm of the serous cells.
Alveoli are all serous. The myoepithe-
lial cells are mainly located in inter-
calated ducts.

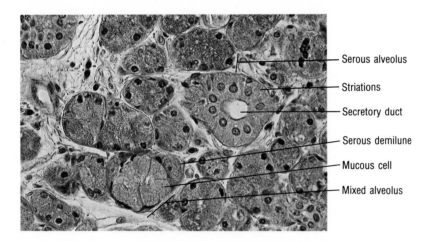

— Serous alveolus

— Striations

— Secretory duct

— Serous demilune

— Mucous cell

— Mixed alveolus

FIGURE 2.
Submandibular gland; human; iron
hematoxylin–aniline blue; ×400. Note
that the alveoli are predominately ser-
ous, but some mixed glands are present.
Faint basal striations can be seen on
the secretory duct cells and some serous
cells.

composed of pyramid-shaped serous cells (see Chap. 2). Each cell has a spherical nucleus and a basophilic cytoplasm filled with granules. The basal portion of the cytoplasm is usually more heavily stained and may have faint striations. Thin, fusiform myoepithelial cells (basket cells) are located between the basal lamina and serous cells; usually only their elongate nuclei may be seen. Intercalated ducts are more abundant than secretory ducts in the parotid glands. **Plate 2, Fig. 1.**

Submandibular gland (submaxillary gland). This gland is smaller than the parotid. It lies below the body of the mandible and is bordered by the digastric, mylohyoid, and styloglossus muscles. The submandibular duct (Wharton's duct) extends upward and anteriorly, passing through the musculature in the floor of the mouth. It terminates on the sublingual papilla just lateral to the attachment of the tongue to the floor of the mouth (the frenulum). Histologically, the organization of the submandibular gland is similar to the parotid gland, having a capsule, septa, stroma, and lobules. It is a *mixed gland* where serous and mucous cells are both present in about 20 percent of the alveoli; the remainder of the alveoli are composed only of serous cells. At the periphery of a mixed alveolus the serous cells, demilunes, form a crescent-shaped cap, which surrounds the mucous cells (Chap. 2). Although all three types of duct segments are present in the duct system, the secretory ducts are longest and therefore more abundant in sections of the gland. **Plate 2, Fig. 2.**

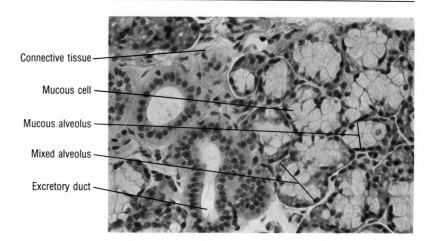

Connective tissue

Mucous cell

Mucous alveolus

Mixed alveolus

Excretory duct

FIGURE 3.
Sublingual gland; human; H&E; ×400.
Note that the alveoli are predominately
mucous, but some mixed ones are also
present.

Sublingual gland. This is the smallest of the three major salivary glands. At the anterior end of the lower jaw, near the symphysis, the oral mucosa is folded into a sublingual fold containing the sublingual gland. The sublingual gland is an aggregation of many glands (8 to 20), most of which have ducts opening separately along the sublingual fold or directly into the submandibular duct. Some fuse into a large sublingual duct which opens near or in common with the submandibular duct at the sublingual papilla (see above). The sublingual gland, unlike the other two salivary glands, lacks a well-defined capsule, but does have septa which divide the glandular parenchyma into lobules. The sublingual is a mixed gland, but differs from the submandibular gland because the branched tubular secretory end pieces are predominately all mucous. Some mixed alveoli are present and contain both mucous cells and serous demilunes. The mucous cells are tall and have a mucous-filled cytoplasm with a flattened basal nucleus (see Chap. 2). Myoepithelial cells are scattered between the secretory cells and basal lamina. The duct system is also quite different in this gland, since the intercalated and secretory ducts are short, quite limited in their distribution, and hard to find in a section of tissue. **Plate 2, Fig. 3.**

VESSELS AND NERVES OF THE SALIVARY GLANDS. The salivary glands are supplied with blood carried by branches of the external carotid artery to capillary plexuses surrounding the ducts and alveoli. The capillaries are drained by venules and veins into the external jugular vein. Lymphatic vessels are also present and drain lymph toward the cervical lymph nodes. A salivary gland is innervated by visceral afferent and efferent nerve fibers. Efferent fibers of the sympathetic and parasympathetic divisions of the autonomic nervous system innervate blood vessels and terminate between glandular cells. These fibers are vasomotor and also influence the quality of the saliva that is produced.

TONGUE. The tongue is anatomically divided into two regions, the *body* and the *root*, each having its own structural and developmental characteristics. The body of the tongue is the highly movable, fleshy portion in the mouth, while the root is less movable, is posterior to the fauces (see below), and forms the anterior wall of the oropharynx. The mass of the tongue is composed of extrinsic and intrinsic skeletal musculature, which is divided into lateral halves by a median fibrous septum. The *extrinsic muscles* originate on bones near the tongue and insert into the tongue proper. Their action is to pull the tongue in different directions; these muscles are the genioglossus, palatoglossus, chondroglossus, styloglossus, and hyoglossus. The *intrinsic muscles* are those contained entirely within the tongue; they are the vertical, transverse, inferior longitudinal, and superior longitudinal muscles. Because they are arranged in three planes at right angles to each other, their actions permit great mobility of the tongue within the mouth. The hypoglossal nerve innervates both the extrinsic and intrinsic muscles, except for the palatoglossus which is innervated by the vagus nerve. The oral mucosa, lining the oral cavity, is continuous over the surfaces of the body and root of the tongue. In addition, the oral mucosa continues posteriorly onto the epiglottic folds and laterally onto the palatine tonsils and walls of the oropharynx. A submucosal layer is lacking on the dorsal surface of the tongue, therefore the fibers in the lower layers of the lamina propria are continuous with the connective tissue surrounding the lingual musculature. On the ventral surface of the body of the tongue, the oral mucosa is smooth and lies on a submucosal layer. The tongue is attached to the floor of the oral cavity by a mucosal fold, the *lingual frenulum*. On the dorsal surface of the tongue the oral mucosa has a prominent V-shaped groove, the *sulcus terminalis*, lying between the anterior two-thirds and posterior one-third of the tongue. The apex of the V is pointed posteriorly and represents the foramen caecum, an embryonic remnant of the early development of the thyroid gland. The region of the tongue posterior to the sulcus terminalis displays many large, irregular bumps. These are lingual tonsils (Chap. 13) and are formed by lymphoid nodules embedded within the submucosal layer. Anterior to the sulcus terminalis, the dorsal and lateral surfaces of the tongue are covered by many tiny *lingual papillae* which stick up from the surface and impart a rough texture. These papillae are mucosal in origin and composed of cores of dense fibroelastic connective tissue, derived from the upper layers of the lamina propria. The papillae are usually covered with a stratified squamous nonkeratinized epithelium, but on certain ones (see below) the epithelium is keratinized. There are four types of lingual papillae: *filiform, fungiform, vallate,* and *foliate*.

Filiform papillae. These form the majority of papillae on the dorsal and lateral surfaces of the tongue. They are tall (about 2 to 3 mm), slender, conical structures terminating in one or several pointed processes. The papillae are organized into chevronlike ranks which parallel the V-shaped sulcus terminalis. At the apex of the tongue, however, they are arranged in transverse lines. The large core of lamina propria, forming the interior of the papilla, is the *primary papilla*. The primary papilla has many smaller papillae, the *secondary papillae*, extending from its upper surface and into the overlying stratified squamous keratinized epithelium. Each of the secondary papilla has a cone-shaped keratinized epithelial cap, or point. **Plate 3, Fig. 1.**

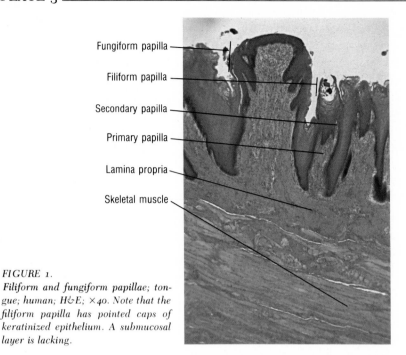

Fungiform papilla —

Filiform papilla —

Secondary papilla —

Primary papilla —

Lamina propria —

Skeletal muscle —

FIGURE 1.
Filiform and fungiform papillae; ton-
gue; human; H&E; ×40. Note that the
filiform papilla has pointed caps of
keratinized epithelium. A submucosal
layer is lacking.

Fungiform papillae. These are less numerous than the filiform papillae and are scattered among them. They occur along the sides and apex of the tongue. The fungiform papillae are somewhat rounded and attached to the lingual surface by a slightly constricted stalk. They are larger than the filiform papillae (about 2 mm tall and 1 mm wide) and appear dark red because of capillaries lying under a translucent stratified squamous epithelium. Although many secondary papillae are present, the overlying epithelium is not formed into points but is smooth. Taste buds may be present in the epithelial walls of the fungiform papillae. **Plate 3, Fig. 1.**

Vallate papillae (circumvallate papillae). There are approximately 7 to 12 of these very large papillae. They are about 1 to 3 mm wide by 1.5 mm tall and lie just anterior to the sulcus terminalis; they parallel the V-shaped groove. The papillae are unique not only because of their large size but because they do not protrude much above the lingual surface. They are separated from the surrounding oral mucosa by a deep moatlike groove which circumscribes each papilla. In a sagittal section a papilla appears as a squared-off cone, with the broader end unattached. Secondary papillae project up into the overlying smooth stratified squamous epithelium. Many taste buds are present in the walls of the vallate papilla, and some in the walls of the groove surrounding the papilla. Prominent serous glands, *von Ebner's glands*, lie below the vallate papillae and have many ducts opening into the bottom of the groove. The glands may be present in the lower layers of the lamina propria, or even extend into regions of the lingual musculature. **Plate 3, Fig. 2.**

Foliate papillae. These are poorly developed in humans but are prominent structures in some mammals, e.g., the rabbit. Foliate papillae are parallel vertical folds of the oral mucosa. They are present along the lateral surfaces at the junction of the body and root of the tongue. Taste buds are located in the stratified squamous epithelium along the sides of the papillae. Small serous glands open into the bottom of the furrows between the foliate papillae. **Plate 3, Fig. 3.**

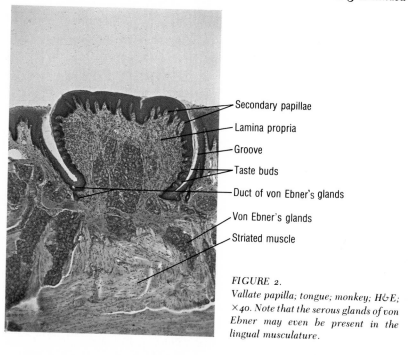

Secondary papillae

Lamina propria

Groove

Taste buds

Duct of von Ebner's glands

Von Ebner's glands

Striated muscle

FIGURE 2.
Vallate papilla; tongue; monkey; H&E;
×40. Note that the serous glands of von
Ebner may even be present in the
lingual musculature.

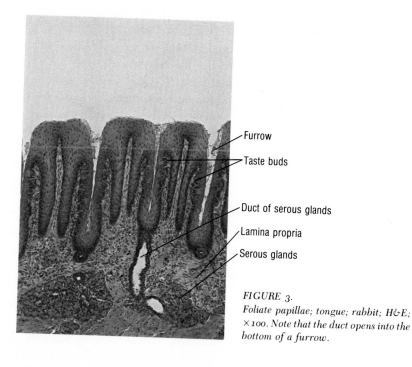

Furrow

Taste buds

Duct of serous glands

Lamina propria

Serous glands

FIGURE 3.
Foliate papillae; tongue; rabbit; H&E;
×100. Note that the duct opens into the
bottom of a furrow.

Lingual glands of the tongue may be located deeply within the lamina propria or in connective tissue amid the deeper lingual muscles. The *seromucous lingual glands* are located on the ventral surface of the tip of the tongue, adjacent to the frenulum. *Serous lingual glands* (von Ebner's glands) have already been described (see above). *Mucous lingual glands* are located at the root of the tongue. They can empty into the pits of lingual tonsils, but mainly they empty onto the surface of the tongue. Mucous glands also are present on the lateral margins of the tongue.

TASTE BUDS. These are large (about 75 μm tall), ovoid, pale structures composed of many tall, fusiform cells. They lie within the stratified squamous epithelium of vallate and foliate papillae. Some taste buds may be found scattered in the epithelium of fungiform papillae, epiglottis, pharynx, and the soft palate. The bottom of the taste bud rests on a lamina propria, while the upper end has a fluid-filled taste pit extending through the overlying epithelium. The taste pit opens onto the surface through a taste pore. Using the electron microscope, five cell types composing the taste buds have been described: two types of *neuroepithelial* cells, *sustentacular* or supporting cells, and *basal* and *peripheral* cells. The latter two are possibly generative cells. Only two types may be distinguished with the light microscope. These are the neuroepithelial cells (no distinction can be made between the two) and the sustentacular cells.

Neuroepithelial cells (gustatory cells, type II cells). These tall, lightly stained, fusiform cells contain an ovoid, moderately dark nucleus. They occupy a central portion of the taste bud and intermingle with the supporting cells. At the apical end of the cytoplasm a few short microvilli extend up into the taste pit. Club-shaped endings of afferent neurons of cranial nerves VII and IX extend into the interior of the bud. These neurons synapse only with the neuroepithelial cells, which have modified synaptic junctions along their surfaces. The neuroepithelial cells are capable of being stimulated by appropriate chemical stimuli and then initiating a nerve impulse at the synaptic points. Impulses reaching specific regions of the cerebral cortex are interpreted as psychological sensations of taste: *salt*, *sweet*, *bitter*, or *sour*. **Plate 4, Fig. 1.**

Sustentacular cells (supporting cells, type I cells). Like the neuroepithelial cells, these cells are tall and fusiform, but may be distinguished by their darker basophilic cytoplasm and somewhat rounded, pale nucleus. The sustentacular cells are distributed throughout the taste bud, but are more numerous at the periphery. The apical end of the sustentacular cell has many long microvilli, "taste hairs" of the earlier literature. The cell secretes granules of glycosaminoglycans which, when released, fill the taste pit surrounding the microvilli. The glycosaminoglycans substances may provide a medium in which chemical compounds dissolve. The dissolved substances eventually reach the neuroepithelial cells and stimulate them. **Plate 4, Fig. 1.**

GUM (gingiva). This is an oral mucosa fused to the underlying periosteum of alveolar bone in the jaw; a submucosal layer and glands are lacking. The gum forms a groove or moatlike collar, the *gingival sulcus*, surrounding each tooth. The sulcus is lined by stratified squamous nonkeratinized epithelium, and the rest of the gum is covered by a stratified squamous keratinized epithelium. At the bottom of the gingival sulcus the epithelium is attached directly to the surface of the tooth (epithelial attachment). In young individuals, the epithelium is attached to an enamel cuticle near the crown. In older persons, as the gums recede, the point of attachment moves toward the root so that the epithelium eventually becomes attached to the cementum. The lamina propria of the gum is a relatively dense layer of fibrous collagenous connective tissue with many tall vascular papillae extending up into the epithelium. Many bundles of collagen fibers (gingival fibers) run through the lamina propria and fasten the gum to the neck and root of the tooth. Nerve fibers are abundant in the lamina propria, and sensory endings are present in both the lamina propria and epithelium of the gums. **Plate 5, Fig. 1.**

TEETH. The human tooth has a *crown*, a *neck*, and one, two, or three *roots*. The crown is exposed, the neck is surrounded by the gingival sulcus, and the roots are contained within an *alveolus*, a bony socket in the jaw. The interior of the tooth is a hollow *pulp cavity*, filled with *dental pulp* (vessels, connective tissue, and nerves).

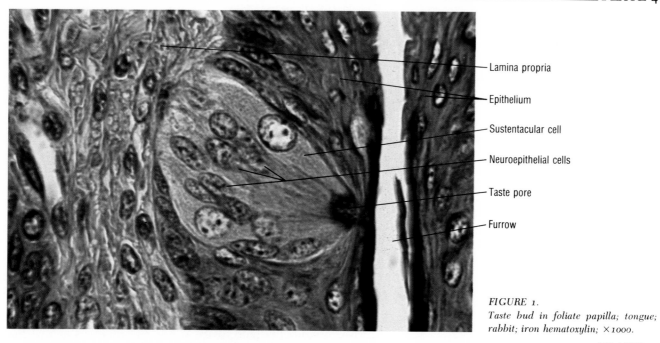

— Lamina propria

— Epithelium

— Sustentacular cell

— Neuroepithelial cells

— Taste pore

— Furrow

FIGURE 1.
Taste bud in foliate papilla; tongue;
rabbit; iron hematoxylin; ×1000.

_____ PLATE 5

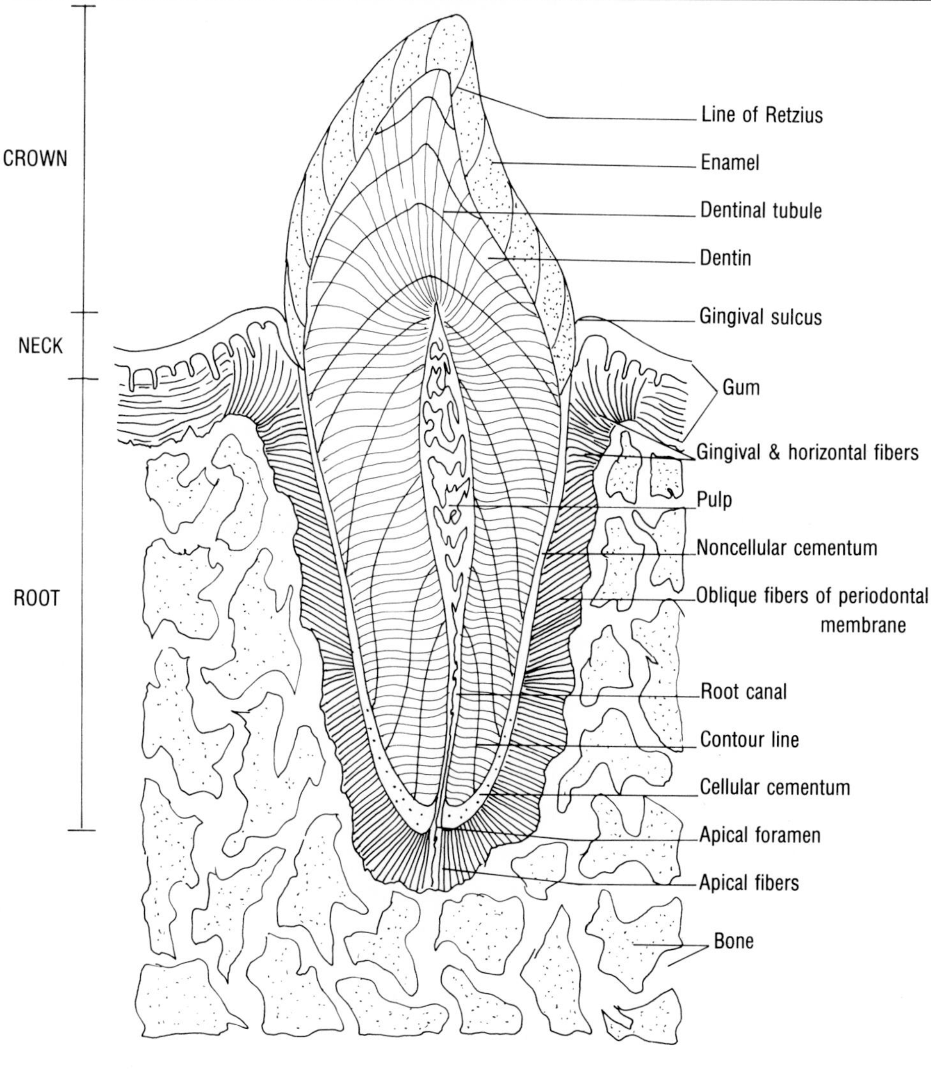

CROWN

NECK

ROOT

— Line of Retzius

— Enamel

— Dentinal tubule

— Dentin

— Gingival sulcus

— Gum

— Gingival & horizontal fibers

— Pulp

— Noncellular cementum

— Oblique fibers of periodontal
    membrane

— Root canal

— Contour line

— Cellular cementum

— Apical foramen

— Apical fibers

— Bone

FIGURE 1.
Drawing of a sectioned tooth.

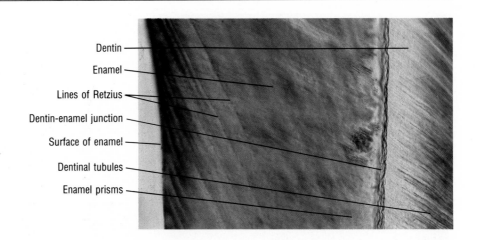

Dentin —
Enamel —
Lines of Retzius —
Dentin-enamel junction —
Surface of enamel —
Dentinal tubules —
Enamel prisms —

FIGURE 1.
Enamel and dentin (longitudinal section); tooth; human; ground and unstained; ×100.

The pulp cavity extends into the roots as narrow *root canals*. At the tips of the roots each canal opens onto a *periodontal membrane* (see below) by an *apical foramen*. Vessels and nerves, running between the dental pulp and periodontal membrane, pass through the apical foramen. The tooth is composed of three hard, calcified tissues: *dentin*, which surrounds the pulp cavity and is discontinuous only at the apical foramen; *enamel*, which covers the dentin at the level of the crown and neck; and *cementum*, a thin superficial layer covering the dentin from the neck down to the apical foramen. The cementum is fastened to the alveolus and gum by gingival fibers (see above), and a fibrous periodontal membrane. **Plate 5, Fig. 1.**

Enamel. This layer is thickest in the crown and thinnest on the neck of the tooth; it is the hardest tissue in the body. About 3 percent of it is composed of organic materials, and the remaining 97 percent is inorganic compounds, of which about 90 percent is calcium phosphate in the form of long, large apatite crystals. These crystals are packed into long, rodlike *enamel prisms* which also contain organic matrix. The long axes of the crystals are parallel to the longitudinal axis of the prisms. The prisms are about 4 μm in diameter and radially arranged. They form a twisted pattern as they extend from the dentin to the surface of the enamel. In a cross section the prisms resemble overlapping hexagonal scales. Each prism is surrounded by a submicroscopic *enamel sheath* composed of organic matrix. The prisms are held together by an interprismatic cement, also composed of apatite crystals and organic matrix, but the axes of the crystals form an angle to the longitudinal axes of the prisms. In addition to the enamel prisms, which can be observed on ground sections of a tooth, another morphological structure of the enamel can be observed, the *lines of Retzius*. These lines are the result of enamel being laid down in successive layers as the tooth develops. They can be seen as concentric lines near the surface of a ground cross section of a tooth. In longitudinal sections they appear as long, dark parallel lines extending diagonally from the surface of the tooth toward the pulp. Depending on the specimen you may find clumps of twisted, poorly calcified enamel prisms lying within an abundant interprismatic cement. These are *enamel tufts*, and they extend from the dentin-enamel junction into the enamel. They represent metabolic disturbances during tooth development. **Plate 5, Fig. 1; Plate 6, Fig. 1.**

Dentin (dentine). This tissue is softer than enamel since it contains proportionately more organic to inorganic compounds—approximately 30 percent organic to 70 percent inorganic. The inorganic compounds are formed into needle- or platelike hydroxyapatite crystals and embedded in an organic matrix of collagen fibers and

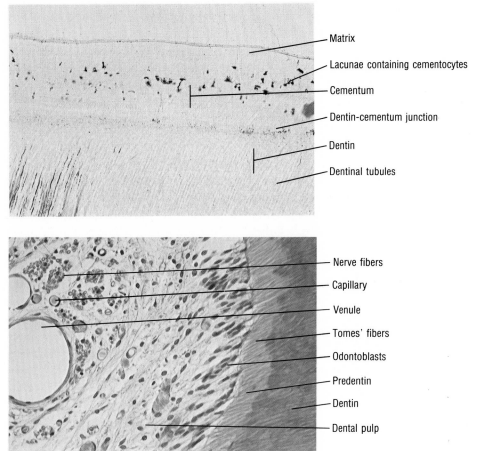

Matrix

Lacunae containing cementocytes

Cementum

Dentin-cementum junction

Dentin

Dentinal tubules

FIGURE 2.
Dentin and cementum (longitudinal section); tooth; human; ground and unstained; ×100.

Nerve fibers

Capillary

Venule

Tomes' fibers

Odontoblasts

Predentin

Dentin

Dental pulp

FIGURE 3.
Odontoblasts and dental pulp (cross section); tooth; human; decalcified and H&E; ×400. Note that the dental pulp is a gelatinous tissue with abundant ground substance.

ground substance. In a ground longitudinal section of a tooth, dentin appears radially striated because of numerous *dentinal tubules*. These tubules extend from the pulp cavity and end blindly at the dentin-enamel junction. Each tubule is an S-shaped structure, about 3 μm at its base and tapering to a narrow blind end. Along its length each dentinal tubule forms branches, some of which anastomose with branches of adjacent tubules. The intertubular dentin contains relatively little organic material in its matrix. The dentin is specialized around each tubule to form a thin, dense, highly calcified peritubular dentinal sheath, the *sheath of Neumann*. Since the sheath will be removed during decalcification, as a tooth is prepared for sectioning, only a clear space, an artifact, will appear in the dentin. The region between the dentin and pulp cavity is lined by a thick epithelioid layer of columnar *odontoblasts*. These are dentin-producing cells and are characterized by their long cytoplasmic progresses, *Tomes' fibers*, which fill the dentinal tubules. A thin band of noncalcified matrix, *predentin*, forms the innermost region of the dentin layer and separates the more peripheral calcified dentin from the pulp cavity. In a stained, decalcified section of a tooth the predentin is lighter than dentin, and the junction between the two appears as an irregular scalloped line. Dentin, like enamel, is deposited in successive layers during tooth development, but unlike enamel, the deposition continues throughout the life of the individual. The result of dentin synthesis will ultimately be to narrow the pulp cavity. The dentin layers may be seen as concentric rings on a ground transverse section of a tooth, the *incremental lines of Owen*. **Plate 5, Fig. 1; Plate 6, Figs. 1, 2,** and **3.**

Cementum. This tissue most closely resembles bone, both physically and chemically, than does either enamel or dentin. Cementum covers a portion of the neck as a thin, acellular layer, but becomes thick and cellular over the surface of the roots. Cementum is composed of a calcified, organic matrix containing collagen fibers, ground substance, and *cementocytes*. The cementocytes are stellate cells which produce the matrix. They are ensconced within cavities, or *lacunae*, in the matrix. As cementum thickens in older teeth, haversian systems may form. Cementum is a dynamic tissue of the tooth; its thickness can be readily increased or decreased in correlation with injury, disease, aging, or tooth movement. **Plate 5, Fig. 1; Plate 6, Fig. 2.**

Periodontal membrane (peridontal ligament). This structure is composed of bundles of dense, irregular collagenous connective tissue. It anchors the neck and root of a tooth to the alveolar bone and gums. Coarse bundles of collagen fibers from the *periodontal membrane* enter the cementum as Sharpey's fibers and become embedded within the matrix. They may appear as clear streaks in the cementum of a ground section of a tooth. Bundles of fibers from the other end of the periodontal membrane are embedded within the matrix of the alveolar bone. At these points of attachment the membrane contains some cementocytes near the cementum, and osteoblasts and osteoclasts near the alveolar bone. Small masses of epithelial cells of the embryonic root sheath, *Hertwig's epithelial sheath*, may be scattered throughout the periodontal membrane; they may form dental cysts. The bundles of collagen fibers in the periodontal membrane are organized into several groups and named according to their position and points of attachment: *gingival fibers* anchor the cementum of the neck and bony crest of the alveolus to the lamina propria of the gum; *circular fibers* encircle the neck of the tooth and support the gingival fibers; *horizontal fibers* (cementoalveolar fibers) lie just below the circular fibers; *oblique fibers* lie below the horizontal fibers and represent the most numerous type of fibers in the periodontal membrane; *apical fibers* are located at the apex of the roots. Although the periodontal membrane will allow some movement of the tooth, the direction of its fibers will prevent the tooth from tilting or being crushed into its alveolus during the process of chewing. The periodontal membrane is well vascularized and contains many lymphatic vessels. It also has numerous sensory nerve fibers and various types of mechanoreceptors which are sensitive to pressure changes. **Plate 5, Fig. 1.**

Dental pulp. The pulp cavity of the tooth is filled with a gelatinous tissue resembling mucous connective tissue (Chap. 3). In addition to the abundant ground substance, thin collagenous fibrils, and fibroblasts, the pulp also contains some mesenchyme cells, lymphocytes, and macrophages. Capillary plexuses are present in the dental pulp and nourish the odontoblasts lining the pulp cavity. These plexuses are supplied by arterioles and drained by venules. Blood and lymphatic vessels pass through the apical foramen. Unmyelinated, postganglionic sympathetic nerve fibers are present in the pulp and innervate smooth muscle fibers of the blood vessels. They bring about vasoconstriction of the vessels. Myelinated afferent fibers, which are intertwined with the sympathetic fibers, give off branches that terminate as bare endings between odontoblast cells or extend for a short distance into the predentin. When the dentin is stimulated, the stimulus is transmitted to these nerve endings. A nerve impulse is formed and carried to the brain, where it is interpreted as pain. **Plate 5, Fig. 1; Plate 6, Fig. 3.**

TOOTH DEVELOPMENT. These are 32 permanent teeth in the adult mouth. Of these, 20 are preceded by deciduous (milk) teeth during their development; the remaining 12, the molars, are not. Since deciduous and permanent teeth have similar developmental patterns, only the deciduous teeth will be described in the following steps and illustrated in **Plate 7, Figs. 1 to 12.**

1. At about 7 weeks of age, an oral epithelium of ectoderm will thicken as a *labial lamina* in the developing upper and lower jaws. The labial lamina will then grow into the underlying mesenchyme of the jaws as a deep vertical plate. This plate follows the curvature of the jaws in both the mandibles and maxillae. **Plate 7, Fig. 1.**

2. As the labial lamina plate grows into the mesoderm, its superficial region will split into two parallel curved layers, an inner gum primordium and an outer lip primordium. These primordia are separated by a labial groove. At the lower unsplit portion of the labial lamina a dental lamina will develop on its gumward side. The dental lamina gives rise to the teeth primordia. As the labial lamina extends deeper into the jaw, the labial groove will deepen and form the vestibule. Durings its development, the vestibule will separate the lips and cheeks from the dental lamina and gums. In the midline of the upper and lower jaws the split is not complete, so that a membrane, the frenulum, is formed. **Plate 7, Fig. 2.**

3. The dental lamina will grow medially into the gum, thereby forming a somewhat horizontal plate which is continuous with and perpendicular to the labial lamina. **Plate 7, Fig. 3.**

4. Early in the third month, a series of knoblike enlargements, the *enamel organs*, will develop on the labial side of the horizontal dental lamina and remain connected by thin stalks. Only ten enamel organs develop in each jaw; they correspond to the number of deciduous teeth. **Plate 7, Fig. 4.**

5. After their formation, each enamel organ enlarges and grows in the direction of a dense mass of ectomesenchyme, the *dental papilla*, which incidentally is derived from neural crest tissue. Eventually, the enamel organ partially surrounds the dental papilla as a thick-walled cup. This entire complex is surrounded peripherally by a *dental sac* of ectomesenchyme, which is continuous with the lower region of the dental papilla. At a later time, the enamel organ produces enamel and will also influence the size, shape, and cusp pattern of the developing crown. The dental papilla eventually produces dentin and forms the pulp, while the dental sac is important in the development of cementum, the periodontal membrane, and bone of the alveolus. **Plate 7, Figs. 5** and **12.**

6. During the third month the enamel organ differentiates into a double-walled sac: the *outer and inner enamel layers*, both of which are composed of simple cuboidal epithelium. These two layers are separated by a mass of loose tissue, the *stellate reticulum*, composed of an abundant ground substance and stellate cells. The outer enamel layer is continuous with the stalk connecting the enamel organ with the dental lamina. It, plus the stellate reticulum, is important in allowing nutrients to reach the inner enamel layer. Through further development, the inner enamel layer becomes folded, establishing the future shape and topography of the crown and cusps, and produces enamel. **Plate 7, Figs. 6** and **12.**

7. The cuboidal tissue of the inner enamel layer will differentiate into several layers of cells: a single layer of columnar, enamel-producing cells, *ameloblasts*, lying on a basement membrane adjacent to the dental papilla; and several layers of cuboidal cells, the *stratum intermedium*, lying between the ameloblasts and stellate reticulum. **Plate 7, Figs. 7** and **12.**

8. By the end of the fourth month, as the enamel organ continues to develop, it induces the peripheral layer of mesenchyme cells of the dental papilla to differentiate into dentin-producing *odontoblasts*. The deeper tissue of the papilla will form the dental pulp. Once differentiated, the odontoblasts deposit *predentin*, an uncalcified organic matrix, just under the basement membrane of the ameloblast layer. Precollagenous fibers (Korff's fibers) extend from the dental papilla into the predentin. The columnar odontoblasts have long, branched tufts of cytoplasm, Tomes' fibers, which also extend

into the predentin. When the predentin reaches a few microns in thickness it calcifies as *dentin*, which contains about 70 percent hydroxyapatite crystals.

As the odontoblasts secrete new layers of predentin, they retreat toward the pulp but leave their ever-lengthening Tomes' fibers embedded within dentinal tubules of dentin. There will always be a thin layer of predentin separating the odontoblasts from the dentin. The junction between the predentin and calcified dentin appears as an irregular border. **Plate 6, Fig. 3; Plate 7, Figs. 8 and 12.**

9. The calcification of predentin and the presence of odontoblasts induce the ameloblasts to secrete enamel on the surface of the dentin. The ameloblasts have tapered cytoplasmic projections, *Tomes' processes*, which extend into the enamel. At the onset of enamel formation, granules appear in the cytoplasm of the ameloblast cells. These granules are the precursors of enamel matrix and contain water, protein, and glycoprotein. Matrix is produced as the granules are released into the extracellular space around the ends of the processes. As the matrix is calcified, long hexagonal crystals of hydroxyapatite are formed and packed into long, thin (3 mm in diameter) enamel prisms. The prisms are joined by interprismatic cement (see above). Each prism, then, is a product of an ameloblast cell and is continuous from the dentin to the ameloblast layer. Each prism increases in length as the secreting ameloblast cell retreats toward the outer enamel layer; the process results in a thickening of enamel. In later development the matrix is almost removed from the prisms, at the expense of the growing crystals and by reabsorption of protein and water by the ameloblast cells. **Plate 7, Fig. 9.**

10. After enamel is deposited on the crown and neck of the developing tooth, the enamel organ elongates to cover the lower portion of the dental papilla as the *epithelial root sheath* (Hertwig's root sheath). Although this sheath does not produce ameloblasts, its tissue induces the differentiation of more odontoblasts from the superficial mesenchymal cells of the papilla. In addition, the sheath influences the growth and shape of the roots and concentrates blood vessels and nerves at the root ends. The number of roots is determined, in part, by the number of dense capillary plexuses developing in regions of the dental papilla. Certain portions of the dental papilla grow actively toward these plexuses and form the definitive roots. In later development, the epithelial root sheath degenerates and may become isolated clumps of epithelial cells lying within the tissues of the periodontal membrane. These clumps of cells are the epithelial nests of Malassez. **Plate 7, Fig. 10.**

11. At about 6 months, just before the eruption of the first deciduous tooth, the dental sac becomes functional around the developing roots:
    a The inner layer of mesenchymal cells, under the influence of the epithelial root sheath, differentiate into cementoblasts and deposit a bonelike *cementum* on the underlying dentin of the root.
    b The outer cells of the sac differentiate into osteoclasts and osteoblasts. The latter produce bone, so that the lower portion of each tooth becomes surrounded by a bony socket or *alveolus*. The alveolar bone will eventually fuse to the bone of the developing jaw.
    c The mesenchyme cells within the interior of the dental sac differentiate into fibroblasts, which produce collagen fibers of the *periodontal membrane*. This membrane will be embedded in cementum on one end, and in alveolar bone on the other end, so that it forms a suspensory ligament that anchors the tooth to the alveolus. **Plate 7, Fig. 11.**

12. A combination of several factors, one of which is the growth of the root, results in the eruption, or "cutting," of the tooth through the gum onto the oral surface.

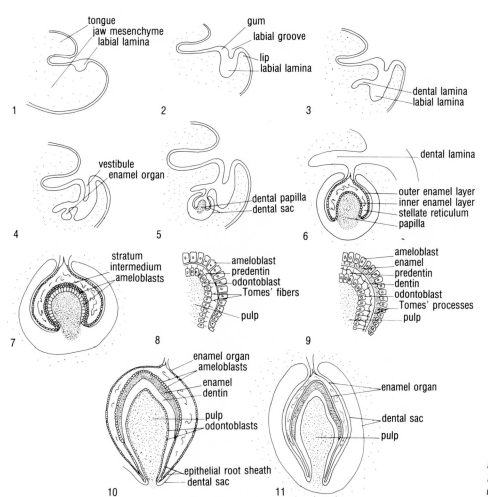

FIGURES 1–11.
Drawings illustrating the stages of tooth development.

13. The deciduous teeth develop from an intact dental lamina and erupt at different times: from 6 months (central incisors) to 24 months (second molar). The enamel organs for the permanent nonmolar teeth also differentiate early, at about 5 to 10 months. They develop from the free edges of a disintegrating dental lamina on the lingual side of the deciduous teeth. They lie dormant for a period of time while the deciduous teeth are present in the mouth. The enamel organs for the permanent nonmolar teeth become active and start to grow at different times, depending on the particular tooth. As a developing permanent tooth elongates, it may exert pressure on the roots of a deciduous tooth, causing a resorption of tissues and subsequent loosening of the tooth. The permanent nonmolar teeth, like the deciduous teeth, erupt at different times: 6 years (central incisors) to 12 years (second premolar). The enamel organs of the permanent molars develop from the free edges of the posterior growing dental lamina as the jaws elongate. These enamel organs develop at different times: from about 6 months to 5 years. The first permanent molars erupt at about 6 years, the second molars at about 11 years, and the third permanent molars erupt at approximately 17 years of age. Once a tooth erupts, the tissues of its enamel organ are lost. The only tissues which continue to grow in an erupted tooth are dentin and cementum.

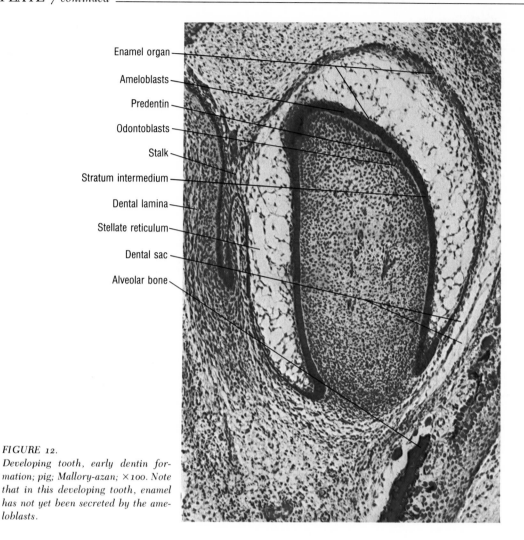

Enamel organ
Ameloblasts
Predentin
Odontoblasts
Stalk
Stratum intermedium
Dental lamina
Stellate reticulum
Dental sac
Alveolar bone

FIGURE 12.
Developing tooth, early dentin formation; pig; Mallory-azan; ×100. Note that in this developing tooth, enamel has not yet been secreted by the ameloblasts.

The digestive tube

The digestive tube is that part of the digestive system where foods are enzymatically digested and absorbed into the bloodstream and lymph. The tube is a continuous structure from the pharynx to anus, but is modified into a number of organs all along its length. The organs of the digestive tube, each with their own specific function, are listed in their anatomical sequence from the superior to the inferior level: esophagus, stomach, duodenum, jejunum, ileum, caecum and appendix, ascending colon, transverse colon, descending colon, sigmoid colon, rectum, and anus. Except for the upper and lower levels, the digestive tube is supported by mesenteries which are attached to the posterior body wall.

TABLE 1
Tunicae

187
The Digestive Tube

Special region	Type tissue	Function
Tunica mucosa		
Epithelium	Stratified squamous simple columnar	Protects; has sensory, secretory, absorptive functions
Lamina propria	Loose and reticular connective tissue	Binds epithelium to wall; carries vessels, nerves
Muscularis mucosae	Usually two layers smooth muscle: inner circular, outer longitudinal	Gives mucosa motility
	Glands	Produce enzymes, and mucous, serous, and seromucous secretions
Tunica submucosa		
	Loose connective tissue, but may be moderately dense	Allows stretching of tube; forms a bed for vessels and nerves
	Occasional glands	Produce serous, mucous, and seromucous secretions
Tunica muscularis externa		
	Usually two layers—inner circular and outer longitudinal smooth muscle around the periphery of tube—but a third oblique layer may be present	Produces peristaltic movements, and imparts muscle tonus to tube
Tunica serosa (visceral peritoneum)		
Mesothelium	Simple squamous epithelium	Prevents adhesion; provides protection
Connective tissue	Loose to moderately dense connective tissue	Embeds large vessels and nerves
Tunica adventitia		
Only connective tissue	Loose to moderately dense connective tissue	Embeds vessels and nerves; is continuous with tissues of adjacent organs

The wall of the digestive tube is composed of four concentric coats or tunicae of tissue. These tunicae are listed in order, going from the inside to the outside of the tube: *mucosa, submucosa, muscularis,* and *serosa* or *adventitia.* Each of these tunicae is composed of characteristic tissues which may be organized into specialized regions with specific functions. **Table 1; Plate 8, Fig. 1.**

Although the organs of the digestive tube are built on a common histological pattern, they may be modified according to their function. The muscularis of the stomach, for example, has three muscular layers which increase the complex muscular movements of mixing food and gastric juices.

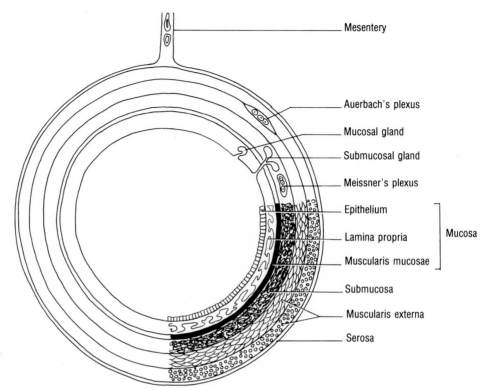

— Mesentery

— Auerbach's plexus

— Mucosal gland

— Submucosal gland

— Meissner's plexus

— Epithelium ⎤

— Lamina propria ⎬ Mucosa

— Muscularis mucosae ⎦

— Submucosa

— Muscularis externa

— Serosa

FIGURE 1.
Schematic drawing of the digestive tube illustrating a general histologic organization as seen in cross section.

ESOPHAGUS. This uppermost portion of the digestive tube is about 2.5 cm long. It is continuous with the laryngopharynx at its upper level and with the stomach at its lower level. It lies on the posterior surface of the trachea and passes through the mediastinum and diaphragm on its way to the stomach. The function of the esophagus is to transport water and masticated food from the mouth to the stomach. As a bolus (ball) of food moves down the esophagus by peristaltic waves, it is lubricated with mucus secreted by submucosal glands. **Plate 8, Fig. 2.**

Mucosa. The mucosa is lined by a stratified squamous nonkeratinized epithelium. This epithelium lies on a lamina propria of loose connective tissue containing many lymphocytes and a few scattered solitary lymphoid nodules. At the extreme upper and lower ends of the esophagus mucous glands are embedded within the lamina propria. The lamina propria forms tall papillae which indent the epithelial layer. At the upper level of the esophagus a muscularis mucosae is present as scattered longitudinal bundles of smooth muscle. This muscle replaces the thick layer of dense, elastic fibers in the mucosa of the laryngopharynx (see Chap. 13). Toward the lower levels, the muscularis mucosae becomes an extremely thick, continuous layer of tissue. The muscularis mucosae departs from the basic pattern (see Table 1) since it has only one layer of longitudinal muscle. **Plate 8, Fig. 2.**

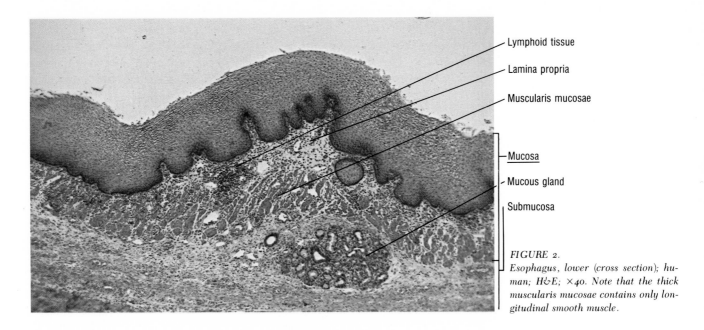

Lymphoid tissue

Lamina propria

Muscularis mucosae

Mucosa

Mucous gland

Submucosa

FIGURE 2.
Esophagus, lower (cross section); human; H&E; ×40. Note that the thick muscularis mucosae contains only longitudinal smooth muscle.

Submucosa. This layer of loose connective tissue is composed mainly of collagen and elastic fibers. The submucosa and the muscularis mucosae will form several temporary longitudinal folds along the surface of the empty esophagus. These folds disappear when the esophagus is dilated. Many small compound tubuloalveolar mucous glands are present in the submucosa. Their ducts penetrate the muscularis mucosae as they run toward the surface of the mucosa. **Plate 8, Fig. 2.**

Muscularis externa. There is a great deal of variation in this musculature from the basic pattern (see above). The inner and outer layers of smooth muscle have many spiral bundles, rather than being strictly circumferential or longitudinal. The muscularis is composed of skeletal muscle in the upper quarter of the tube, but will gradually be replaced by smooth muscle in the second quarter, so that in the lower half only smooth muscle will be present.

Adventitia. This is a layer of loose connective tissue which blends with the connective tissue of adjacent structures. It contains large vessels and nerves associated with the esophagus. The abdominal part of the esophagus below the diaphragm is covered by a serosa rather than an adventitia.

STOMACH. This is a large, curved, pouchlike structure lying in the upper portion of the abdomen just below the diaphragm. The curved convex border on the left side of the stomach is the *greater curvature*, while the small concave border on the right side is the *lesser curvature*. These curvatures are the points where the visceral peritoneum of the stomach is attached to the lesser omentum on the right and the greater omentum and gastrosplenic ligament on the left. An upper cardiac orifice connects the stomach with the esophagus and a lower pyloric orifice connects the stomach with the duodenum. Both of these openings are surrounded by sphincter muscles. The expanded left side of the stomach is the *body*, while the tapered right side is the *pyloric region*. That portion of the body which is above and to the left of the cardiac orifice is the *fundus*, and the area immediately surrounding the orifice is the *cardia*. The stomach secretes gastric juices containing enzymes (pepsin, rennin, and lipase), hydrochloric acid, and mucus. The gastric juices are mixed with masticated food as peristaltic waves move along the stomach wall. As the food becomes partially digested, it is converted into a semifluid mass, *chyme*. The intermittent movement of chyme into the duodenum is regulated by a strong pyloric sphincter muscle. Temporary longitudinal folds of the mucosa, *rugae*, are present in the empty stomach. These folds, like those in the esophagus, flatten when food fills the stomach.

Mucosa. The mucosa is thin at the cardia, about 0.3 mm, and progressively thickens to 1.5 mm at the pyloric end of the stomach. The stratified squamous epithelium of the esophagus terminates abruptly at the cardia, and a simple columnar epithelium continues as the mucosal lining. The epithelium is composed of tall *surface mucous cells* which produce mucus to lubricate and protect the mucosal surface. The cells have an ovoid or flattened basal nucleus. The cytoplasm may appear unstained and foamy, or filled with pale granules of neutral polysaccharides. The surface mucous cells dip down into the numerous *gastric pits* or *foveolae* which indent the mucosal surface. These pits are the openings to simple tubular or branched tubular glands which fill the mucosa and extend down to the muscularis mucosae. The loose connective tissue of the *lamina propria* is sparse between these glands, but is more abundant around the gastric pits. In addition to reticular and elastic fibers, the lamina propria contains lymphocytes, lymphoid tissue, plasma cells, leucocytes, mast cells, and fibroblasts. Although the *muscularis mucosae* usually has an inner circumferential and outer longitudinal layer of smooth muscle, it may have an outer third circular layer in some regions of the stomach. Slips of muscle from the inner layer extend up into the lamina propria to surround the glands. They function to express their secretory products into the lumen of the stomach.

Of the four tunicae of the stomach, the mucosa is the most variable. Three regional variations exist because of the presence of one of three possible types of glands, *cardiac*, *gastric*, and *pyloric*, and their associated gastric pits. These three regions of the stomach mucosa are indicated below.

Cardiac mucosa. The surface of the mucosa is pitted by numerous wide foveolae extending into the upper one-third to one-half of the mucosa. Tall surface mucous cells line the gastric pit, but at the bottom of the pit the cells are very short. The bottom of each pit is open and serves as a duct for several *cardiac glands* opening into it. The glands are simple or compound tubular structures which are slightly coiled. They fill the remaining mucosa by extending down to the muscularis mucosae. The cardiac glands are composed of small mucus-producing cells lying on a basal lamina. These columnar cells have a pale basophilic, granulated cytoplasm, and a basal nucleus which is round or somewhat flattened. These cells are believed to be comparable in their cytology and function to the seromucous cells in the pyloric glands and neck mucous cells in the gastric glands (see below). Although the cardiac glands are predominately composed of these cells, some argentaffin cells (see below) may also be present. **Plate 9, Fig. 1.**

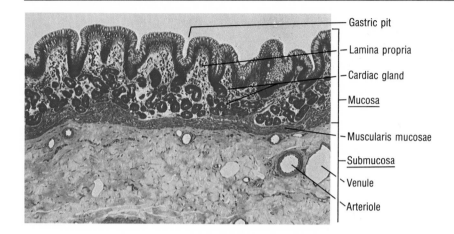

Gastric pit

Lamina propria

Cardiac gland

Mucosa

Muscularis mucosae

Submucosa

Venule

Arteriole

FIGURE 1.
Cardiac mucosa (longitudinal section); stomach; rhesus monkey; H&E; ×100. Note that the gastric pits are wide and extend into the upper one-half of the mucosa.

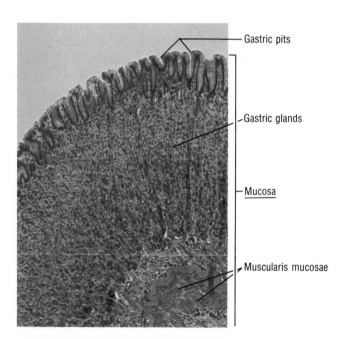

Gastric pits

Gastric glands

Mucosa

Muscularis mucosae

FIGURE 2.
Fundic mucosa (longitudinal section); stomach; human; H&E; ×100. Note that the gastric pits are narrow and extend into about one-fourth of the upper mucosa. The glands are relatively straight.

Fundic and body mucosa. Gastric pits are more numerous in the body and fundus than in the cardiac region. They are narrower and only extend into the upper one-fourth of the mucosa. They are lined by surface mucous cells, and several *gastric glands* open into the bottom of each pit. The glands are simple, branched, relatively straight tubular structures which extend down to the muscularis mucosae. The gastric glands produce some mucus, hydrochloric acid, and enzymes. Each gland has three anatomical regions: an upper, short, constricted neck; a lower, long, straight body; and a somewhat expanded, coiled, blind terminal end. Four cell types are present in these glands, and all line on a basal lamina: parietal cells, chief cells, neck mucous cells, and argentaffin cells. **Plate 9, Fig. 2.**

Parietal cells

Chief cells

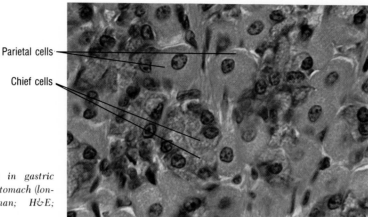

FIGURE 3.
Parietal and chief cells in gastric glands; fundic mucosa of stomach (longitudinal section); human; H&E; ×1000.

PARIETAL CELLS (oxyntic cells). In general, the parietal cells are relatively less numerous in the glands near the cardiac region but become more abundant toward the pyloris. These are large, deeply stained, spherical or pyramidal acidophilic cells. They are more abundant in the neck than the body or terminal end of the gland. The cells are interspersed with neck mucous cells in the neck and chief cells in the lower portions of the gland. At the lower levels, the parietal cells may bulge from the gland out into the surrounding lamina propria. Usually the cells have one spherical nucleus centrally located in the cytoplasm, but sometimes there are two nuclei. The cytoplasm has a system of secretory canaliculi which open onto the lumen of the gland. They are formed by an infolding of the plasma membrane at the apex of the cell. The canaliculi may appear as light streaks 1 to 2 μm wide in the cytoplasm. The cells secrete hydrochloric acid, with a pH of about 2.0, into the lumen of the gland. **Plate 9, Fig. 3.**

CHIEF CELLS (zymogenic cells, peptic cells). The chief cells are abundant in glands near the cardiac region, but become progressively less numerous toward the pyloric end of the stomach. They are low columnar serous cells forming most of the body and terminal end of a gland. The cells have a basophilic cytoplasm, the apical end of which is filled with basophilic zymogen granules. In some preparations the granules may not be preserved so that the cytoplasm appears vacuolated. The round nucleus is located either near the center of the cell or at its base. Mitochondria, ribosomes, and the endoplasmic reticulum form a series of faint basophilic basal striations which may be seen with the light microscope. The zymogen granules are composed of pepsinogen, a preenzyme. Pepsinogen will be converted to pepsin when released into the lumen of the gland and comes into contact with hydrochloric acid. Pepsin is important in the digestion of proteins into smaller peptones and proteoses. The chief cells also secrete limited amounts of gastric lipase, which digests fats. In most young animals milk protein is digested or coagulated by rennin, but in humans renninlike pepsin probably assumes this function. **Plate 9, Fig. 3.**

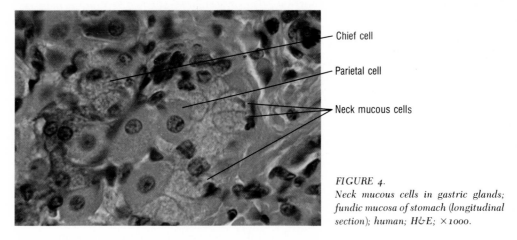

— Chief cell

— Parietal cell

— Neck mucous cells

FIGURE 4.
Neck mucous cells in gastric glands;
fundic mucosa of stomach (longitudinal
section); human; H&E; ×1000.

NECK MUCOUS CELLS. These cells are interspersed with parietal cells in the necks of glands, near the gastric pits. Occasionally neck mucous cells may extend varying distances into the body of the gland and are found lying between the chief cells. Near the cardiac region they are relatively scarce, but become more numerous toward the pyloric end of the stomach. These cells are cytologically and functionally similar to the seromucous cells of the cardiac and pyloric glands. They are unlike the surface mucous cells in the epithelium because they are smaller, somewhat basophilic, and produce a different type of mucus: acid glycosaminoglycans rather than neutral glycosaminoglycans. These irregularly shaped or columnar cells have an ovoid or flattened basal nucleus. Depending on the preparation of the tissue, the cytoplasm may be vacuolated or filled with pale basophilic mucigen granules. The mucus functions as a lubricant to protect the lining of the mucosa from enzymes and acids. Unfortunately, in routine preparations these seromucous cells may resemble the chief cells, but they do not stain as intensely, have somewhat flattened basal nuclei, and may be irregular·in shape. **Plate 9, Fig. 4.**

ARGENTAFFIN CELLS (enterochromaffin cells). Although five types of argentaffin cells have been distinguished with the electron microscope, all the cells appear similar with the light microscope. The cells may be found in the mucosal lining at all levels of the digestive tube, but are more common in the small intestine. They are located deeply within the gastric gland, lying singly between the chief cells. They are triangular cells with their broad, granular-filled bases lying on a basement membrane. Argentaffin cells have an irregularly shaped nucleus which lies closer to the lumen than the more basal granules, although this is not obvious in some specimens. The tiny acidophilic granules stain pink with H&E. The granules may be stained brown with potassium dichromate (enterochromaffin granules), or appear black by reacting with silver stains (argentaffin or argyrophilic granules). Although all the argentaffin cells can secrete a vasoconstrictive hormone, serotonin, each type may also be able to synthesize specific hormones, depending on the type of cell and its location. Argentaffin cells in the pyloric glands may produce gastrin and those in the duodenal mucosa may produce secretin; both hormones are important in the digestive processes. See **Plate 12, Fig. 2.**

Mucosa of the pyloric region. The gastric pits are less numerous than those in the body and fundus, but are wider and deeper. They extend about one-half the depth of the mucosa, and the glands fill the remaining one-half, down to the muscularis mucosae. The muscularis mucosae is unique because it has a third outer layer of circular or spiral smooth muscle. Several *pyloric glands* open into the bottom of a gastric pit. Each gland is a simple, branched, convoluted tubular structure with a very wide lumen. Like the glands in the cardiac region, the tubules are so coiled that many cross sections may be seen filling the lamina propria. Although a gland may contain an occasional parietal cell and several argentaffin cells (see above), the predominant cell type is a small, columnar, pale basophilic seromucous cell. The cytoplasm is granulated or vacuolated and contains an ovoid or flattened basal nucleus. These cells may be the same type as found in the cardiac glands or neck mucous cells in the gastric glands (see above). The function of these cells is to produce mucus and possibly a pyloric protease. **Plate 10, Figs. 1 and 2.**

Regeneration of mucosal cells in the stomach. At the bottom of the gastric pits and upper necks of the glands there is an active mitotic zone. Here, undifferentiated epithelial cells with large pale nuclei and prominent nucleoli divide and differentiate into other cell types: surface and neck mucous cells, parietal cells, chief cells, and argentaffin cells. The surface mucous cells have a short life: about 4 days. They are replaced by new cells produced deep in the gastric pits which then migrate to the surface. The neck mucous cells have a longer life and are replaced by new cells which differentiate in the upper portion of the gland, just below the gastric pits, and then migrate downward. The other types of cells (parietal, chief, and argentaffin) have the slowest turnover rate and are probably also derived from the cell pool, just under the gastric pits.

Submucosa. This is a layer of loose connective tissue which lies under the muscularis mucosae and binds the mucosa to the muscularis externa. The submucosa extends into the longitudinal folds, rugae, of the stomach (see above). The tissue is composed of the typical cells and fibers normally associated with loose connective tissue. It provides a bed for blood and lymphatic vessels, venous plexuses, nerves, and nerve plexuses. **Plate 10, Figs. 1 and 2.**

Muscularis externa. This is a prominent outer tunic which departs from the common plan of the digestive tube by having three layers of smooth muscle rather than two: an inner oblique, a middle circular, and an outer longitudinal. The *longitudinal muscle* layer is divided into superior and inferior regions, which overlap at the middle level of the stomach. The muscle fibers of the superior region are continuous with those of the esophagus, and its fibers also fan out over the upper and middle level of the body and fundus. The fibers of the inferior region begin at the middle level of the body and continue inferiorly over the pyloric end of the stomach. They contribute fibers to the pyloric sphincter muscle and are continuous with the musculature of the duodenum. The *circular muscle* layer is the most prominent and best developed layer of the muscularis. It, like the longitudinal muscle layer, is continuous with the esophageal musculature, but terminates as the pyloric sphincter. The *oblique musculature* is a less developed layer than the outer two, and its distribution is limited only to the body of the stomach. It is best developed near the lesser curvature and cardiac regions. The extensive musculature of the stomach facilitates mixing and movement of chyme into the duodenum. **Plate 10, Fig. 1.**

Serosa (visceral peritoneum). This outermost layer is a serous membrane, composed of loose connective tissue and covered by a mesothelium. The serosa covers most of the stomach, except for a small region under the diaphragm. At the lesser and greater curvatures the two opposing layers of serosa fuse and are continuous with the greater and lesser omenta. The omenta have a core of loose connective tissue

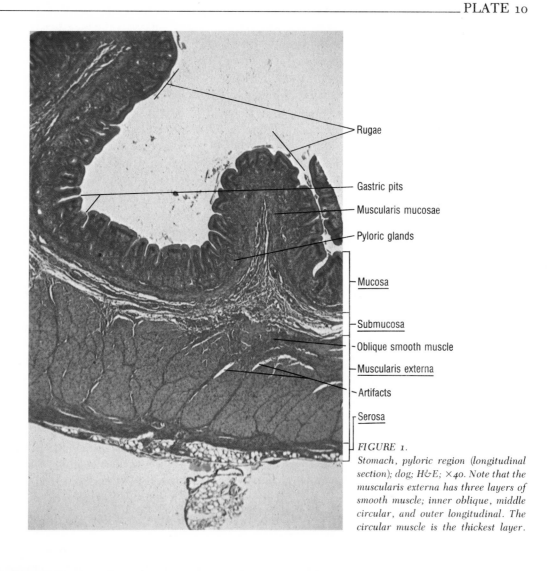

Rugae

Gastric pits

Muscularis mucosae

Pyloric glands

Mucosa

Submucosa

Oblique smooth muscle

Muscularis externa

Artifacts

Serosa

FIGURE 1.
Stomach, pyloric region (longitudinal section); dog; H&E; ×40. Note that the muscularis externa has three layers of smooth muscle; inner oblique, middle circular, and outer longitudinal. The circular muscle is the thickest layer.

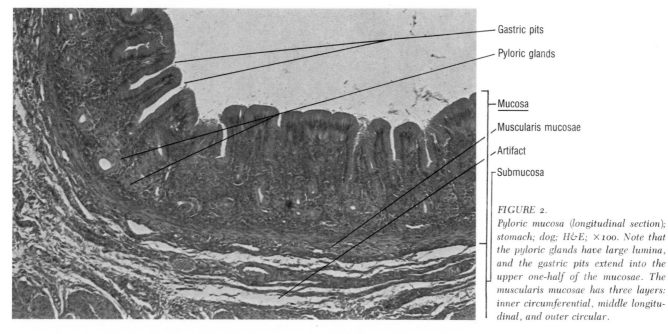

Gastric pits

Pyloric glands

Mucosa

Muscularis mucosae

Artifact

Submucosa

FIGURE 2.
Pyloric mucosa (longitudinal section); stomach; dog; H&E; ×100. Note that the pyloric glands have large lumina, and the gastric pits extend into the upper one-half of the mucosae. The muscularis mucosae has three layers: inner circumferential, middle longitudinal, and outer circular.

containing adipose tissue, blood and lymphatic vessels, and nerves. They are lined on both surfaces with mesothelium. **Plate 10, Fig. 1.**

SMALL INTESTINE. This lower portion of the digestive tube extends from the pyloris to the large intestine. It is a relatively narrow, long tube about 5 m in length, and is divided into three anatomical regions: upper duodenum, middle jejunum, and lower ileum. The duodenum is about 20 cm long; two-fifths of the remaining small intestine is jejunum, and three-fifths is ileum. The duodenum and lower portion of the ileum are attached directly to the posterior abdominal wall, while the jejunum and remainder of the ileum are suspended from the abdominal wall by mesenteries. Food is enzymatically digested as it moves by peristalsis through the small intestine from the stomach to the large intestine. The products of digestion are absorbed through the intestinal wall and enter the vascular and lymphatic vessels. Although the small intestine has the typical four tunicae as found in the rest of the digestive tube (mucosa, submucosa, muscularis, and serosa), certain anatomical structures are unique to this area. These structures are prominent folds of the intestinal lining, the plicae and villi, which provide an increased surface area for absorption. Rather than describe each level of the small intestine, since there is a great deal of anatomical similarity, only the regional modifications of the tunicae will be stressed.

Mucosa. The mucosal layer is folded into a number of structures which increase the surface area: the *plicae circulares* (valves of Kerckring), *villi*, and *crypts of Lieberkühn*. The plicae are tall (about 8 mm), permanent, semicircular folds of both the mucosa and submucosa. They are absent in the upper portion of the duodenum and lower portion of the ileum. Numerous tiny (0.5 to 2.0 mm), mucosal, fingerlike villi cover the mucosa and extend above its surface into the lumen of the intestine. The crypts of Lieberkühn (intestinal crypts) are folds of the mucosa lying between the bases of the villi and almost reaching the muscularis mucosae. The crypts are intestinal glands. They produce intestinal juices containing enzymes. The villi are characteristic for each region of the small intestine. In the duodenum they are low and leaflike, in the jejunum they are low and have clubbed ends, and in the ileum they are tall and slender. Each villus is lined by a simple columnar epithelium and has a core of highly vascular lamina propria containing a closed central lacteal (lymphatic capillary). The lacteal is continuous with a plexus of lymphatic vessels at the base of the villus. The *lamina propria* is a loose connective tissue composed of reticular fibers, along with some elastic and collagen fibers. The typical cells for a loose connective tissue are present, but lymphocytes, plasma cells, mast cells, and eosinophils are usually quite abundant. Solitary lymphoid nodules may be found along the small intestine, but aggregate nodules (Peyer's patches, see Chap. 10) are present in the ileum opposite the attachment of the mesentery. The *muscularis mucosae* is composed of two layers of smooth muscle: the inner circular layer and the outer longitudinal layer. Some fibers of the inner layer extend up into the villi, giving them motility. The simple columnar *epithelium* lining the mucosa covers the villi and extends down into the crypts of Lieberkühn. It rests on a thin basement membrane and contains several types of cells: *absorptive cells, goblet cells, Paneth cells, argentaffin cells,* and *undifferentiated cells*. **Plate 11, Fig. 1; Plate 13, Fig. 2.**

ABSORPTIVE CELLS. These are tall cells, about 25 μm. The cytoplasm is moderately basophilic and contains an elongate nucleus located near the base of the cell. A striated border formed by many tall microvilli is present at the apex of the cell. The microvilli increase the surface area of these cells through which many digested substances are absorbed. The digested components of proteins, carbohydrates, and nucleic acids are absorbed and then released to networks of blood capillaries within the villus. Digested fat has a unique pathway, and its products eventually enter the

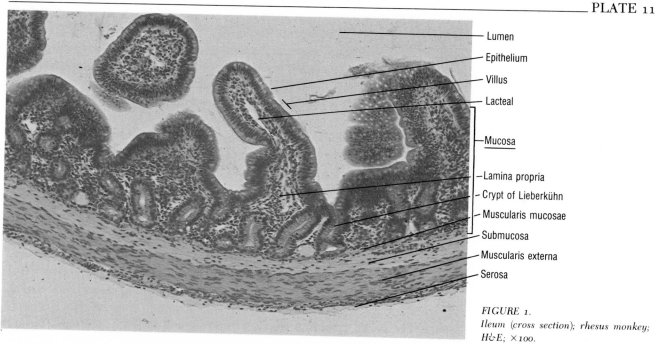

— Lumen
— Epithelium
— Villus
— Lacteal
— Mucosa
— Lamina propria
— Crypt of Lieberkühn
— Muscularis mucosae
— Submucosa
— Muscularis externa
— Serosa

FIGURE 1.
Ileum (cross section); rhesus monkey;
H&E; ×100.

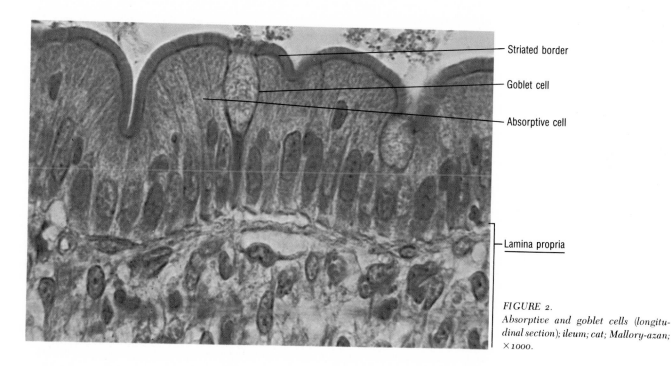

— Striated border
— Goblet cell
— Absorptive cell
— Lamina propria

FIGURE 2.
Absorptive and goblet cells (longitudinal section); ileum; cat; Mallory-azan; ×1000.

lacteals. The striated border is covered by a glycocalyx or glycoprotein coat, which is not visible with the light microscope. This is a protective coat. It also may absorb some enzymes and their substrates, so that digestion occurs here as well as in the lumen of the small intestine. The striated border has also been found to be the site of certain enzymes (aminopeptidase, sucrase, maltase, and fructase) which continue the digestion of proteins and carbohydrates started in the mouth and stomach. **Plate 11, Fig. 2.**

GOBLET CELLS (unicellular exocrine gland; see Chap. 2). These are prominent goblet-shaped cells scattered among other cell types in the epithelium. In the upper region of the cell the basophilic cytoplasm surrounds a pale or poorly stained, vacuolated mass of mucigen. A flattened nucleus lies in the slender, stalklike stem of the cell, close to the basement membrane. As mucus is secreted at the apex of the cell, it lubricates and protects the surface of the mucosa. These cells become more numerous toward the lower levels of the small intestine, and are quite abundant in the upper portions of the crypts of Lieberkühn. **Plate 11, Fig. 2.**

PANETH CELLS. These cells appear singly or in clumps in the epithelium lining the bottom of the crypts of Lieberkühn. These pyramidal cells sit on a basement membrane with their apical ends extending toward the lumen of the crypt. A large, oval nucleus lies in the basal portion of a basophilic cytoplasm, while large, acidophilic, secretory granules appear in a supranuclear position near the lumen. Although the synthesis of intestinal enzymes (peptidases) has been suggested for these cells, evidence is lacking. **Plate 12, Figs. 1 and 2.**

ARGENTAFFIN CELLS. These cells lie in the epithelium of the crypts of Lieberkühn, but occasionally they can be found on the villi. They are small, oval or pyramidal cells which are usually sandwiched between other epithelial cells and the basement membrane. Their tiny acidophilic granules are located below the irregularly shaped nucleus and lie close to the base of the cell. Although the granules are acidophilic and stain pink with H&E, they also react with silver and chromate stains and may then appear black or brown. These cells commonly produce serotonin, but also secrete secretin in the duodenum. Refer to the section on the stomach for further morphology and function of the argentaffin cells. **Plate 12, Fig. 2.**

UNDIFFERENTIATED CELLS. These cells are located in the epithelium, deep in the crypts of Lieberkühn. They are undifferentiated columnar cells with large, oval, pale nuclei. In some cells, however, the nuclei may appear in some stage of mitosis (see Chap. 1). These cells readily divide and differentiate into either absorptive, goblet, Paneth, or argentaffin cells. All of them except Paneth cells migrate up the walls of the crypt and surface of the villus to be shed at its tip. The turnover rate for all these cells, except Paneth cells, is about 2 to 4 days. The turnover rate for the Paneth cells is on the order of several weeks. **Plate 12, Figs. 1 and 2.**

Submucosa. This is a prominent layer of moderately dense, loose connective tissue lying between the muscularis mucosae and the muscularis externa. It contains a relatively abundant amount of elastic fibers along with some adipose tissue. The submucosa forms a connective tissue bed for blood and lymphatic vessels, nerves, and a prominent autonomic Meissner's plexus. The submucosa of the duodenum is unique since it contains a large duodenal gland, *Brunner's gland*. This is a compound, branched, convoluted tubuloalveolar gland composed of many lobules. Portions of the gland may extend into the plicae circulares or general mucosal areas. The secretory portion of the gland contains seromucous cells (see Chap. 2). These columnar cells have an ovoid or flattened basal nucleus. The cytoplasm may be clear or vacuolated, and filled with secretory granules or droplets. Brunner's gland is most well developed at the pyloric-duodenal junction and upper duodenum. It diminishes in size and usually is lost before the jejunum is reached. Occasionally the glands of Brunner extend as far as the pyloric region of the stomach and upper region of the jejunum. Its several excretory ducts penetrate the muscularis mucosae and are lined with cuboidal epithelium. They open into the bottom of the crypts of Lieberkühn. Their secretion is a viscid, alkaline fluid (pH 8.2 to 9.3). It is high in bicarbonate compounds which provide an alkaline pH for the intestinal enzymes, and which may

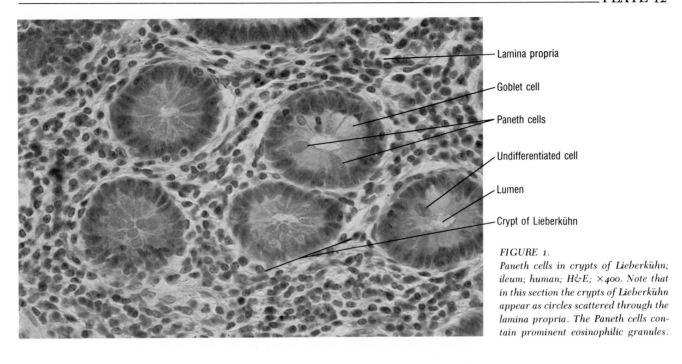

Lamina propria

Goblet cell

Paneth cells

Undifferentiated cell

Lumen

Crypt of Lieberkühn

FIGURE 1.
Paneth cells in crypts of Lieberkühn; ileum; human; H&E; ×400. Note that in this section the crypts of Lieberkühn appear as circles scattered through the lamina propria. The Paneth cells contain prominent eosinophilic granules.

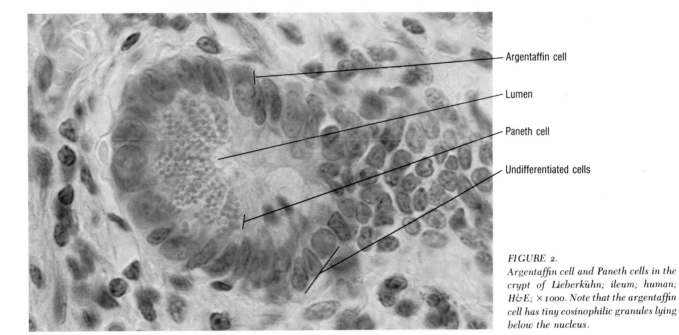

Argentaffin cell

Lumen

Paneth cell

Undifferentiated cells

FIGURE 2.
Argentaffin cell and Paneth cells in the crypt of Lieberkühn; ileum; human; H&E; ×1000. Note that the argentaffin cell has tiny eosinophilic granules lying below the nucleus.

protect the mucosal surface from the acidic chyme. The secretions may also contain a proteolytic enzyme and *enterokinase*. The latter is an enzyme which activates *pancreatic trypsinogen* to *trypsin*, another proteolytic enzyme. **Plate 13, Figs. 1** and **2.**

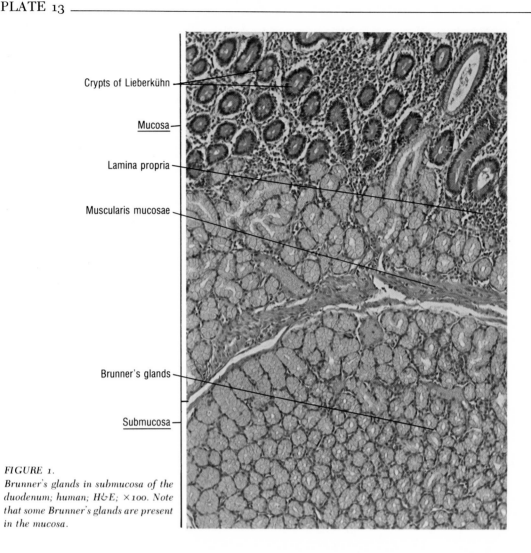

Crypts of Lieberkühn

Mucosa

Lamina propria

Muscularis mucosae

Brunner's glands

Submucosa

FIGURE 1.
Brunner's glands in submucosa of the
duodenum; human; H&E; ×100. Note
that some Brunner's glands are present
in the mucosa.

MUSCULARIS EXTERNA. The muscularis is organized according to the basic plan for the digestive tube: an outer longitudinal and an inner circular layer of smooth muscle. The two layers of muscle are separated by an extensive autonomic myenteric plexus, *Auerbach's plexus* (see below), which is usually easily seen in the small intestine. **Plate 11, Fig. 1; Plate 13, Fig. 2.**

SEROSA. This outermost layer is a loose connective tissue layer containing adipose tissue, blood and lymphatic vessels, and nerves. Its surface is covered by a mesothelium. The serosa is continuous with mesenteries which anchor the small intestine to the posterior abdominal wall. **Plate 11, Fig. 1.**

LARGE INTESTINE. This lower part of the digestive tube is continuous with the ileum and extends to the anus. It is about 1.5 m in length and twice the diameter of the small intestine. The large intestine is composed of the following organs, which are given in their anatomical order from the ileum to the anus: *ileocaecal valve and caecum, vermiform appendix, colon* (ascending, transverse, descending, and sigmoid), *rectum,* and *anal canal.* Although the large intestine is built on the same general plan as the small intestine, it lacks villi and plicae. The large intestine also

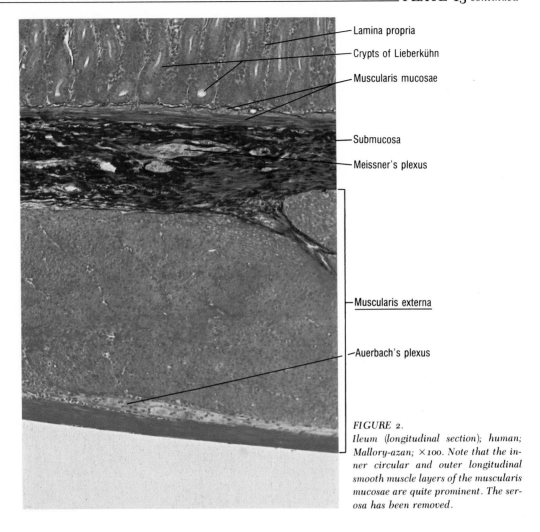

— Lamina propria
— Crypts of Lieberkühn
— Muscularis mucosae
— Submucosa
— Meissner's plexus
— Muscularis externa
— Auerbach's plexus

FIGURE 2.
Ileum (longitudinal section); human; Mallory-azan; ×100. Note that the inner circular and outer longitudinal smooth muscle layers of the muscularis mucosae are quite prominent. The serosa has been removed.

contains structures unique to it; e.g., longitudinal bands of smooth muscle, *teniae coli*, in the colon. The function of the large intestine is to extract water and vitamins from undigested waste and lubricate the fecal mass as it moves by peristalsis to the anus.

Ileocaecal valve and caecum. Below the junction where the ileum joins the large intestine there is a blind pouch, the *caecum*, which is the beginning of the large intestine. This pouch is about 6 cm long by 7 cm wide. Its walls are similar to those described for the colon (see below). The *ileocaecal valve* is a pair of long, parallel, crescent-shaped lips surrounding the opening between the ileum and caecum. It controls the unidirectional movement of waste substances between the small and large intestine. The valves are folds of the mucosal and submucosal layers. Each valve contains a thickened core of smooth muscle; this is derived mainly from the circular layer of the muscularis externa, but some longitudinal fibers are also incorporated into the valve musculature. The mucosa of the ileum covers the surface of the valves exposed to the ileum, while the surfaces that are exposed to the large intestine have a mucosal layer typical of the colon (see below).

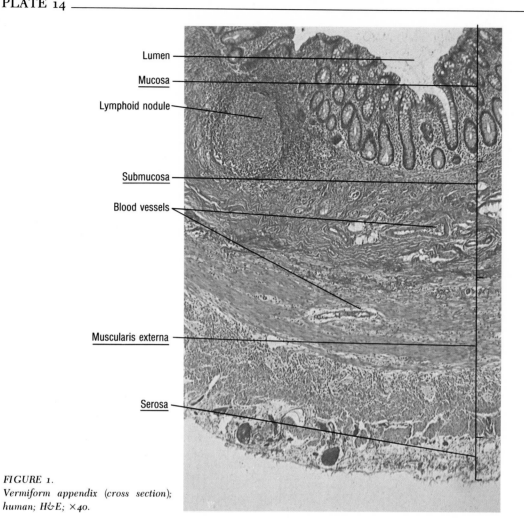

Lumen

Mucosa

Lymphoid nodule

Submucosa

Blood vessels

Muscularis externa

Serosa

FIGURE 1.
Vermiform appendix (cross section);
human; H&E; ×40.

Vermiform appendix. The appendix is a narrow, blind, tubelike structure that usually lies behind the caecum and lower portion of the ascending colon, about 2 cm below the ileocaecal junction. It is variable in diameter and length, but in the adult its average length is about 10 cm. In cross section it has thick walls and appears irregular in outline. The relatively small, irregularly shaped lumen may be filled with intestinal contents or obliterated. **Plate 14, Fig. 1.**

MUCOSA. This layer is relatively thick and contains a moderate number of irregular crypts of Lieberkühn, some of which may not reach the muscularis mucosae. The crypts are lined with columnar absorptive cells, many argentaffin cells, and some goblet and Paneth cells (refer to the section on the small intestine for the cytology of these cells). The lamina propria is composed of loose connective tissue containing great numbers of solitary lymphoid nodules. Some of these nodules may encroach onto the submucosa. Usually pale germinal centers (see Chap. 10) will be present in the nodules, and several types of leucocytes may be found in the lamina propria.

Although the muscularis mucosae is composed of inner circular and outer longitudinal layers of smooth muscle, they are discontinuous and may be difficult to observe in a section of appendix. **Plate 14, Fig. 1.**

SUBMUCOSA. This is a relatively thick layer of moderately dense, loose connective tissue. It contains blood and lymphatic vessels and nerves. Because of the poorly developed muscularis mucosae and the large lymphoid nodules, the boundary between the mucosa and submucosa may be difficult to observe. **Plate 14, Fig. 1.**

MUSCULARIS EXTERNA. This is a weak layer of musculature composed of two relatively thin layers of inner circular and outer longitudinal muscle; no teniae are present (see below). **Plate 14, Fig. 1.**

SEROSA. The serosa is continuous with that of the large intestine, and is typically composed of loose connective tissue containing vessels and nerves. It is lined with mesothelium. **Plate 14, Fig. 1.**

Colon. Although the colon is anatomically divided into four regions (ascending, transverse, descending, and sigmoid), only the description for the ascending colon will be given since all these regions are histologically quite similar. The walls of the ascending colon are continuous with those of the caecum and are composed of four histologic layers: mucosa, submucosa, muscularis, and serosa.

MUCOSA. The mucosa is not folded into plicae or villi, which are characteristic of the small intestine, but contains many crypts of Lieberkühn. The crypts are distinct from those in the small intestine, because they are deeper, more numerous, and closely packed; they also have relatively more goblet cells. The simple columnar epithelium lining the mucosal surface is composed of tall absorptive and goblet cells which dip down into the crypts. The deeper portions of the crypts of Lieberkühn also contain undifferentiated cells and argentaffin cells; Paneth cells usually are not present. Although the absorptive cells have striated borders, like those in the small intestine, they do not contain enzymes. Regeneration of epithelial cells in the mucosa is similar to that described above for the small intestine. The epithelium of the colon will be replaced about every 5 days by the processes of regeneration. The loose connective tissue of the lamina propria is usually not prominently visible because it is squeezed in between the numerous crypts. Numerous large, solitary lymphoid nodules, many scattered lymphocytes, and eosinophils will be scattered throughout the lamina propria. The prominent *muscularis mucosae* can be distinguished with its inner circular and outer longitudinal layers of smooth muscle. **Plate 15, Figs. 1 and 2.**

SUBMUCOSA. The histologic organization of this prominent layer is similar to those at other levels of the digestive tube. It is a moderately dense connective tissue layer containing blood and lymphatic vessels and nerves. Occasionally large masses of adipose tissue may be present.

MUSCULARIS EXTERNA. The outer longitudinal layer of smooth muscle in the muscularis externa departs from the basic pattern of the digestive tube. Most of this muscle is formed into three thick, parallel, longitudinal bands, *teniae coli,* which are equidistant from each other and extend the length of the caecum and colon. The teniae are interconnected by a thin layer of muscle, representing the remainder of the longitudinal muscle fibers of the muscularis. Since the teniae are shorter than the colon, the wall of the latter is folded into a series of accordianlike pleats, the *plicae semilunares coli,* and between the pleats are sacculations, the *haustra.* The inner circular layer of smooth muscle is periodically "invaded" by some of the longitudinal fibers, which may also contribute to the formation of haustra.

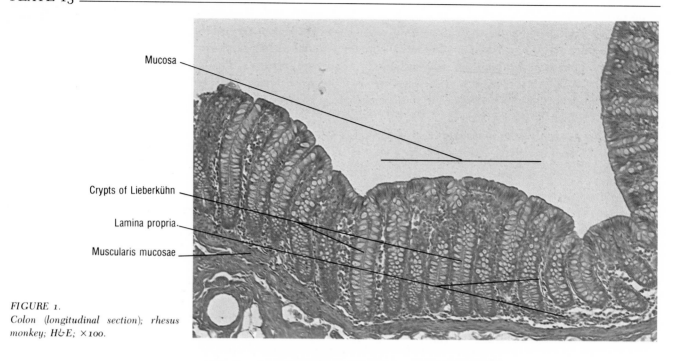

Mucosa

Crypts of Lieberkühn

Lamina propria

Muscularis mucosae

FIGURE 1.
Colon (longitudinal section); rhesus
monkey; H&E; ×100.

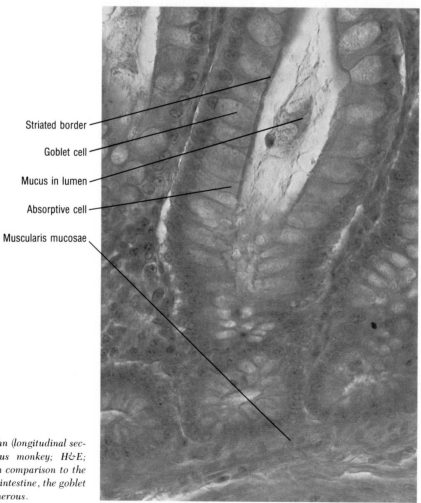

Striated border

Goblet cell

Mucus in lumen

Absorptive cell

Muscularis mucosae

FIGURE 2.
Crypt of Lieberkühn (longitudinal section); colon; rhesus monkey; H&E;
×400. Note that in comparison to the
crypts in the small intestine, the goblet
cells are more numerous.

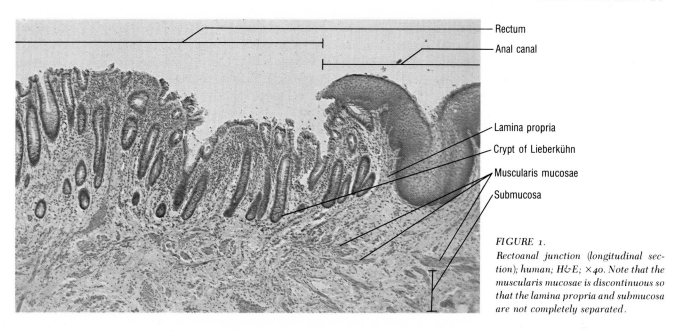

Rectum

Anal canal

Lamina propria

Crypt of Lieberkühn

Muscularis mucosae

Submucosa

FIGURE 1.
Rectoanal junction (longitudinal sec-
tion); human; H&E; ×40. Note that the
muscularis mucosae is discontinuous so
that the lamina propria and submucosa
are not completely separated.

SEROSA AND ADVENTITIA. Depending on the region of the colon, whether it is pressed against the posterior abdominal wall (ascending colon), free within the abdominal cavity (transverse colon), or retroperitoneal (descending colon), the outermost tunica may be a serosal or adventitial layer. Although the serosa is present on an exposed surface and the adventitia is present on an unexposed surface, these tunicae are histologically somewhat similar. The serosa is a layer of loose connective tissue containing blood and lymphatic vessels and nerves. It is lined with a mesothelium. The serosa is also formed into small lobelike structures filled with adipose tissue, the *appendices epiploicae.* The adventitia lacks a mesothelial lining and appendices epiploicae; otherwise it resembles the serosa histologically.

Rectum. This lower region of the digestive tube is continuous from the sigmoid colon to the anal canal, and is approximately 12 cm long. It extends from the level of the third sacral vertebra down through the pelvic diaphragm, forming the floor of the pelvic cavity. Except for the differences listed below, the four tunicae of the rectum (mucosa, submucosa, adventitia, and muscularis) are similar to those of the colon. The rectum is distinct from the colon because the crypts of Lieberkühn have relatively more goblet cells and the teniae coli and appendices epiploicae are lacking. Also, the lining of the rectum is formed into temporary longitudinal folds and permanent horizontal folds. The permanent folds are composed of the mucosa and submucosa, plus some smooth muscle fibers from one or both layers of the muscularis externa. The temporary folds are formed only by the mucosa. **Plate 16, Fig. 1.**

Anal canal. The anal canal is continuous with the lower end of the rectum and terminates at the anus. In the adult it is about 3.5 cm in length and somewhat flattened. Although the walls of the anal canal are composed of a mucosa, submucosa, muscularis externa, and adventitia, the histologic organization of these tunicae departs drastically from the basic plan of the digestive tube. **Plate 16, Fig. 1.**

MUCOSA. At the rectoanal junction the crypts of Lieberkühn become short and disappear; none are present in the anal canal. The simple columnar epithelium of the rectum abruptly changes into a stratified cuboidal type at the rectoanal junction. Below this junction, in the anal canal, the cuboidal epithelium becomes stratified squamous and nonkeratinized. At the anal orifice, where the epithelium is continuous with the epidermis of the skin, it becomes keratinized. The mucosa is formed into a number of longitudinal folds, *anal columns*, distributed around the periphery of the anal canal. These columns fuse at their lower ends to form a series of blind pouches, the *anal valves*, each of which contains a cavity or *anal sinus*. At the level of the anal columns, the muscularis mucosae becomes fragmented and disappears, and so the connective tissue layers of the lamina propria and submucosa can no longer be distinguished as separate layers. At the anus, where the lamina propria becomes continuous with the dermis of the skin, hair follicles and circumanal glands (odoriferous sweat glands) are present (see Chap. 11). **Plate 16, Fig. 1.**

SUBMUCOSA. At all levels of the anal canal the submucosa is highly vascularized, and prominent plexuses of hemorrhoidal veins are embedded within the loose connective tissue. Also, Pacinian corpuscles and many nerves are present in the submucosa. **Plate 16, Fig. 1.**

MUSCULARIS EXTERNA. At the rectoanal junction, the inner layer of circular smooth muscle becomes a thickened *internal sphincter muscle*, surrounding the upper two-thirds of the anal canal. The outer layer of longitudinal fibers blend with skeletal fibers of the levator ani. Together they form a longitudinal coat just peripheral to the internal sphincter muscle. As this outer coat extends down the length of the anal canal, its muscle fibers are eventually replaced by fibroelastic tissue. A prominent layer of skeletal muscle, the *external sphincter*, lies peripheral to this longitudinal coat of smooth muscle and fibroelastic tissue. It runs parallel to the coat as it extends from the rectoanal junction to the anus.

ADVENTITIA. This layer is not distinct; it blends with the surrounding fibroelastic tissue of the longitudinal coat between the internal and external sphincter muscles.

BLOOD AND LYMPHATIC VESSELS OF THE DIGESTIVE TUBE. These vessels enter the serosa or adventitia of the digestive tube, either directly or by being carried within a mesentery. The *arteries* form submucosal plexuses which send arterioles to the mucosa and muscularis mucosae. These arterioles are continuous with capillary networks in the mucosa, supplying blood to special mucosal structures, such as villi, glands, and etc. The capillary networks are drained by venules and then veins, the pattern of which approximates that of the arteries. Venous blood is drained from the upper mucosal areas into deep mucosal plexuses. The blood is then drained into deeper plexuses of larger vessels in the submucosa. Venous blood is collected from these plexuses by larger veins, which accompany the arteries as they pass through the muscularis externa and serosa.

The distribution of lymphatic vessels corresponds closely to the venous pattern. Large, blind lymphatic capillaries drain lymph from the mucosa into deep mucosal plexuses. The lymph is then drained into deeper submucosal plexuses of larger lymphatic vessels. Lymph from these submucosal plexuses, as well as plexuses in the muscularis, will be drained by yet larger lymphatic vessels which pass through the serosa or adventitia. The lymphatic vessels which drain fat-filled lymph (chyle) from the small intestine are designated as *lacteals*. During digestion, fat is absorbed into the central lacteals. A central lacteal is a large, blind lymphatic capillary running in the core of a villus from the tip to its base. Each lacteal is then drained, according to the pattern already described for lymphatic vessels in the mucosa. Duodenal villi have two or more intercommunicating central lacteals, while villi in the other parts of the small intestine usually have only one per villus.

NERVES OF THE DIGESTIVE TUBE. The digestive tube is well innervated by the autonomic nervous system: visceral afferent fibers, postganglionic sympathetic and parasympathetic fibers, and preganglionic parasympathetic fibers. The latter innervate many ganglionated plexuses located in the submucosa, *Meissner's plexus*, and between the circular and longitudinal smooth muscle layers of the muscularis externa, the *myenteric plexus of Auerbach* (see **Plate 13, Fig. 2**). Both these plexuses contain mostly parasympathetic ganglion cells, postganglionic parasympathetic fibers, association neurons, some postganglionic sympathetic fibers, and some preganglionic parasympathetic fibers. Although the ganglion cells are easily identified (see Chap. 6), it is difficult to distinguish between the parasympathetic and sympathetic fibers. The efferent fibers of the sympathetic and parasympathetic nerves innervate glands and the smooth muscle of villi, blood vessels, muscularis mucosa, and muscularis externa. The visceral afferent fibers are believed to innervate the epithelium. Sympathetic nerves will influence a decrease in muscular activity and peristalsis, constrict blood vessels, and inhibit secretions, while the parasympathetic nerves will bring about the opposite effects.

Major digestive glands: Liver and pancreas

The pancreas and liver are large glands lying outside of the digestive tube. They secrete digestive substances which enter the tube through ducts.

PANCREAS. This is an elongate organ, about 20 cm long. It is divided into a broad *head*, moderately wide *body*, and narrow *tail*. The pancreas is a retroperitoneal organ lying posterior to the stomach and extending horizontally from the duodenum to the spleen. It is surrounded by a poorly developed capsule of loose connective tissue, and is subdivided into lobules by septa extending from the capsule. The lobules of the pancreas are composed of two types of glandular tissue: *exocrine* and *endocrine*. The exocrine tissues secrete digestive enzymes which are carried by a system of ducts to the lumen of the duodenum. The endocrine tissues secrete hormones directly into the blood, the function of which is to regulate carbohydrate metabolism. **Plate 17, Figs. 1 and 2.**

Exocrine pancreas. The exocrine pancreas comprises compound tubuloalveolar glands embedded within a delicate stroma of reticular tissue. Depending on how they were sectioned, the alveoli may appear as ovoid, round, or pear-shaped structures packed within a lobule. The exocrine pancreas becomes secretive during psychic (vagal stimulation) and gastric phases (gastrin production) of digestion. It is most productive when chyme enters the duodenum. The acidity of chyme and its contents of organic acids stimulates the production and release of two hormones, *secretin* and *pancreozymin (cholecystokinin)*, possibly by the action of argentaffin cells in the duodenal mucosa. Secretin influences the pancreas (possibly duct cells) to produce copious amounts of fluids rich in bicarbonates. These bicarbonates raise the pH of the duodenal contents, which is important for the digestive activity of the pancreatic enzymes. Pancreozymin stimulates the alveolar cells to secrete inactive enzymes as zymogen granules and active enzymes in a nongranular form. The zymogen granules contain several inactive proteolytic enzymes: trypsinogen, chymotrypsinogen, and carboxypeptidase. After their entrance into the duodenum, trypsinogen reacts with enterokinase, an enzyme produced in the mucosa, which transforms trypsinogen to trypsin. Trypsin then activates the other proteolytic enzymes. These enzymes digest proteins, peptones, proteoses, and peptides. Lipase, amylase, and nuclease are secreted in an active nongranular form. Amylase digests polysaccharides, lipase hydrolyzes triglycerides into fatty acids and glycerol, and the nucleases digest ribonucleoprotein and deoxyribonucleoprotein.

ALVEOLUS. Each alveolus is composed of serous cells lying on a basement membrane. Each alveolar cell is pyramid-shaped and has a basophilic cytoplasm. The lighter-stained apical portion of the cell, adjacent to the lumen of the gland, is usually filled with acidophilic zymogen granules. The deeper-stained basal portion displays a series of faint longitudinal striations. These striations are produced by the vertical orientation of mitochondria and extensive folding of the plasma membrane. A large, round nucleus lies near the base of the cell. It is moderately heavy with chromatin and contains one or several nucleoli. **Plate 17, Figs. 1 and 2.**

DUCTS. Each alveolus drains directly into a long, extensively branched, narrow, intralobular *intercalated duct*. These ducts are surrounded by a basement membrane and lined with a simple cuboidal epithelium. At the junction between the alveolus and intercalated duct, many alveolar cells form a peripheral collar around the duct. The appearance of these junctions in cross section is a peripheral ring of alveolar cells surrounding a lumen filled with pale cuboidal cells of the duct, *centroalveolar cells* (centroacinar cells). The intercalated ducts are continuous with the wider *interlobular ducts*. These latter ducts are located in the connective tissue between lobules. The smaller ducts are lined with a simple cuboidal epithelium but the larger ones have a low columnar epithelium. The interlobular ducts join the large pancreatic duct, the *duct of Wirsung*, and the smaller accessory duct, the *duct of Santorini*, if it is present. The duct of Wirsung usually unites with the ductus choledochus (common bile duct) as the two ducts penetrate the duodenal wall. The union forms a short, wide *hepatopancreatic ampulla*, which opens into the duodenum through a major duodenal papilla. The accessory duct opens independently into the duodenum through a minor duodenal papilla located about 2 cm away from the major papilla. The ampulla, lower portions of the ductus choledochus, and pancreatic ducts are surrounded by a coat of smooth muscle, the *sphincter of Oddi*, which regulates the flow of bile and pancreatic juices into the duodenum. The epithelium of these large pancreatic ducts is tall columnar with occasional goblet cells. The ducts have a layer of fibroelastic connective tissue surrounding the epithelium. **Plate 17, Fig. 1.**

Endocrine pancreas. The endocrine portion of the pancreas are the *islets of Langerhans.* They are small, pale-stained, subspherical to irregular masses of tissue scattered throughout the exocrine tissue. There are about 0.5 to 2 million islets of Langerhans in the pancreas. Each islet is highly vascularized, and is composed of clumps of polygonal glandular cells embedded within a sparse network of reticular tissue. The reticular tissue also partially separates the islets from the exocrine tissue. In humans, three types of granular parenchyma cells can be distinguished with special stains. Unfortunately H&E is not one of these, so the cells in an H&E preparation appear as pale, undistinguished cords of tissue lying within a vascularized reticular network. Using special techniques, such as fixing with Zenker's fluid and using Mallory-azan stain, the following cell types may be distinguished. **Plate 17, Figs. 1 and 2.**

ALPHA CELLS (A cells). These are large, moderately abundant cells located at the periphery of the islets. Their large, red, uniform, spherical granules are insoluable in alcohol. The cells produce *glucagon*, a hormone which increases the level of blood sugar by causing *glycogenolysis*, a breakdown of glycogen to glucose in the liver. Glucagon also increases the rate of *gluconeogenesis*, a conversion of fats and proteins to carbohydrates.

BETA CELLS (B cells). These are small, very numerous cells located in the interior of the islet. Their small, brownish orange cytoplasmic granules are soluble in alcohol. These cells produce insulin, which has the opposite effect of glucagon. Insulin decreases the level of blood sugar by stimulating glycogenesis in the liver and skeletal muscle, where glucose is converted to glycogen, and by facilitating movement of glucose through the membranes of certain cells.

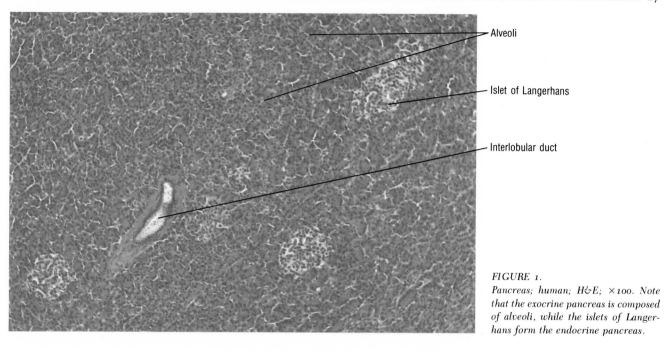

Alveoli

Islet of Langerhans

Interlobular duct

FIGURE 1.
Pancreas; human; H&E; ×100. Note
that the exocrine pancreas is composed
of alveoli, while the islets of Langer-
hans form the endocrine pancreas.

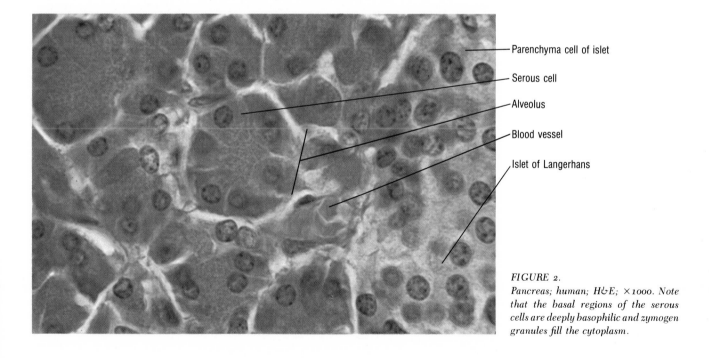

Parenchyma cell of islet

Serous cell

Alveolus

Blood vessel

Islet of Langerhans

FIGURE 2.
Pancreas; human; H&E; ×1000. Note
that the basal regions of the serous
cells are deeply basophilic and zymogen
granules fill the cytoplasm.

DELTA CELLS (D cells). These cells resemble the alpha cells and are also located at the periphery of the islet. Delta cells are usually larger than the alpha cells and their larger granules stain blue. There are very few of these cell types. They may represent alpha cells in some stage of secretory activity or undergoing regressive transformations.

C CELLS. These are small, unstained, ungranulated cells scattered among the beta cells within the interior of the islets. The C cells are present in certain species (e.g., guinea pig) but not in humans. They fall into the same speculative category as the delta cells; they may be reserve cells which could differentiate into alpha or beta cells.

Blood and lymphatic vessels of the pancreas. Arterial branches from the splenic arteries and anterior and posterior pancreaticoduodenal arteries follow the interlobular connective tissue into the gland. Smaller vessels then extend into the lobules and form capillary plexuses around the alveoli, or invade the islets of Langerhans to form extensive capillary networks among the islet tissues. The capillaries are drained first by venules and then veins, which approximate the arterial pattern of vessel distribution. The venous blood will be drained into the hepatic portal, splenic, and superior mesenteric veins. *Lymphatic* capillaries are present only in the exocrine pancreas. They are drained by larger lymphatic vessels which accompany blood vessels in the connective tissue. These large vessels terminate in lymph nodes located in various regions: between the pancreas and spleen, between the pancreas and duodenum, and near the celiac artery.

Nerves of the pancreas. Sympathetic postganglionic fibers from the celiac ganglion and parasympathetic preganglionic fibers from the vagus innervate the exocrine pancreas. In addition, parasympathetic ganglia and sometimes Pacinian corpuscles are present in the interlobular septa. The endocrine pancreas also is innervated by both sympathetic and parasympathetic fibers. The automatic nervous system will control the vasomotor activities of the blood vessels and to a small degree will regulate secretion.

LIVER. The liver is a large gland weighing about 1.5 kg. It lies between the stomach and diaphragm and extends into the upper lateral regions of the abdomen. It is divided into two unequal principal lobes: a large right and a smaller left lobe. The right lobe has two smaller lobes on its inferior and posterior surface: the quadrate and caudate lobes. The liver is anchored to the anterior body wall and diaphragm by the falciform ligament and to the diaphragm by the coronary ligament. Blood vessels (hepatic portal vein and hepatic artery), lymphatic vessels, bile duct, and nerves enter and leave the inferior surface of the liver through a deep transverse fissure, the *porta hepatis*. The porta is located between the quadrate and caudate lobes.

The liver is both an exocrine gland (secretes bile) and an endocrine gland (releases metabolic substances directly into the blood). Some of the numerous functions performed by the liver are listed below:

Interconversion of digested molecules (glucose, amino acids, fatty acids, and glycerol).

Elimination of nitrogenous compounds as urea, which is synthesized in the liver as a by-product of amino acid metabolism.

Storage of blood.

Synthesis of globulin, heparin, prothrombin, vitamin A, fats, and proteins.

Metabolism and degradation of drugs and poisons.

Phagocytosis (by Kupffer cells), removing foreign material, inactive or old cells and erythrocytes, and microorganisms.

Storage of carbohydrates and fats.

Maintenance of the proper blood sugar level by glycogenolysis and glycogenesis.

Secretion of bile, which contains fluids, bile salts (to emulsify fats), and waste materials in the form of bilirubin glucuronide.

Old or damaged erythrocytes are removed from the blood by phagocytes in splenic cords and sinusoids mainly in the liver, and marrow. As the erythrocytes are digested, hemoglobin is degraded into iron and heme components. If the concentration of plasma iron is high, the degraded iron may be stored within the macrophages as an iron-protein complex, ferritin. If the concentration is low, the iron will be transported by transferrin, an iron-binding globulin, to the hematopoietic tissues of the bone marrow and utilized in the synthesis of new hemoglobin. Also, with a low plasma concentration, ferritin will release its stored iron into the blood where it will combine with transferrin. Iron, therefore, is conserved by the body and used over and over; only small amounts of iron are eliminated in the urine and feces. The heme is converted to the pigment bilirubin within the macrophages and then released into the blood. Eventually bilirubin is taken up by the liver cells and transformed into highly soluable bilirubin glucuronide. In this form, it is excreted into the bile. As bile enters the small intestine, bilirubin glucuronide is reduced to urobilinogen by bacterial action. Most of the urobilinogen is excreted with the feces in the form of stercobilin, but a small amount of it is reabsorbed from the intestine back into the blood. Some urobilinogen will be reexcreted in the bile, but the remainder will be excreted by the kidneys as urobilin.

The liver, except the region in contact with the diaphragm, is covered by a visceral peritoneum. The peritoneum is continuous with a thin collagenous connective tissue capsule, *Glisson's capsule*. In the region of the porta hepatis, thin septa of connective tissue extend from Glisson's capsule to divide the liver parenchyma into *lobes* and *lobules*. The parenchyma is a latticework of perforated plates composed of hepatic cords and sinusoids. The lobules are polygonal or hexagonal and about 1 to 2 mm in diameter; they are not well defined in humans. Each septum carries a branch of the hepatic portal vein, a branch of the hepatic artery, and a bile duct. This anatomic triad, along with some lymphatic vessels, is designated as a *portal canal* and may be seen between the angles of the lobules. The relationship is such that one portal canal is shared by three adjacent hexagonal lobules. The boundaries of the lobules are indistinct, and the liver parenchyma appears to be continuous between them. Sparse strands of connective tissue, carrying small branches of the canal system, are located between the lobules. Each lobule contains a longitudinal vessel, the *central vein*, which is a branch of the hepatic vein. The parenchyma is organized into a radiating pattern of hepatic cords extending from the central vein to the periphery of the lobule. Blood, carried by small branches of the hepatic artery and hepatic portal vein, enters the sinusoids at the periphery of the lobule and flows towards the central vein. It is collected first by sublobular and then hepatic veins. **Plate 18, Figs 1** and **2.**

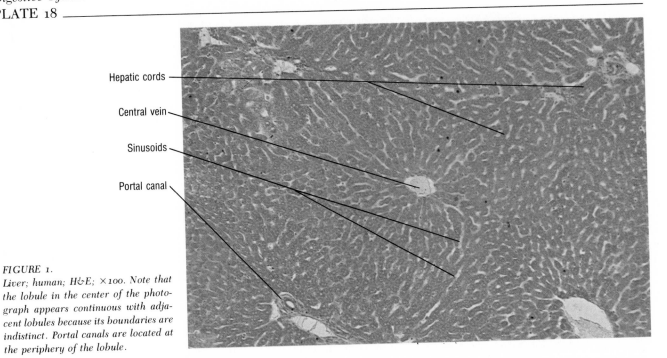

Hepatic cords

Central vein

Sinusoids

Portal canal

FIGURE 1.
Liver; human; H&E; ×100. Note that the lobule in the center of the photograph appears continuous with adjacent lobules because its boundaries are indistinct. Portal canals are located at the periphery of the lobule.

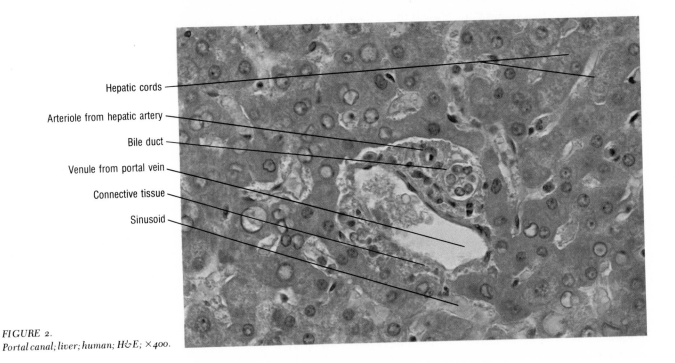

Hepatic cords

Arteriole from hepatic artery

Bile duct

Venule from portal vein

Connective tissue

Sinusoid

FIGURE 2.
Portal canal; liver; human; H&E; ×400.

The lobule discussed above can be designated as a *classical lobule* (hepatic lobule), which is only one of the three possible but compatible interpretations of liver lobules; the other two are the portal lobule and the liver acinus. The classical lobule illustrates a possible endocrine function. As blood flows from the periphery to the center of the lobule, it receives metabolic substances produced and released by the liver cells. The *portal lobule* is an illustration of an exocrine gland, because

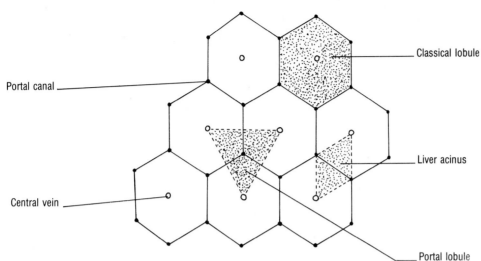

Portal canal

Central vein

Classical lobule

Liver acinus

Portal lobule

FIGURE 3.
Diagram illustrating the possible types of liver lobules.

bile secretions flow from its periphery to the center and are collected by a duct. Geographically, the portal lobule occupies a triangular area within three central veins; a portal canal lies in the center of the lobule. The concept *liver acinus* (functional unit) is an interpretation which explains the intricacies of liver metabolism and patterns of regeneration. The liver acinus is the tissue of adjacent triangular segments of two classical lobules which are separated by the horizontal branches of the portal canal. The acinus extends between two central veins and the area may be diamond-shaped, ovoid, or irregularly shaped. **Plate 18, Fig. 3.**

Hepatic cells (parenchymal cells). These cells form the liver cords and are large, polygonal cells with one or two pale, spherical nuclei. The nuclei may be variable in size, contain scattered clumps of chromatin, and one to several nucleoli. Hepatic cells are unique in that endomitosis is common: there may be a single large polyploid nucleus; two nuclei; or several nuclei (refer to Chap. 1, **Plate 2, Fig. 2**). The appearance of the cytoplasm is variable, since it depends on the physiologic condition of the cells and the types of fixatives used in the preparation of the sections. In sections taken from nonfasted animals, the cytoplasm appears as a basophilic network containing irregular spaces. Ribosomes are responsible for the basophilic condition, while dissolved fats and glycogen granules account for the vacuoles and irregular spaces. In fasted animals the cytoplasm loses its basophilia and becomes acidophilic. **Plate 19, Fig. 1.**

Sinusoids. These large (9 to 12 μm diameter), irregular, vascular channels forming the spaces between the hepatic cords are lined with two types of cells: *endothelial and Kupffer cells* (see Chaps. 3 and 9). **Plate 19, Fig. 1.**
ENDOTHELIAL CELLS. These are extremely flat, fenestrated cells with a relatively small, flattened, dark-stained nucleus. The cells do not form a continuous lining so gaps are present between them. The spaces, both in the cytoplasm and sinusoidal lining, facilitate the movement of small molecules from the blood to liver cells over perisinusoidal spaces (Disse's space). **Plate 19, Fig. 1.**
KUPFFER CELLS. (stellate cells). Another term for these cells is the fixed macrophage (see Chap. 3). These irregularly shaped or stellate cells extend into the sinusoidal lumen more than the endothelial cells. They contain a small to medium-sized, oval

TABLE 2
Hepatic vascular pattern

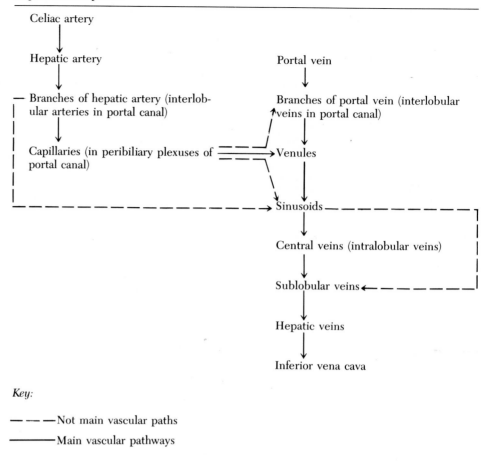

Key:

— — — Not main vascular paths

———— Main vascular pathways

nucleus which stains moderately dark and is usually indented on one side. Since the cell is highly phagocytic the vacuolated cytoplasm may be filled with debris, aged erythrocytes, or granules of *hemosiderin*. Hemosiderin is a golden-brown iron-containing pigment derived from the degradation of hemoglobin. As hemoglobin is degraded, the iron may be formed into ferritin, an iron-containing protein, and stored in macrophages as pigment granules of hemosiderin. In diseases, where there is a rapid destruction of erythrocytes, much hemosiderin will be present in many macrophages (alveolar phagocytes, Kupffer cells, etc.). **Plate 19, Fig. 1.**

Blood and lymphatic vessels of the liver. The diagram of the hepatic vascular pattern in Table 2 supplements the description of hepatic circulation given above. From the diagram it can be seen that the liver is supplied by two vascular sources, the hepatic artery and the portal vein. It is drained by the hepatic veins. The sinusoids carry mixed arterial and venous blood to the hepatic cells. The hepatic artery provides a smaller amount of blood to the liver (about 25 percent) than the portal vein (about 75 percent).

Lymph is formed in the perisinusoidal spaces. It percolates toward the periphery of a lobule and then into the connective tissues of a portal canal. Although a connection between the perisinusoidal spaces and lymphatic capillaries has not been demonstrated, lymph is collected by lymphatic capillaries within the portal

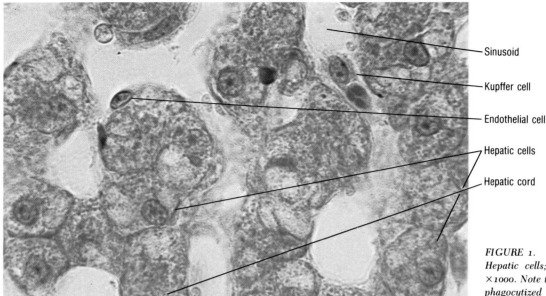

Sinusoid

Kupffer cell

Endothelial cell

Hepatic cells

Hepatic cord

FIGURE 1.
Hepatic cells; human; Mallory-azan;
×1000. Note that the Kupffer cell has
phagocytized some erythrocytes. The
cytoplasm of the hepatic cells is gran-
ular and vacuolated.

canal. As lymph is transported to the hilus of the liver, it is carried by a system of progressively larger lymphatic vessels.

Nerves of the liver. Unmyelinated nerve fibers of the autonomic nervous system and ganglion cells are present in the connective tissue of the capsule and portal canals. Sympathetic postganglionic fibers innervate the smooth muscle of the arteries, while bile ducts are innervated by both sympathetic and parasympathetic postganglionic fibers. Innervation of hepatic cells has not been demonstrated, and so the major physiologic influence of the autonomic system is to regulate the flow of liquids within the blood vessels and biliary ducts.

Biliary system. The biliary system is a continuous labyrinth of ducts. It carries bile from the liver cells to the gallbladder where it is stored, and to the duodenum where it emulsifies fats for digestion. The components of the biliary system, from hepatic tissues to the extrahepatic regions, are indicated in **Plate 19, Fig. 2**, and listed below.

1. *Bile canaliculi.* This is a continuous system of microscopic tubules formed by plasma membranes of adjacent hepatic cells. The canaliculi drain bile toward the periphery of the classic lobule where they are continuous with larger bile ductules. Although the canaliculi are about 1.0 μm in diameter, they may be seen in routine H&E preparations. They are quite prominent as a network of tubules in silver-stained preparations. **Plate 20, Fig. 1.**

2. *Bile ductules* (canals of Hering). These are small (2 to 15 μm diameter) tubules, located within the peripheral connective tissue of the lobules, which drain the canaliculi. The tubules are composed of small, pale-strained, fusiform cells containing dark, elongated nuclei; near the bile ducts the cells become somewhat cuboidal.

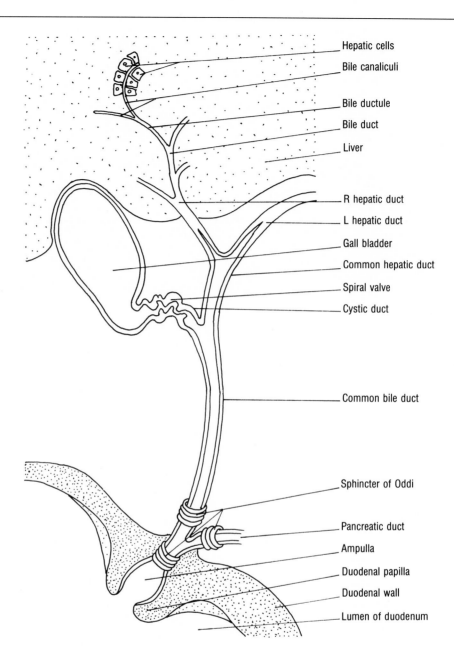

Hepatic cells
Bile canaliculi
Bile ductule
Bile duct
Liver
R hepatic duct
L hepatic duct
Gall bladder
Common hepatic duct
Spiral valve
Cystic duct
Common bile duct
Sphincter of Oddi
Pancreatic duct
Ampulla
Duodenal papilla
Duodenal wall
Lumen of duodenum

FIGURE 2.
Drawing of the biliary system.

3. *Bile Ducts* (interlobular ducts). These ducts are located in the portal canals and drain the ductules. The smaller ones are about 16 μm in diameter, but they anastomose to become larger as they approach the hilus of the liver. The smaller bile ducts have a simple low cuboidal epithelium, while the larger ducts have a low columnar epithelium. The epithelium of the ducts rest on a basal lamina which is surrounded by bundles of dense, irregular collagenous connective tissue. Some smooth muscle may also be found in the walls of the larger ducts.

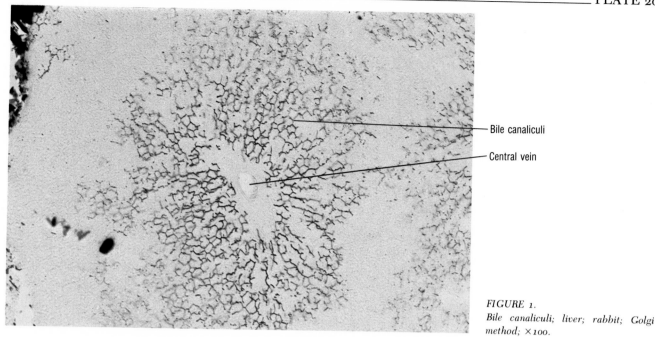

— Bile canaliculi

— Central vein

FIGURE 1.
Bile canaliculi; liver; rabbit; Golgi method; ×100.

4. *Extrahepatic bile ducts.* These ducts drain the interlobular ducts and the lobes of the liver. They fuse to form the large left and right *hepatic ducts*, which in turn fuse to form the *common hepatic duct*. The common hepatic duct fuses with the *cystic duct*, draining the gallbladder, and both ducts form the *common bile duct* (ductus choledochus). The common bile duct usually joins the pancreatic duct, and the two terminate as an enlarged hepatopancreatic ampulla. The ampulla then opens into the duodenum at the apex of a duodenal papilla. The histology of these extrahepatic passages is quite similar: each has a mucosal lining and a fibroelastic coat containing various amounts of scattered smooth muscle (see below).

MUCOSA. The simple columnar epithelium is composed of tall cells. The lamina propria is a loose connective tissue containing many elastic fibers and numerous lymphocytes. Tubuloalveolar mucus glands are present and open into the lumen. The mucosa is folded, but in the cystic duct, near the gallbladder, it forms the spiral *valve of Heister* which contains some smooth muscle. Blood and lymphatic vessels and nerves are also present in the mucosa.

FIBROELASTIC COAT. All the extrahepatic passages contain a peripheral coat of collagen and elastic fibers and some scattered smooth muscle cells. In the common bile duct the smooth muscle is organized into longitudinal, oblique, and circular layers. These layers are incomplete and scatttered at the upper levels, but become more prominent at the lower end of the common bile duct. At the lower end, the circular muscles form a prominent sphincter choledochus. This sphincter muscle, along with sphincters of the pancreatic duct (sphincter pancreaticus) and the ampulla, form the *sphincter of Oddi*. When the sphincter of Oddi is relaxed, bile may enter the duodenum to emulsify fats, but if the sphincter is contracted, bile flows into the cystic duct and is stored in the gallbladder.

Gallbladder. The gallbladder is a pear-shaped pouch about 8 cm in length by 3 cm wide at its broadest part. It lies within a recess on the inferior surface of the right hepatic lobe, and may be connected to the liver by connective tissue or a mesentery. The gallbladder is anatomically divided into an expanded fundus, a narrower body, and a thin neck which is continuous with the cystic duct. Although the gallbladder is continuous with the cystic duct, its histologic organization is more complex. The wall of the gallbladder is composed of three well-defined layers: *mucosa, muscularis,* and *serosa.* The function of the gallbladder is to store bile and concentrate it by absorbing fluids through the epithelial layer of the mucosa. The gallbladder contracts as a response both to the hormone produced in the duodenal mucosa, cholecystokinin, and to the autonomic nervous system. As it contracts, the sphincter of Oddi relaxes and bile enters the duodenum via the common bile duct. **Plate 19, Fig. 2.**

MUCOSA. The mucosa is formed into many temporary folds in the empty bladder, but it flattens out when the bladder is filled. In the neck, however, the mucosa forms a number of oblique, permanent folds, similar to those in the cystic duct (see above). These folds contain some smooth muscle fibers and form a spiral valve of Heister. This valve probably maintains a patent lumen during extensive pressure changes in the gallbladder. The simple columnar epithelium is composed of tall, pale, eosinophilic cells with an oval basal nucleus. The apical borders of the cells are faintly striated, indicating the presence of absorptive microvilli. The cells lie on a delicate basement membrane, which may not be visible in most preparations. The lamina propria is composed of a highly vascularized loose connective tissue containing solitary lymphoid nodules. At the level of the neck, simple tubuloalveolar mucous glands may be found in the lamina propria. Occasionally, diverticula of the mucosa, *Rokitansky-Aschoff sinuses,* may extend into the outer walls of the gallbladder. They appear as large, irregular cavities lined with simple columnar epithelium, and they open onto the lumen of the gallbladder. These sinuses represent abnormalities in the mucosal lining and may become inflamed. **Plate 20, Fig. 2.**

MUSCULARIS. This is a relatively thin, irregular network of smooth muscle tissue embedded within a connective tissue coat of collagen, elastic, and reticular fibers. The muscle bundles are randomly oriented in longitudinal, circular, and oblique directions throughout the muscularis. **Plate 20, Fig. 2.**

SEROSA. This is a moderately dense loose connective tissue layer, surrounding the muscularis. It contains collagen and elastic fibers, fibroblasts, macrophages, fat cells, blood and lymphatic vessels, and nerves. On the exposed surface of the gallbladder the tissue is covered by a mesothelium. In places where the gallbladder is touching the inferior surface of the liver, the outer tunica is an adventitia and its connective tissue is continuous with Glisson's capsule. In some specimens *Luschka ducts* may be present in the adventitial layer. They are located on the hepatic surface of the gallbladder, near the neck. These tubular structures resemble small, interlobular bile ducts and therefore should not be confused with the Rokitansky-Aschoff sinuses. Luschka ducts may be continuous with the bile ducts of the liver, but are nonfunctional since they do not open into the gallbladder. It is believed that they represent aberrant, vestigial, embryonic structures. **Plate 20, Fig. 2.**

Blood and lymphatic vessels. The cystic artery has branches which supply blood to the muscularis and prominent capillary plexuses in the serosa and mucosa. On the hepatic surface of the gallbladder, small veins drain blood into hepatic veins located within the liver. The remainder of the gallbladder is drained by the cystic vein, which joins the right branch of the hepatic portal vein. *Lymphatic vessels* form extensive plexuses in the mucosa and serosa. Plexuses on the hepatic surface of the gallbladder also receive some lymphatic vessels from the liver. Lymph is drained from these plexuses, by large lymphatic vessels, toward lymph nodes near the neck of the gallbladder.

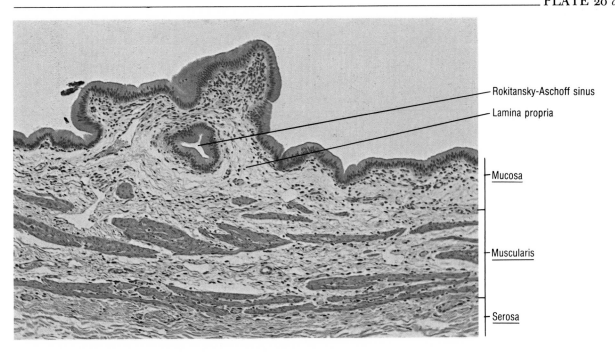

Rokitansky-Aschoff sinus

Lamina propria

Mucosa

Muscularis

Serosa

FIGURE 2.
Gallbladder; human; H&E; ×100. Note that there is no submucosa. The muscularis is a network of smooth muscle bundles scattered through a bed of fibroelastic tissue.

Nerves. Sympathetic and parasympathetic nerve fibers innervate the smooth muscle tissue of the muscularis while sympathetic fibers innervate blood vessels. Plexuses of these fibers are prominent in the connective tissue of the mucosa and muscularis. In addition, visceral afferent nerves are present in the gallbladder.

Respiratory System 13

External respiration is the movement of inspired and expired air between the environment and the lungs. It is made possible by an interconnecting system of air passages which warms, moistens, and removes foreign particles from the air. Internal respiration is concerned only with the diffusion of oxygen and carbon dioxide between air in the lungs and blood in the pulmonary vessels. The histology of the air passages will be considered in sequence, in going from the superficial to the deepest anatomical levels. These are the nasal cavity, pharynx (nasopharynx, oropharynx, laryngopharynx), larynx, trachea, bronchi, and the bronchial tree within the lungs.

Nasal cavity

The nasal cavity is a large chamber extending from the external nares to the more posterior choanae or internal nares. The choanae form a boundary between the nasal cavity and the lower nasopharynx. The vomer bone forms a part of the floor of the nasal cavity while the ethmoid bone forms portions of the roof and lateral walls. The ethmoid bone consists of a cribiform plate (roof), a perpendicular plate (dividing the nasal cavity into left and right halves), and two lateral masses (composed of shelflike conchae and deep recesses, the meatuses). Parts of the nasal, palatine, sphenoid, maxillary, lacrimal, and frontal bones also contribute to the structure of the nasal cavity.

The nasal cavity has three anatomical regions: the anterior *vestibule*, lined with skin containing hair, sweat, and sebaceous glands; a more posterior *olfactory region*, lined with sensory olfactory mucosa; and a most posterior *respiratory region*, lined with a respiratory mucosa. Many cavities in the skull (paranasal sinuses) are connected with the nasal cavity and lined with a modified respiratory mucosa. In all regions, the mucosa is firmly anchored to the skeletal components by a periosteum or perichondrium.

RESPIRATORY MUCOSA. This tissue is composed of a pseudostratified columnar ciliated epithelium with scattered goblet cells. The epithelium rests on a prominent basement membrane lying on a lamina propria of moderately dense, irregular

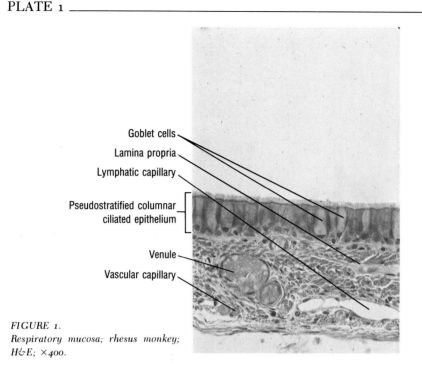

Goblet cells

Lamina propria

Lymphatic capillary

Pseudostratified columnar
ciliated epithelium

Venule

Vascular capillary

FIGURE 1.
Respiratory mucosa; rhesus monkey;
H&E; ×400.

collagenous connective tissue. The lamina propria has many lymphocytes and compound branched tubuloalveolar glands containing serous and mucous cells. The glands have short ducts opening onto the epithelial surface. The smaller ducts are usually lined with secretory cells, while larger ones have cuboidal nonsecretory cells. In the deeper levels of the lamina propria, just above the perichondrium or periosteum, there is an extensive vascular supply. The vessels normally carry blood to the respiratory surface to warm inspired air. In certain regions venous plexuses can become engorged with blood and influence the mucosa to become turgid and extend into the nasal cavity. The engorged mucosa may be effective in closing certain passages and rerouting the airflow through others. **Plate 1, Fig. 1.**

OLFACTORY MUCOSA. The olfactory mucosa resembles respiratory mucosa, except that the pseudostratified columnar epithelium is thicker and lacks cilia and goblet cells. Also, the epithelium is pigmented and has three specialized cell types: *olfactory, sustentacular,* and *basal cells.* Branched tubuloalveolar serous glands (Bowman's glands) are located in the lamina propria. The secretory cells are low pyramidal with cytoplasmic granules, and the cells lining the duct are low cuboidal. **Plate 1, Figs. 2 and 3.**

Olfactory cells. These are fusiform bipolar sensory neurons with modified upper and lower cytoplasmic processes. The upper process is a short dendrite terminating as a clump (6 to 10) of long, nonmotile cilia (olfactory hairs) on the epithelial surface. The lower process is a nonmyelonated axon passing through the lamina propria with other axons to form the olfactory nerve. The large, spherical nucleus lies at the middle of the cell and, with similar nuclei, occupies the middle level of the epithelium. These nuclei lie between the oval sustentacular cell nuclei, located at the upper level of the epithelium, and the small, oval basal cell nuclei, at the lower level. **Plate 1, Fig. 3.**

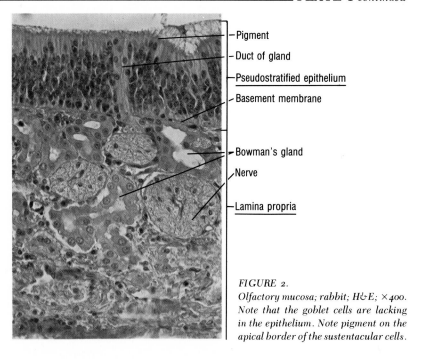

—Pigment
—Duct of gland
—Pseudostratified epithelium
—Basement membrane

—Bowman's gland
/Nerve

—Lamina propria

FIGURE 2.
*Olfactory mucosa; rabbit; H&E; ×400.
Note that the goblet cells are lacking
in the epithelium. Note pigment on the
apical border of the sustentacular cells.*

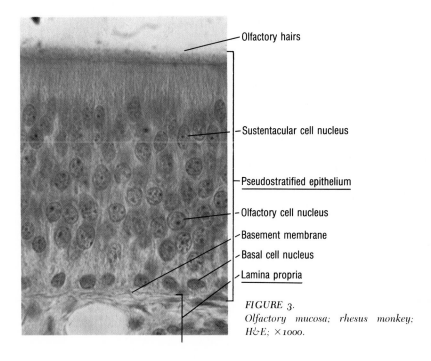

—Olfactory hairs

—Sustentacular cell nucleus

—Pseudostratified epithelium
—Olfactory cell nucleus
—Basement membrane
—Basal cell nucleus
—Lamina propria

FIGURE 3.
*Olfactory mucosa; rhesus monkey;
H&E; ×1000.*

Sustentacular cells. These cells support the olfactory cells and are the most numerous type in the epithelium. They are columnar cells with a narrow base and a wider upper portion, and contain golden brown lipofuscin granules. The cells appear to be striated because of the presence of long microvilli. The oval nuclei are in the uppermost level of the epithelium, just above the olfactory cell nuclei. **Plate 1, Fig. 3.**

Basal cells. These relatively scarce cells are located at the bottom of the epithelium. They appear as small, pyramidal cells with dark basophilic cytoplasm and thin, branched processes. The dark, small, round nuclei form the lowest layer of nuclei in the epithelium. These cells may be precursors to the olfactory and sustentacular cells. **Plate 1, Fig. 3.**

Pharynx

The pharynx or throat, is a common chamber for both the respiratory and digestive systems, since air, food, and water pass through it. It communicates with the mouth, nasal cavity, larynx, eustachian tubes, and esophagus. It is a tubelike structure bordered superiorly by parts of the occipital and sphenoid bones; inferiorly by the esophagus; posteriorly by the cervical vertebra; anteriorly by the nasal cavity, mouth, and larynx; and laterally by the eustachian tubes, which communicate with the middle ear cavities. At the upper levels the pharynx is anchored to bone by a thin layer of relatively dense fibrous connective tissue, but at the lower levels it is connected to the vertebral column and other adjacent structures by loose connective tissue. In going from a superior to more inferior levels the pharynx is divided into three regions: *nasopharynx, oropharynx,* and *laryngopharynx.* Histologically the wall of the nasopharynx resembles the wall of the respiratory region of the nasal cavity, while the oropharynx and laryngopharynx both show similarities to the esophagus. The pharyngeal wall is organized into several superimposed layers. From the innermost to the outermost layer, there is a *mucosa* (composed of an epithelium and a lamina propria of connective tissue), *submucosa, muscularis,* and *adventitia.*

NASOPHARYNX. This is the upper level of the pharynx and is continuous with the posterior region of the nasal cavity. The nasopharynx lies above a fleshy, soft palate which separates it from the mouth. Pharyngeal tonsils (adenoids) are located in the dorsal midline of the nasopharynx, and openings of the eustachian tubes are present in its dorsolateral walls. **Plate 2, Fig. 1.**

Mucosa. The *epithelium* in the upper levels of the nasopharynx is pseudostratified columnar ciliated with a few scattered goblet cells. At the lower levels, where the edge of the soft palate touches the pharyngeal wall during the act of swallowing, the epithelium is stratified squamous and nonkeratinized. A small patch of stratified columnar ciliated or nonciliated epithelium is present in a transitional zone between the pseudostratified and stratified squamous epithelium. A prominent basement membrane is found under the epithelium only in the nasopharynx.

The *lamina propria* is a relatively dense layer of connective tissue containing some collagen fibers, many elastic fibers, blood and lymphatic vessels, and nerves. Diffuse lymphoid tissue and pharyngeal tonsils (see above) will also be present in the lamina propria. The elastic fibers form a very dense layer at the outermost portion of the lamina propria, which would be the equivalent of a muscularis mucosae in the esophagus (see Chap. 12). Small, compound branched tubuloalveolar glands extend from the epithelium down into the lamina propria. The glands are of the mucous type in the lower levels of the nasopharynx lined with stratified squamous epithelium, but they are of the mixed type in the upper levels and their ducts are lined with ciliated epithelium.

Submucosa. This layer of loose connective tissue is only present in the lateral walls of the nasopharynx. It contains lymphoid tissue, small mucous glands, blood and lymphatic vessels, and nerves.

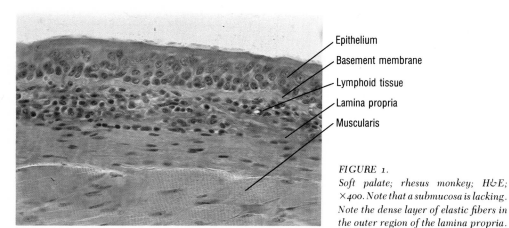

Epithelium
Basement membrane
Lymphoid tissue
Lamina propria
Muscularis

FIGURE 1.
Soft palate; rhesus monkey; H&E;
×400. Note that a submucosa is lacking.
Note the dense layer of elastic fibers in
the outer region of the lamina propria.

Muscularis. The muscularis is a relatively thick layer of striated muscle, where the fibers are organized into an inner longitudinal and outer circular layers.

Adventitia. At the upper level of the nasopharynx, where it is attached to the skull, the adventitia is a thin layer of relatively dense fibrous connective tissue, but at the lower levels it becomes less dense and indistinct.

OROPHARYNX. This region of the pharynx lies inferiorly to the nasopharynx and is continuous with it. It is located between the palatopharyngeal and palatoglossal arches and the cranial part of the epiglottis. The arches are two pairs of lateral folds at the entrance of the throat, separating the mouth from the pharynx; the passage between them is the fauces. A pair of *palatine tonsils* lie in the lateral walls of the oropharynx in tonsillar recesses between the palatopharyngeal and palatoglossal arches. Many small elevations, *lingual tonsils*, are located on the root of the tongue which extend back into the oropharynx.

Mucosa. The *epithelium* is stratified squamous and nonkeratinized; it lies on an indistinct basement membrane. The *lamina propria* is similar to that described in the nasopharynx, except small papillae of connective tissue lie below the epithelium, and solitary lymphoid nodules and mucous glands are present.

Submucosa. This layer is not present; therefore the lamina propria is attached directly to the muscularis.

Muscularis. This is similar to the nasopharynx (see above).

Adventitia. This is a relatively thin layer of loose connective tissue containing blood and lymphatic vessels and nerves.

LARYNGOPHARYNX. This most inferior region of the pharynx is continuous with the oropharynx and is located between the cranial part of the epiglottis and the esophagus.

Mucosa. Similar to the oropharynx (see above).

Submucosa. This is present as a layer of loose connective tissue containing small mucous glands, diffuse lymphoid tissue, blood and lymphatic vessels, and nerves.

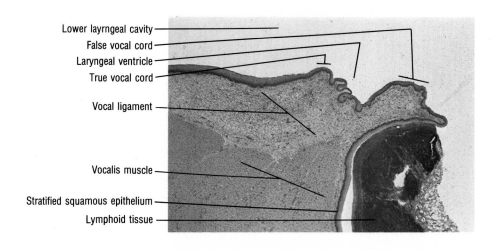

Lower layrngeal cavity
False vocal cord
Laryngeal ventricle
True vocal cord

Vocal ligament

Vocalis muscle

Stratified squamous epithelium

Lymphoid tissue

FIGURE 2.
Larynx (upper frontal section); cat;
H&E; ×40.

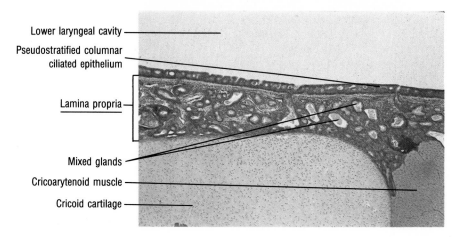

Lower laryngeal cavity
Pseudostratified columnar
ciliated epithelium

Lamina propria

Mixed glands

Cricoarytenoid muscle

Cricoid cartilage

FIGURE 3.
Larynx (lower frontal section); cat; H&
E; ×40. Note that a submucosa is lack-
ing. Ciliated ducts in the epithelium
drain the glands in the lamina propria.

Close to the esophagus, it becomes a more prominent layer. In places, the glands may extend into the muscularis.

Muscularis. Same as described in the nasopharynx (see above).

Adventitia. Similar to the oropharynx (see above).

Larynx

The larynx is located at the lower level of the pharynx (laryngopharynx). It is an irregularly shaped box lying between the trachea and pharynx. It functions as a valve, allowing only air to move between the pharynx and trachea, and is important in the production of vocal sounds. The laryngeal cavity, just below the flaplike epiglottis, is partially divided into three cavities (upper vestibule, middle ventricles, and lower larynx) by two parallel pairs of mucosal folds. The upper pair of folds (false vocal cords) separate the vestibule and ventricles, and the lower pair (true vocal cords or vocal folds) separate the ventricles from the lower larynx. The lower larynx is continuous with the lumen of the trachea. The laryngeal cavity is lined by a mucosa and its walls are composed of cartilagineous plates embedded in connective tissue. The plates are joined by ligaments and muscles. **Plate 2, Figs. 2 and 3.**

LARYNGEAL CARTILAGES. There are three large, single cartilages (thyroid, cricoid, and epiglottis) and three pairs of small ones (arytenoid, corniculate, and cuneiform). Only the epiglottis, corniculate, cuneiform, and arytenoid tips are composed of elastic cartilage, while the others are of hyaline cartilage. The cartilages provide strength to the larynx and maintain it as a hollow organ.

LARYNGEAL MUSCLES. Two types of skeletal muscles, extrinsic and intrinsic, are associated with the larynx. Extrinsic muscles insert on parts of the larynx from adjacent neck anatomy and their action will move the larynx during the process of swallowing. The intrinsic muscles interconnect the cartilages and constantly regulate the diameter of the laryngeal passages. They also place tension on the vocal cords which changes the pitch of the vocal sounds.

LARYNGEAL MUCOSA. The epithelium is stratified squamous and nonkeratinized at the upper levels of the larynx, but at the lower levels (below the vocal cords) it is pseudostratified columnar ciliated and contains goblet cells. The lamina propria contains collagen and elastic fibers, many small, mixed compound tubuloalveolar glands, lymphocytes, and some solitary lymphoid nodules. A submucosa is lacking.

The true vocal cords are folds of the mucosa, but here the lamina propria contains much elastic tissue, which is organized into cords (the vocal ligaments) and covered by stratified squamous nonkeratinized epithelium. An intrinsic striated muscle, the vocalis muscle, runs parallel and lateral to each vocal cord.

Trachea and primary bronchi

The trachea is a short (11 cm), moderately wide (2.5 cm) fibroelastic tube, supported and held open by C-shaped cartilages. It extends from the base of the larynx to the lungs where it divides into left and right primary bronchi. Jugular veins, carotid arteries, and vagus nerves lie lateral to the trachea. The esophagus rests on its posterior wall, and the isthmus of the thyroid crosses its anterior surface at the upper level. The wall of the trachea is divided into three layers: the inner mucosa, middle submucosa, and outer adventitia. **Plate 3, Figs. 1** and **2.**

Mucosa. The epithelium is pseudostratified columnar ciliated and has goblet cells scattered through it. Although six different types of epithelial cells may be identified with the electron microscope, only three can be readily identified with the light microscope: ciliated cells, goblet cells, and basal cells (see Chap. 2). The epithelium lies on a thick basement membrane containing a network of reticular and elastic fibers. The lamina propria is a relatively thin layer of reticular, collagen, and elastic fibers, blood vessels, small nerves, lymphatics, fibroblasts, lymphocytes, and some lymphoid tissue. In the outer region of the lamina propria, elastic fibers are organized into a dense longitudinal network, the *elastic membrane*. This membrane extends from the larynx down to the tertiary bronchi, separating the lamina propria from the submucosa.

Submucosa. This is a poorly organized layer of loose connective tissue containing mainly collagen fibers and some elastic fibers. It binds the lamina propria to the adventitia. Large nerves, vessels, fat cells, and many small, mixed compound tubuloalveolar glands are present. Short excretory ducts may be lined with cuboidal or low pyramidal cells which open onto the mucosal surface.

Adventitia. This layer of loose connective tissue is peripheral to the submucosa and continuous with the fascia of neck musculature and tissues of the mediastinum. In addition to the blood vessels, lymphatic vessels, lymph nodules, and nerves, the inner region of the adventitia contains 16 to 20 C-shaped or branched hyaline

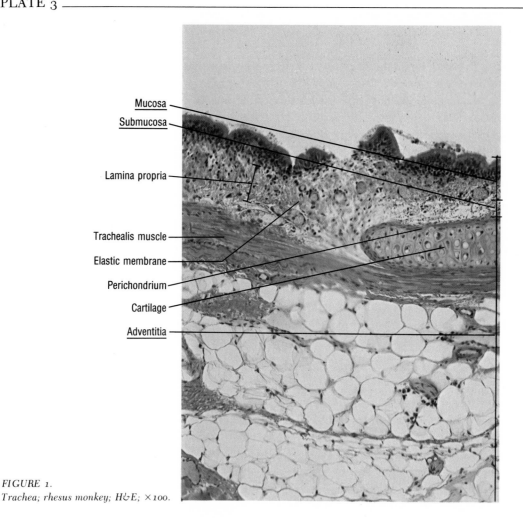

Mucosa
Submucosa

Lamina propria

Trachealis muscle

Elastic membrane

Perichondrium

Cartilage

Adventitia

FIGURE 1.
Trachea; rhesus monkey; H&E; ×100.

cartilage rings, evenly spaced along the length of the trachea. These cartilages are set off from the loose connective tissue of the adventitia by a fibroelastic membrane running between adjacent cartilages and continuous with the perichondrial layer. Between the open ends of each incomplete cartilage ring, the fibroelastic membrane is mixed with circumferentially oriented smooth muscle fibers, the *trachealis muscle*, which may represent an incomplete muscularis.

Compared to the trachea, the *primary bronchi* have a similar histologic organization, but differ in that the adventitial layer has fewer cartilaginous rings. The primary bronchi are approximately 1.2 to 1.8 cm in diameter.

Lungs

The paired lungs are conical lobed organs lying in the pleural cavities of the thorax. The pleural cavities are separated by a broad septum of connective tissue, the mediastinum, which is in the midline of the thorax and extends from the vertebral column anteriorly to the sternum, and from the diaphragm superiorly to the thoracic inlet. The mediastinum supports the esophagus, the heart and its associated vessels,

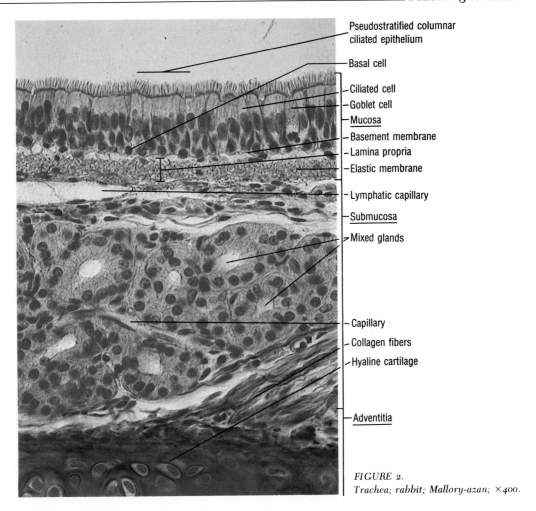

Pseudostratified columnar ciliated epithelium

Basal cell

Ciliated cell

Goblet cell

Mucosa

Basement membrane

Lamina propria

Elastic membrane

Lymphatic capillary

Submucosa

Mixed glands

Capillary

Collagen fibers

Hyaline cartilage

Adventitia

FIGURE 2.
Trachea; rabbit; Mallory-azan; ×400.

the thymus, the inferior end of the trachea, bronchi, and the roots of the lungs. On the medial mediastinal surface of each lung is a depression, the *hilus*, which receives the primary bronchi, large blood and lymphatic vessels, and nerves. The lung is covered by visceral pleura, a mesothelium lying on a dense layer of elastic and collagen fibers containing some smooth muscle. The lobes of the lung are divided into tiny, irregular lobules by connective tissue septa (interlobular septa) extending from the visceral pleura. The lobules consist of reticular and fibroelastic tissue, blood and lymphatic vessels, nerves, air passages, and alveoli.

As the bronchi extend into the lungs, they give rise to the air passages of the bronchial tree. Deeper in the lungs these air passages branch extensively and become smaller in diameter, and their walls become progressively thinner. The walls of the air passages in the upper regions of the bronchial tree are generally organized like the primary bronchi: an inner mucosa, middle submucosa, and outer adventitia. Given in their anatomic order, the structures of the bronchial tree concerned *only* with movement of air in the lungs are: the *secondary bronchi*, *tertiary bronchi*, *bronchioles*, and *terminal bronchioles*. The deeper structures concerned with *both* movement of air and gas exchange are the *respiratory bronchioles, alveolar ducts, alveolar sacs,* and *alveoli*.

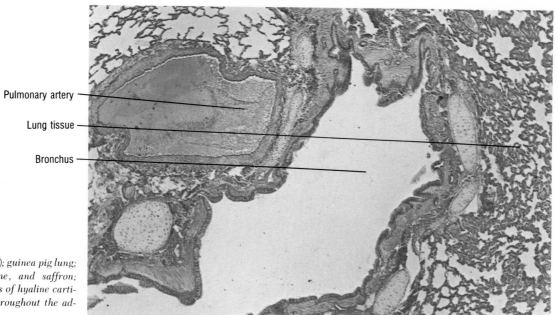

Pulmonary artery

Lung tissue

Bronchus

FIGURE 1.
Bronchus (secondary); guinea pig lung; hematoxylin, phloxine, and saffron; ×40. Note that plates of hyaline cartilage are scattered throughout the adventitia.

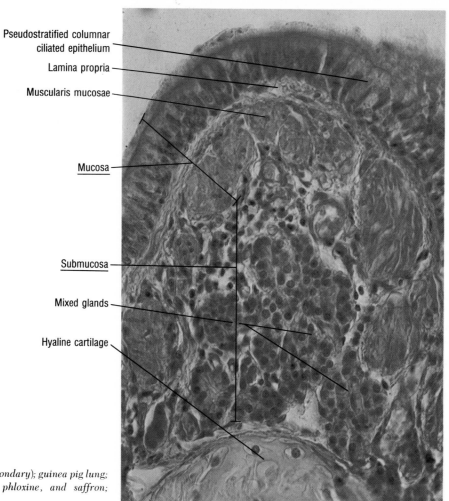

Pseudostratified columnar ciliated epithelium

Lamina propria

Muscularis mucosae

Mucosa

Submucosa

Mixed glands

Hyaline cartilage

FIGURE 2.
Bronchus (secondary); guinea pig lung; hematoxylin, phloxine, and saffron; ×400.

BRONCHI. (secondary and tertiary). These structures are larger than 1 mm in diameter, but smaller than the primary bronchi. **Plate 4, Figs. 1 and 2.**

Mucosa. In going from the larger secondary bronchus to the smaller tertiary bronchus, the tall pseudostratified columnar ciliated epithelium gradually becomes simple columnar ciliated. Goblet cells are abundant at all levels. The thin lamina propria is composed of reticular, elastic, and collagen fibers. The elastic membrane of the primary bronchi is represented here only by a few elastic fibers in the outer region of the lamina propria. It is mainly replaced by a prominent ring of spirally to circularly oriented smooth muscle tissue, the muscularis mucosae.

Submucosa. This layer is relatively consistent in both the secondary and tertiary bronchi, although it becomes thinner and has fewer glands at the lower levels. It is composed of a loose connective tissue containing compound tubuloalveolar seromucous glands with simple cuboidal epithelium lining their ducts, lymph nodules, capillaries, lymphatic vessels, and small nerves.

Adventitia. In the *secondary bronchi*, the adventitia is composed of a loose connective tissue in which a relatively dense fibroelastic membrane connects irregular hyaline cartilage plates. The C-shaped rings, characteristic of the primary bronchi, are no longer present. In the *tertiary bronchi*, the plates are smaller and scarcer, and portions of them may be filled with elastic fibers.

BRONCHIOLES AND TERMINAL BRONCHIOLES. Bronchioles range from about 0.5 to 1 mm in diameter. The smallest are designated as *terminal bronchioles*. Bronchioles are distinguished from bronchi by an absence of cartilage plates and glands. The muscularis mucosae is prominent, but the submucosa and adventitia are difficult to separate as distinct histologic layers. In the lower levels of the bronchial tree cartilage is no longer needed to keep the smaller air passages open, since elastic tissue is effective in maintaining this function. **Plate 5, Figs. 1 and 2.**

Mucosa. The largest bronchioles have a simple columnar ciliated epithelium containing some goblet cells. In the smaller bronchioles and terminal bronchioles, goblet cells are replaced by nonciliated Clara cells, which probably secrete a surfactant to reduce surface tension. These are serous cells which have a basophilic cytoplasm surrounding a large, round nucleus. The apical ends of the Clara cells are somewhat convex and bulge into the lumen of the bronchiole. The remaining epithelial cells appear as patches of low columnar or cuboidal ciliated epithelium among the Clara cells.

The muscularis mucosae is prominent and well developed in the larger bronchioles, but becomes discontinuous in the terminal bronchioles. The lamina propria contains reticular, elastic, and collagen fibers and becomes less prominent at the lower levels.

Submucosa and adventitia. The loose connective tissues of both of these layers blend so that it is difficult to identify them as separate entities. Although the composition of the tissue is relatively uniform at the upper and lower levels of the bronchioles, it becomes thinner at the lower levels. There are no glands, lymph nodules, cartilage, or fibroelastic membranes in either of these layers. Blood and lymphatic vessels and nerves are present.

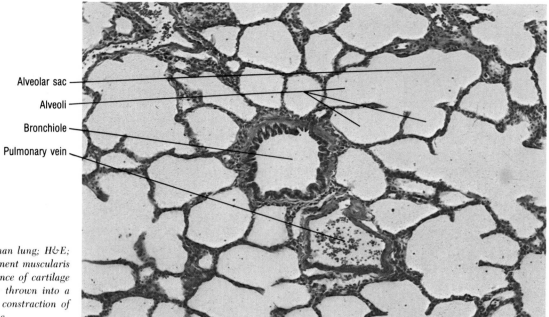

Alveolar sac

Alveoli

Bronchiole

Pulmonary vein

FIGURE 1.
Small bronchiole; human lung; H&E;
×100. Note the prominent muscularis
mucosae and the absence of cartilage
plates. The mucosa is thrown into a
series of folds by the constraction of
the muscularis mucosae.

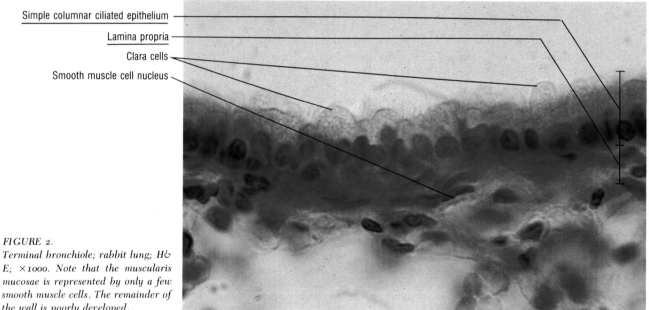

Simple columnar ciliated epithelium

Lamina propria

Clara cells

Smooth muscle cell nucleus

FIGURE 2.
Terminal bronchiole; rabbit lung; H&
E; ×1000. Note that the muscularis
mucosae is represented by only a few
smooth muscle cells. The remainder of
the wall is poorly developed.

RESPIRATORY BRONCHIOLES. These are the smallest bronchioles (0.1 to 0.5 mm
in diameter). They are thin-walled, short, branched tubes which are continuous with
the terminal bronchioles and give rise to alveolar ducts. Alveoli project from the
walls of the respiratory bronchioles and are scattered along their length. The wall

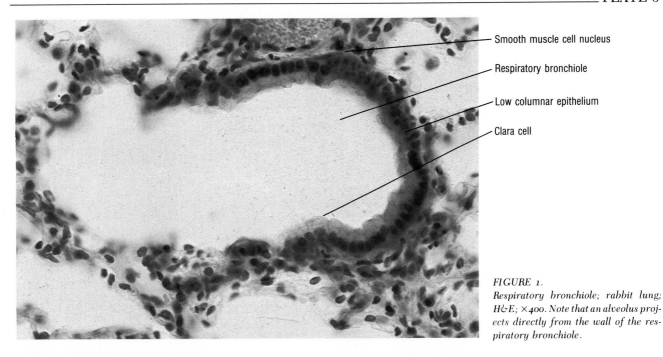

Smooth muscle cell nucleus

Respiratory bronchiole

Low columnar epithelium

Clara cell

FIGURE 1.
Respiratory bronchiole; rabbit lung;
H&E; ×400. Note that an alveolus proj-
ects directly from the wall of the res-
piratory bronchiole.

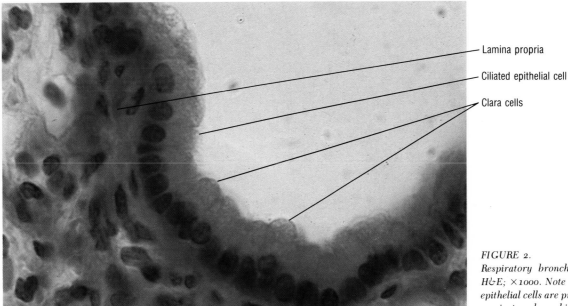

Lamina propria

Ciliated epithelial cell

Clara cells

FIGURE 2.
Respiratory bronchiole; rabbit lung;
H&E; ×1000. Note that a few ciliated
epithelial cells are present in the larger
respiratory bronchioles.

is lined by a simple cuboidal or low columnar epithelium containing Clara cells (see above). Some scattered ciliated cells are present in the larger ducts. The remainder of the wall is composed of blood and lymphatic vessels, nerves, and smooth muscle cells scattered between collagen and elastic fibers. **Plate 6, Figs. 1** and **2.**

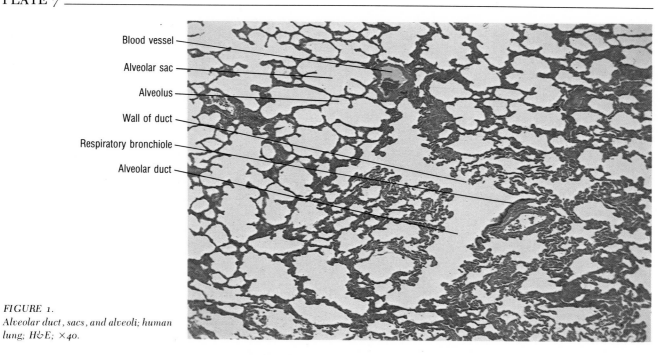

Blood vessel
Alveolar sac
Alveolus
Wall of duct
Respiratory bronchiole
Alveolar duct

FIGURE 1.
Alveolar duct, sacs, and alveoli; human
lung; H&E; ×40.

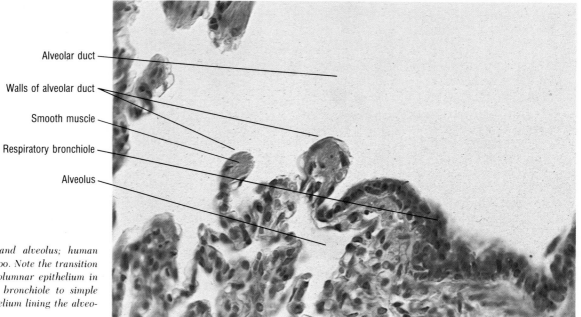

Alveolar duct
Walls of alveolar duct
Smooth muscle
Respiratory bronchiole
Alveolus

FIGURE 2.
Alveolar duct and alveolus; human
lung; H&E; ×400. Note the transition
of the simple columnar epithelium in
the respiratory bronchiole to simple
squamous epithelium lining the alveo-
lar duct.

ALVEOLAR DUCTS. These are thin-walled, long, narrow (0.1 mm in diameter) tubes which are continuous with respiratory bronchioles. Their walls are perforated by numerous openings leading to alveoli and alveolar sacs. The discontinuous wall, between alveoli and sacs, may appear as spherical clumps of tissue covered with an indistinct simple squamous epithelium. The clumps contain smooth muscle, elastic and collagen fibers, vessels, and nerves. The smooth muscle forms a ring around the entrance of an alveolus or alveolar sac leading to an alveolar duct. **Plate 7, Figs. 1 and 2.**

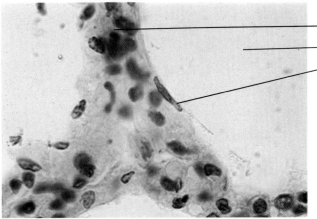

— Alveolar septum

— Alveolar cavity

— Squamous alveolar cell

FIGURE 1.
Squamous alveolar cell; Human lung;
H&E; ×1000.

ALVEOLAR SAC. This is an aggregation of alveoli, all of which open onto a common lumen. The lumen of the sac may open directly onto an alveolar duct or an antrum, which is a terminal branch of an alveolar duct. Where alveoli are pressed together, their adjacent walls form an alveolar septum. The cavities of adjacent alveoli are interconnected by tiny (about 12 μm diameter) alveolar pores in the septum and may be important as auxiliary ventilating pathways. **Plate 5, Fig. 1; Plate 7, Fig. 1.**

ALVEOLI. An alveolus is a small (100 to 300 μm), thin-walled chamber opening either into an alveolar sac, alveolar duct, or respiratory bronchiole (see above). The wall is covered with a simple squamous epithelium and composed of a loose network of reticular fibers, elastic fibers, and some collagen fibers containing fibroblasts, macrophages, and lymphocytes. Numerous capillaries wind through the fibers and lie close to the alveolar epithelium. The basal laminae of cells in the alveolar epithelium and endothelial cells in the capillaries fuse to form an extremely thin layer over which gasses may diffuse. Three types of cells can be distinguished in the alveolar epithelium; squamous alveolar cells, great alveolar cells, and alveolar phagocytes. **Plate 5, Fig. 1; Plate 7, Figs. 1 and 2; Plate 8, Figs. 1, 2, and 3.**

Squamous alveolar cells (membranous pneumocytes, type I cells). The cells are large but extremely thin, so the cytoplasm is indistinguishable. The small, flat nuclei can only be seen as widely separated structures in any one section. The diffusion of gases between alveolar air and blood within the capillaries occurs through these cells. **Plate 8, Fig. 1.**

Great alveolar cells (granular pneumocytes, type II cells). These cells, like the squamous alveolar cells, sit directly on a basal lamina. They are relatively numerous both on the surface or deep within niches of the alveolar wall. In the latter case, the cells appear below the squamous alveolar cells. The cells are irregularly shaped or cuboidal, may bulge into the lumen, and may appear separately or in groups. The cytoplasm is pale acidophilic and vacuolated, and contains tiny (0.2 to 1.0 μm diameter) inclusions. Microvilli are present and may be seen as a faint striated border. The large, round, vesicular, pale-stained nucleus is quite prominent.

The cytoplasmic inclusions, or cytosomes, are tiny oval bodies composed of phospholipids, proteins, and gylcosaminoglycans. As these substances are released, they form a thin film over the surface of the epithelium. The phospholipids are surfactants which reduce surface tension and resist collapse of the alveolus. **Plate 8, Fig. 2.**

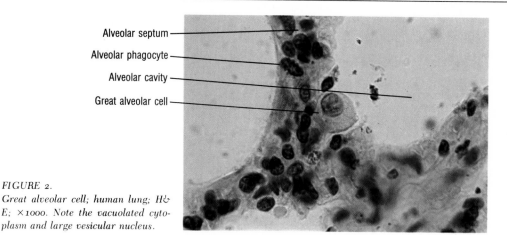

Alveolar septum
Alveolar phagocyte
Alveolar cavity
Great alveolar cell

FIGURE 2.
Great alveolar cell; human lung; H&
E; ×1000. Note the vacuolated cyto-
plasm and large vesicular nucleus.

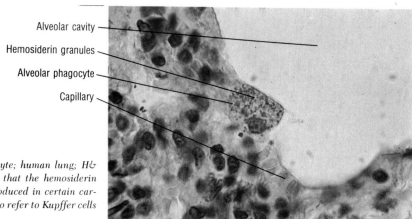

Alveolar cavity
Hemosiderin granules
Alveolar phagocyte
Capillary

FIGURE 3.
Alveolar phagocyte; human lung; H&
E; ×1000. Note that the hemosiderin
granules are produced in certain cardiac diseases (also refer to Kupffer cells
in Chap. 12).

Alveolar phagocytes (dust cells). The cells of this type resemble wandering macrophages (see Chap. 3) and scavenge the epithelium as they migrate over its surface.
The irregular, amoeboid, vacuolated cytoplasm is usually filled with ingested particles
mostly from inspired air, or hemosiderin granules (see page 214). The relatively
small, moderately dark-stained nucleus is usually eccentrically positioned in the cytoplasm. Although the origin of alveolar phagocytes is uncertain, some studies indicate
that they probably are derived from monocytes or macrophages which have migrated
to the alveolar epithelium from tissues in the alveolar wall. Once the phagocytes
become filled with debris, they may either move up the respiratory tubes to be
expectorated or migrate through the alveolar wall tissue to reach the lymphatic
system. **Plate 8, Fig. 3.**

BLOOD AND LYMPHATIC VESSELS. Pulmonary arteries carry venous blood from the
right ventricle of the heart to the lungs. They follow the tubes of the bronchial tree
and terminate as capillary beds in the alveolar walls. After an exchange of oxygen
and carbon dioxide between alveolar air and blood, pulmonary venules collect
oxygenated blood from the capillaries, and then veins carry it from the alveoli to the
left atrium of the heart. In addition, these veins carry oxygenated blood from visceral
pleura and alveolar ducts as well as unoxygenated blood from bronchial veins. The

smaller venules and veins do not follow the bronchial tree, but are isolated in connective tissue septa within the lungs; only the larger pulmonary veins accompany the bronchi and pulmonary arteries.

Bronchial arteries carry blood from the aorta to the bronchial tree, as deep as the respiratory bronchioles. These vessels lie within submucosal tissues and supply the lamina propria with plexuses of capillaries. The plexuses are then drained by bronchopulmonary (bronchial) veins into the pulmonary veins. Bronchial arteries also anastomose directly with pulmonary arteries and, via shunts, indirectly with pulmonary veins. The extrapulmonary bronchi (outside the lungs), visceral pleura, and the hilar region of the lungs are drained by bronchial veins directly into the azygos vein on the right side. On the left side, they drain into the superior intercostal or accessory hemiazygos veins. Histologically, all bronchial vessels are typical systemic vessels (see Chap. 9). The extrapulmonary vessels lie on the bronchial tubes, while the intrapulmonary vessels lie mainly within the walls of the bronchial tubes.

There are two *lymphatic drainage systems* which are interconnected in certain regions of the lung: the superficial and deep systems. The superficial lymphatic system drains the visceral pleura and interlobular septa, while the deep system drains the alveolar ducts and all upper portions of the bronchial tree. These structures are first drained by plexuses of lymphatic capillaries which become prominent lymphatic collecting vessels as lymph is moved toward the hilus. Although the two systems interconnect at various points, they become confluent at the hilus and enter the hilar lymph nodes.

NERVES. Sympathetic nerves and parasympathetic branches of the vagus nerve innervate glands and smooth muscles of the bronchial tree. The parasympathetic nerves control the constriction of air passages, and sympathetic nerves bring about the opposite effect, a dilation.

Urinary System 14

The urinary system is composed of urine-producing organs, the *kidneys*, and urinary passages: *ureters*, *bladder*, and *urethra*. The kidneys filter and selectively reabsorb substances from the blood. The resulting filtrate, urine, is collected by calyces and renal pelves and then transported to the urinary bladder by paired ureters. Elimination of urine from the bladder occurs through the urethra. Except for the urethra, the anatomy of the urinary system is similar in both the male and female.

The kidneys maintain homeostasis of the body by regulating ion concentration, pH, and the volume of body fluids. They also function to eliminate waste metabolic end products, mainly nitrogenous substances such as urea.

Kidneys

The kidneys are paired retroperitoneal organs, located in the dorsal lumbar region of the body. They are about 11 cm long by 5 cm wide and have a medial concave surface, the *hilus*. The space at the hilus is the slitlike *renal sinus*, through which blood and lymphatic vessels, nerves, and the ureter enter the kidney. Each kidney is covered externally by a dense, irregular collagenous connective tissue *capsule*. The renal parenchyma is organized into an outer *cortex* and an inner *medulla*. Under a low power of the light microscope the stained cortex appears dark and granular, while the medulla is pale and striated. The medullary tissue forms approximately 8 to 18 conical *renal pyramids*. Their apices, or *papillae*, point medially toward the hilus and are drained by minor calyces. Some medullary tissue, the *medullary rays*, extend from the base of each pyramid laterally into the cortex. Although the cortex is a continuous peripheral layer of the kidney, some of its tissue extends medially, as *renal columns*, between adjacent pyramids. A pyramid and its peripherally associated cortex is considered a lobe, but its superficial boundaries can only be determined in the fetal stage. Each lobe is composed of many vascularized tubular *nephrons*, which are the basic excretory units and form the parenchyma of the kidney. Small blood vessels, the peritubular capillaries, are intimately associated with the nephrons and are important in the excretory function. **Plate 1, Fig. 1.**

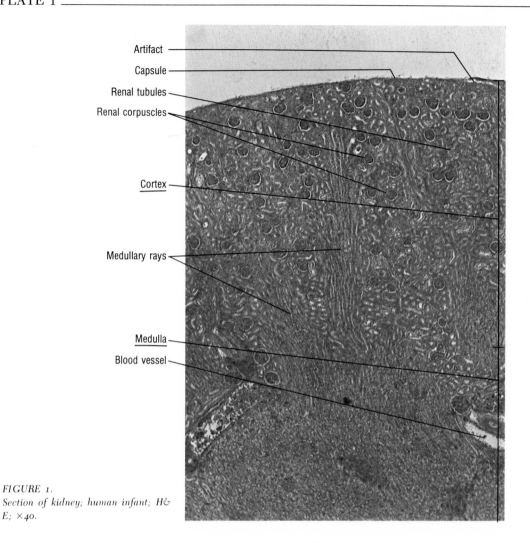

Artifact
Capsule
Renal tubules
Renal corpuscles
Cortex
Medullary rays
Medulla
Blood vessel

FIGURE 1.
Section of kidney; human infant; H&
E; ×40.

NEPHRON. The nephron is composed of several distinct histologic segments which are indicated in **Table 1** and **Plate 1, Fig. 2.** These segments are present in the cortex, medulla, medullary rays, and renal columns. The position of the nephron in the cortex (peripheral to or near the corticomedullary junction) will influence its structure and relative amounts of the segments. The major variations are apparent in Henle's loop. If the nephron lies high in the cortex, it may have a short, thick Henle's loop which may not extend far into the medulla, or have a short, thin segment on the descending limb of Henle's loop. A nephron that lies near the medulla will have a long, thin segment of Henle's loop that dips far into the medulla. You may find all variations between these extremes. Nephrons and their associated blood vessels lie in a renal interstitium of delicate fibers, fibroblasts, and fluids.

In Table 1 the segments of the nephron are listed in order, as urine is produced in the renal corpuscle and passes toward the collecting tubules for excretion. The regions of the kidney are also indicated where the segments are most commonly located. The loop of Henle has a structural U-shaped loop where that portion of the nephron turns back on itself. Actually, the collecting tubules should not be considered as part of the nephron since they have a different embryonic origin, the *ureteric bud*, while segments of the nephron are derived from *metanephrogenic tissue*.

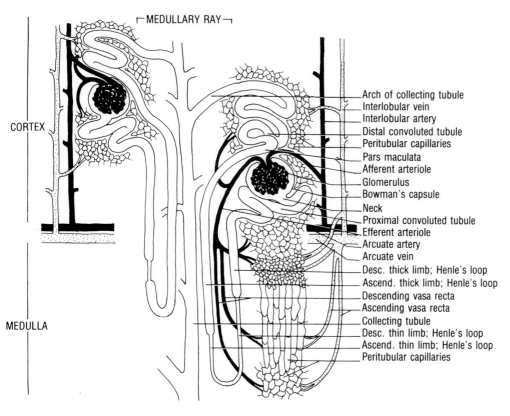

┌MEDULLARY RAY┐

CORTEX

MEDULLA

Arch of collecting tubule
Interlobular vein
Interlobular artery
Distal convoluted tubule
Peritubular capillaries
Pars maculata
Afferent arteriole
Glomerulus
Bowman's capsule
Neck
Proximal convoluted tubule
Efferent arteriole
Arcuate artery
Arcuate vein
Desc. thick limb; Henle's loop
Ascend. thick limb; Henle's loop
Descending vasa recta
Ascending vasa recta
Collecting tubule
Desc. thin limb; Henle's loop
Ascend. thin limb; Henle's loop
Peritubular capillaries

FIGURE 2.

Schematic drawing of a cortical nephron (left) and juxtaglomerular nephron (right) in the human kidney. Note that not all of the vasa recta or pericapillary tubules are shown. Arteries are thick black lines, capillaries are thin black lines, and veins are stippled. (The drawing was modified from J. Fourman and D. Moffat, The Blood Vessels of the Kidney, Blackwell Scientific Publications, Oxford, 1971.)

TABLE 1
Histologic segments of the nephron

Renal corpuscle	Glomerulus (cortex)	
	Bowman's capsule (cortex)	
Neck (cortex)	Proximal convoluted tubule (cortex)	
Proximal tubule	Straight descending limb, thick segment (medulla, medullary ray)	
Thin segment of	Descending limb, thin segment (medulla)	Loop of
Henle's loop	Ascending limb, thin segment (medulla)	Henle
	Straight ascending limb, thick segment (medulla, medullary ray, cortex)	
Distal tubule	Pars maculata (cortex)	
	Distal convoluted tubule (cortex)	
Collecting tubule	Collecting tubules (medulla, medullary ray)	

Renal corpuscle. This is a large spherical body lying in the cortex of the kidney. It is composed of a vascular *glomerulus* which is surrounded by a double walled cup, *Bowman's capsule.* The corpuscles are scattered throughout the cortex and separated from each other by tubular segments of the nephrons. Each renal corpuscle is responsible for a high filtration pressure of blood and subsequent collection of the filtrate. The filtrate, or urine, is similar in composition to plasma, except it lacks the large proteins. **Plate 1, Fig. 1; Plate 2, Figs. 1, 2, and 3.**

Glomerulus

Bowman's capsule

Renal tubules

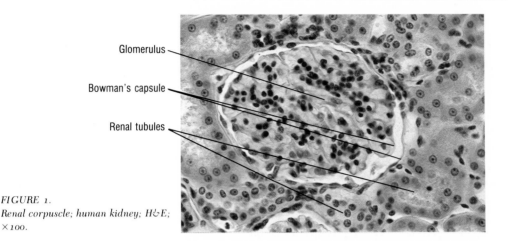

FIGURE 1.
Renal corpuscle; human kidney; H&E;
×100.

GLOMERULUS. This is composed of several lobes of capillary plexuses which join afferent and efferent arterioles (see below). At the base of each lobe there is a group of supporting cells, the *mesangium*, the function of which is unknown. The mesangium is difficult to distinguish in routine preparations and is composed of small cells (possibly pericytes) embedded within an amorphous matrix. The cells have a small, dark nucleus and fibrous cytoplasmic processes which may contact the endothelium of a capillary. Most, but not all of the endothelial cells have tiny (800 Å diameter) open pores in their cytoplasm to facilitate filtration. The afferent arterioles enter and efferent arterioles leave the renal corpuscle at a common point, the *vascular pole*. By their contraction and restriction of blood flow, the efferent arterioles can sustain a high filtration pressure within the capillary plexuses. **Plate , Fig. .**

BOWMAN'S CAPSULE. This capsule is a double-layered cup of simple squamous epithelium. It almost completely surrounds the glomerulus, except at the vascular pole. Both epithelial layers lie on a basement membrane. The inner *visceral layer* covers the glomerular capillaries while the outer *parietal layer* is separated from the visceral layer by a cavity, *Bowman's space*. The visceral layer, which is more difficult to distinguish, is composed of specialized *podocyte* cells. **Plate 2, Fig. 1; Plate 2, Fig. 2.** These are stellate cells which project into Bowman's space and only their cytoplasmic processes rest on the basement membrane. Podocyte cells have a large, pale, irregularly shaped nucleus. Cytoplasmic processes, the *pedicels*, form a loose interdigitating network along the basement membrane through which molecules with a molecular weight of less than 70,000 may be filtered from the blood. The filtrate, or urine, is collected in Bowman's space. Urine averages about 180 liters/day filtration from both kidneys, but about 99 percent is reabsorbed by various segments of the nephrons, leaving about 1.5 liters/day total volume to be excreted.

Neck. This is a continuation of the parietal layer of Bowman's capsule. It is drawn out into a relatively short, narrow neck of cuboidal cells. The neck is opposite the vascular pole and forms the urinary pole. **Plate 1, Fig. 2; Plate 2, Fig. 3.**

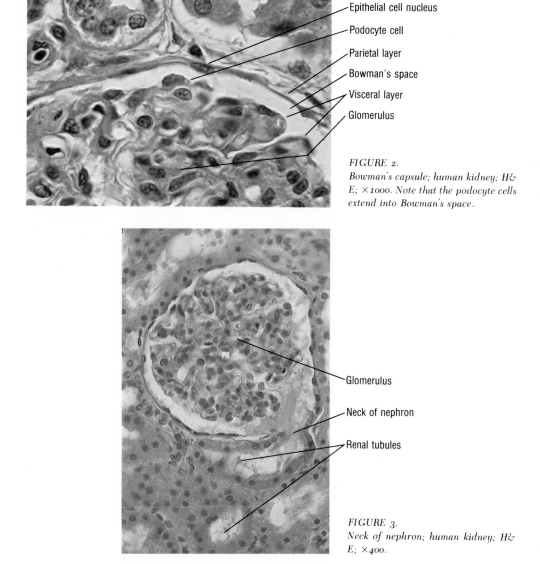

Epithelial cell nucleus

Podocyte cell

Parietal layer

Bowman's space

Visceral layer

Glomerulus

FIGURE 2.
Bowman's capsule; human kidney; H&
E; ×1000. Note that the podocyte cells
extend into Bowman's space.

Glomerulus

Neck of nephron

Renal tubules

FIGURE 3.
Neck of nephron; human kidney; H&
E; ×400.

Proximal tubule. This portion of the nephron is continuous with the neck and is divided into (1) a *proximal convoluted tubule*, and (2 a *straight, thick descending limb of the loop of Henle*. Histologically, it is usually difficult to distinguish between these two segments, except for location in the kidney and height of the epithelium. The proximal convoluted tubule is only present in the cortex, near the renal corpuscles, and has a tall epithelium. The straight, thick descending limb occurs in the medullary ray and medulla and has a similar but lower epithelium lining the tubule.

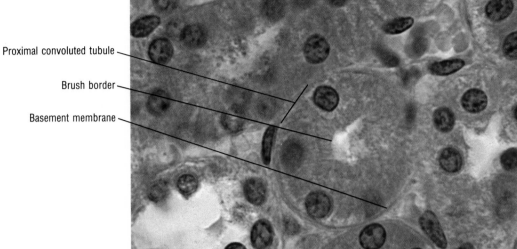

Proximal convoluted tubule

Brush border

Basement membrane

FIGURE 1.
Proximal convoluted tubule; human kidney; H&E; ×1000. Note the few tall epithelial cells composing the tubule wall, and the deep acidophilic cytoplasm.

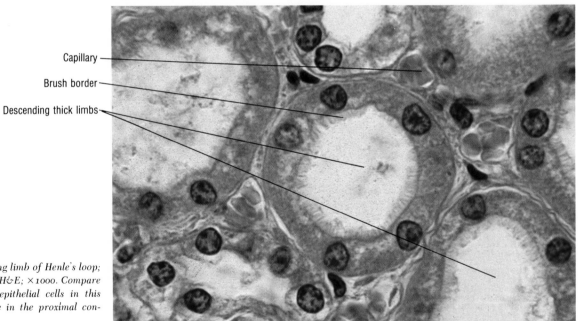

Capillary

Brush border

Descending thick limbs

FIGURE 2.
Thick descending limb of Henle's loop; human kidney; H&E; ×1000. Compare the height of epithelial cells in this tubule to those in the proximal convoluted tubule.

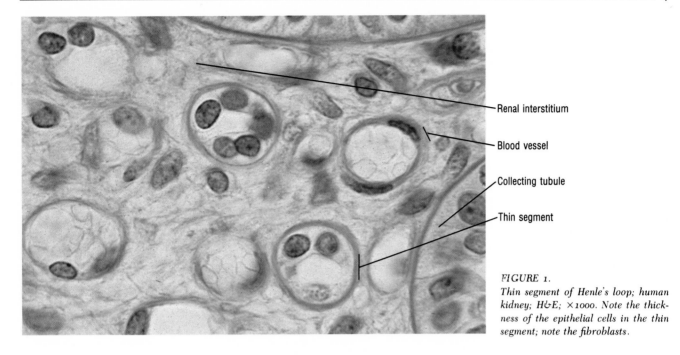

Renal interstitium

Blood vessel

Collecting tubule

Thin segment

FIGURE 1.
Thin segment of Henle's loop; human kidney; H&E; ×1000. Note the thickness of the epithelial cells in the thin segment; note the fibroblasts.

In cross section the tubules may appear somewhat irregular and are approximately 30 to 60 μm in diameter. There are three to four pyramid-shaped epithelial cells sitting on a porous basement membrane. Each cell has an abundant, deeply stained, acidophilic cytoplasm. Detail is usually lacking, and cell boundaries cannot be seen because they are difficult to preserve. The basal portion of the cytoplasm may have faint longitudinal striations (formed by mitochondria), while the apical portion has a fuzzy brush border (microvilli). The nucleus is large and round, and is centrally positioned in the cytoplasm; it has a prominent nucleolus. **Plate 1, Fig. 2; Plate 3, Figs. 1 and 2.**

Thin segment of Henle's loop. This segment of a nephron is highly variable, depending on the position of the nephron in the cortex. It may be absent, short, or long with descending and ascending limbs. It is the portion of the nephron where a U-shaped loop is formed as the tubule turns back on itself. The thin segment is located in the medulla, and even though ascending and descending limbs may be present, they cannot be distinguished histologically. In cross section, the thin segment appears much like a capillary, but the simple squamous epithelial cells forming the tubules are thicker (1 to 2 μm) and more numerous (three to five), and the pale cytoplasm appears more prominent. Also, the tubule is wider than a capillary, about 20 μm in diameter. **Plate 1, Fig. 2; Plate 4, Fig. 1.**

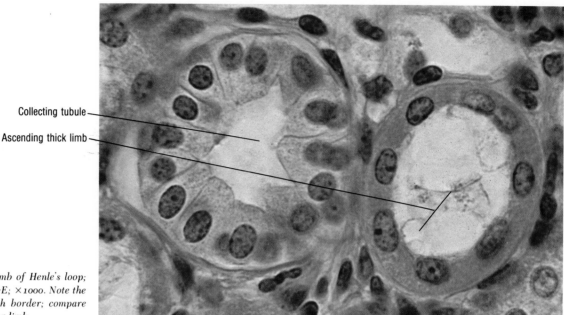

Collecting tubule

Ascending thick limb

FIGURE 2.
Thick ascending limb of Henle's loop;
human kidney; H&E; ×1000. Note the
absence of a brush border; compare
with the descending limb.

Distal tubule. The distal tubule is continuous with the thin segment of Henle's loop. It has three morphological regions, each with specific excretory functions. The three regions are: (1) straight, thick ascending limb of Henle's loop; (2 pars maculata; (3) distal convoluted tubule. **Plate 1, Fig. 2.**

STRAIGHT, THICK ASCENDING LIMB OF HENLE'S LOOP. This tubule is continuous with the thin segment of Henle's loop and is wider (20 to 50 μm). It is located in the cortex, medullary rays, and medulla. Compared to the proximal tubule, a cross section of the straight, thick ascending limb of Henle's loop is more irregular in outline and has a wider lumen; it has many (five to eight) low cuboidal cells; the cytoplasm is less acidophilic; plasma membranes are more distinct; and the cells lack brush borders. **Plate 1, Fig. 2; Plate 4, Fig. 2.**

PARS MACULATA. This region of the distal tubule is located in the cortex, near the afferent arteriole, as it enters the renal corpuscle. It is characterized by a cluster of tall, narrow epithelial cells whose crowded nuclei appear as a compact group, the *macula densa.* The cells of the macula densa, along with modified smooth muscle cells of adjacent afferent arterioles, the *juxtaglomerular cells,* form part of a juxtaglomerular apparatus. The juxtaglomerular cells are large, elongate, and usually poorly stained. Their pale basophilic cytoplasm lacks myofibrils but contains secretory granules and a rounded nucleus. **Plate 5, Fig. 1.**

When there is a decrease in plasma volume, the juxtaglomerular apparatus becomes functional by regulating the release of *renin,* an enzyme produced and stored in the juxtaglomerular cells. Renin will initiate a series of biochemical changes in which a plasma protein, angiotensinogen, is converted to a decapeptide, angiotensin I. Angiotensin I is then converted by a second enzyme (produced in the lungs) to angiotensin II, an octapeptide which is a vasoconstrictor. Angiotensin II is also a hormone which stimulates aldosterone production in the zona glomerulosa of the adrenal cortex. Aldersterone will bring about sodium reabsorption and potassium excretion by the distal convoluted tubules. The combined physiologic characteristics

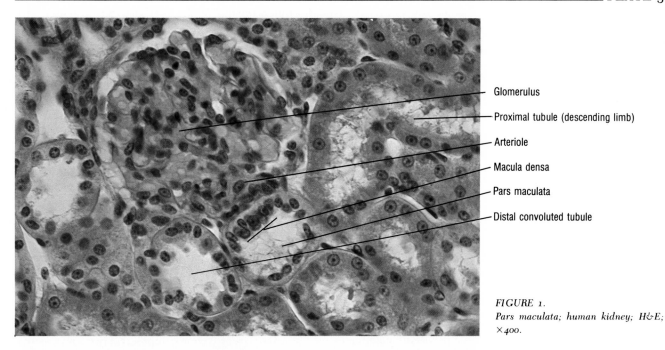

— Glomerulus

— Proximal tubule (descending limb)

— Arteriole

— Macula densa

— Pars maculata

— Distal convoluted tubule

FIGURE 1.
Pars maculata; human kidney; H&E; ×400.

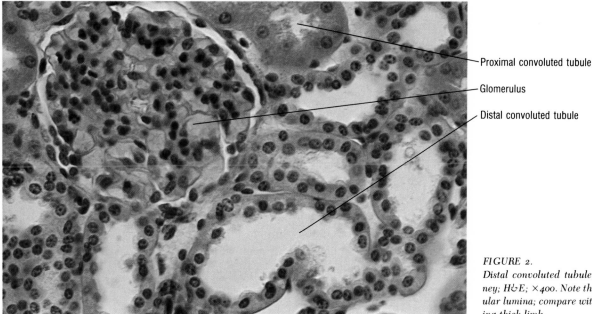

— Proximal convoluted tubule

— Glomerulus

— Distal convoluted tubule

FIGURE 2.
Distal convoluted tubule; human kidney; H&E; ×400. Note the wide, irregular lumina; compare with the ascending thick limb.

of angiotensin II are effective in counteracting fluid loss from the body and a corresponding decrease in blood pressure.

DISTAL CONVOLUTED TUBULE. Histologically, this most distal portion of the nephron is somewhat like the straight, thick ascending limb of Henle's loop (see above); and it is therefore difficult to distinguish between the two. The convoluted tubule, however, is located in the cortex near the renal corpuscles, has a larger lumen, and is quite irregular in outline because of its convolutions. **Plate 1, Fig. 2; Plate 5, Fig. 2.**

Collecting tubules. These tubules collect urine from many distal convoluted tubules in the cortex and carry it through the renal pyramids to the papillae, where it is collected by the minor calyces. The collecting tubules are arched in the cortex and straight and unbranched in the outer regions of the medulla, but are somewhat branched and unite with other collecting tubules near the renal papilla.

In cross section the tubules are circular, and are about 50 to 250 μm in diameter. The epithelium is low cuboidal in the small collecting tubules but tall columnar in the larger ones. The largest tubules within the papilla are the *papillary ducts of Bellini*, which are lined with transitional epithelium. **Plate 6, Fig. 3.** A majority of the epithelial cells, *principal cells*, lining the collecting tubules have distinct, sharp boundaries, pale cytoplasm, bulging convex apical ends, and a prominent, round nucleus containing a nucleolus. Some of the cells, *dark cells*, have a deep acidophilic cytoplasm and are scattered among the principal cells. The dark cells occur in collecting tubules within the cortex and outer medullary regions of the kidney and may be important in the acidification of urine. **Plate 6, Figs. 1 and 2.**

FORMATION OF URINE: ITS CONCENTRATION AND DILUTION. Nephrons lie within an osmotic gradient in the renal tissue where the osmotic pressure (sodium ion concentration) is lowest in the cortex and highest in the renal papillae. The importance of this gradient is to concentrate urine by osmotically withdrawing water as the urine passes through the thin segments of the descending limb of Henle's loop, distal convoluted tubules, and collecting tubules. The osmotic gradient is established and maintained by a countercurrent system composed of two components, working in concert and simultaneously: portions of Henle's loop, *countercurrent multipliers*, and the vasa recta blood vessels, *countercurrent exchangers*. The thin and thick segments of the ascending limb of Henle's loop are the countercurrent multipliers. They pump only sodium ions into renal interstitial spaces, since their epithelium is impermeable to water. These ions, along with sodium ions diffusing from the descending limb of Henle's loop, form the source for the osmotic gradient.

Efferent arterioles of nephrons located near the medullary border run deep into the medulla. They accompany the loop of Henle and, in a similar fashion, form a loop with descending (arteriolae rectae) and ascending (venae rectae) limbs. These are the vasa recta and function as countercurrent exchangers. They maintain the osmotic gradient by not allowing sodium to be removed from the concentrated areas of the renal interstitium. As blood flows down the descending limbs of the vasa recta, deep in the medulla, it becomes increasingly concentrated as sodium ions diffuse into it from the concentrated interstitial fluids. As the blood flows toward the cortex in the ascending limbs, through less concentrated regions, the sodium ions diffuse back out of the blood and remain within the renal interstitium. The specific steps for the formation of urine are outlined in the following steps.

1 Blood is carried into the glomerulus by afferent arterioles. Within the glomerular capillaries the hydrostatic blood pressure is about 90 mmHg, the colloidal osmotic pressure of blood is about 25 mmHg, and the capsular hydrostatic pressure is about 15 mmHg; therefore the net filtration pressure is about 50 mmHg. With this high pressure, substances in the plasma are filtered through the endothelial fenestrae and basal lamina of the glomerular capillaries, then through the podocyte fenestrae of Bowman's capsule, and finally into Bowman's space. The filtrate, or urine, will be of the same composition as the plasma, except for the large proteins, since molecules of 70,000 molecular weight or less are filterable. The urine is isoosmotic to blood plasma and contains glucose, amino acids, acetoacetic acid, ascorbic acid, inorganic ions, urea, creatine, and water.

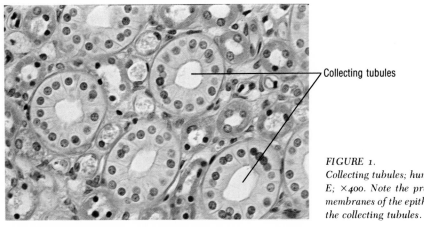

Collecting tubules

FIGURE 1.
Collecting tubules; human kidney; H&E; ×400. Note the prominent plasma membranes of the epithelial cells lining the collecting tubules.

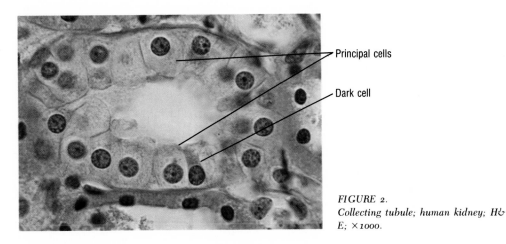

Principal cells

Dark cell

FIGURE 2.
Collecting tubule; human kidney; H&E; ×1000.

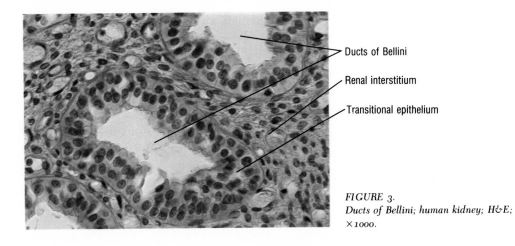

Ducts of Bellini

Renal interstitium

Transitional epithelium

FIGURE 3.
Ducts of Bellini; human kidney; H&E; ×1000.

2 As urine passes through the *proximal tubule* (proximal convoluted tubule and straight, thick descending limb of Henle's loop), most of the substances are reabsorbed by the epithelium. Here, they pass into the renal interstitium of the cortex and eventually enter the peritubular capillaries surrounding the tubules. Although the urine becomes concentrated, it remains isotonic to the fluids of the renal interstitium. Reabsorption occurs by: (1) *active transport* (using energy to move substances across the plasma membrane) of glucose, amino acids, small proteins, acetoacetic acid, water-soluble vitamins, and most ions; (2) *passive diffusion* of water (osmotic gradient), urea and uric acid (concentration gradient), and chloride ions (electrical gradient). Chloride ions are electrically attracted to sodium ions in the interstitial fluids and move passively through the walls of the tubule, while water moves by osmosis. As water leaves the urine, urea and uric acid become so concentrated that some of these nitrogenous waste products diffuse back into the plasma. In addition to reabsorption, the proximal tubule secretes hydrogen ions, organic acids, and bases.

3 As the urine flows down the *descending limb of the thin segment of Henle's loop*, it becomes more concentrated and hypertonic compared to the urine in the proximal tubule. This concentration occurs as water diffuses into the interstitial fluids of the medulla which have a higher osmolarity than urine. In the deepest portion of the medulla, where the osmolarity of interstitial fluids is greatest, the highly concentrated urine is isotonic to these fluids.

4 As the urine flows through the *ascending thin limb of Henle's loop*, it becomes dilute and hypotonic to the interstitial fluids. This happens because the epithelium is impervious to water but sodium ions are actively pumped into the renal interstitium.

5 As urine flows up the *straight, thick ascending limb of Henle's loop*, it remains dilute and hypotonic, since only sodium ions and not water are removed. This is similar to the condition in the ascending thin limb.

6 The dilute urine, as it flows through the *distal convoluted tubules* and *collecting tubules*, may or may not be concentrated according to the physiologic needs of the body. The permeability of the epithelium to water is under the control of the antidiuretic hormone (ADH), released by the neurohypophysis of the pituitary gland (see Chap. 17). In the presence of a high concentration of this hormone in the blood, the epithelial cells lining these tubules become very permeable to water. As water is osmotically drawn into the renal interstitium, the urine becomes concentrated and hypertonic. If there is an absence or low concentration of ADH, the cells are impermeable to water and the urine remains dilute and hypotonic.

The distal convoluted tubules also reabsorb sodium and excrete potassium ions, and are important for the regulation of the acid-base balance of body fluids. This regulation involves a simultaneous absorption of sodium and bicarbonate ions and excretion of hydrogen ions. Although urine is normally acidic because of the hydrogen ions, phosphate buffers and ammonia (secreted by the tubule epithelium) prevent it from becoming too acidic.

BLOOD AND LYMPHATIC VESSELS OF THE KIDNEY. Segmental branches of the renal artery leave the renal sinus and enter the renal columns as interlobar arteries. They run peripherally between adjacent pyramids toward the junction between the cortex and medulla. Here they branch, giving rise to horizontal arcuate arteries. The arcuate arteries then give off radial interlobular vessels to the cortex, which supply the capsule and renal corpuscles. Afferent arterioles, derived from the interlobular arteries, form plexuses of capillaries, the *glomeruli*. The glomerular capillaries converge, giving rise to efferent arterioles, and leave the renal corpuscles at the vascular poles. **Plate 1, Fig. 2.**

The *vascular supply of the renal medulla* is formed mainly by efferent arterioles coming from glomeruli located near the medulla (juxtamedullary nephrons), although some come from glomeruli located near the intermediate and outer regions of the cortex (cortical nephrons). As an efferent arteriole from a juxtamedullary glomerulus extends toward the medulla, it first gives off branches to capillary plexuses in the cortex and then divides into many branches, *descending vasa recta* (arteriolae rectae). These are relatively straight, thin-walled vessels which resemble capillaries but are larger in diameter. They extend to different depths within the medulla, supplying networks of peritubular capillaries which surround Henle's loop and the collecting tubules. The venous ends of the peritubular capillaries are drained by many ascending vasa recta (venae rectae), which carry the blood either to arcuate or interlobular veins. The endothelium of the ascending vasa recta is discontinuous, thin, and fenestrated, while that of the descending vasa recta is continuous, thick, and nonfenestrated. The histologic and anatomic organization of these vascular limbs, as well as their proximity to each other, facilitates the rapid exchange of diffusable susbstances which is essential for them to function as countercurrent exchangers (see above). **Plate 1, Fig. 2.**

The *vascular supply of the cortical region* is formed by efferent arterioles coming from the cortical glomeruli. These arterioles branch as they extend into the cortical region. They give rise to networks of peritubular capillaries which surround the proximal and distal convoluted tubules. The venous ends of these capillary networks are drained by stellate and interlobular veins. The stellate veins drain only the outer regions of the renal cortex and are continuous with the interlobular veins. As venous blood leaves the interlobular veins it is drained by arcuate veins, which are drained in turn by interlobar veins. The interlobar veins become confluent, forming the renal vein, which drains blood into the inferior vena cava. **Plate 1, Fig. 2.**

Lymphatic vessels are present as plexuses beneath the capsule and surround the renal tubules and blood vessels. The plexuses are drained through a set of several large collecting vessels which accompany large blood vessels as they exit at the hilus.

NERVES OF THE KIDNEY. Nerves accompany the blood vessels as they enter the kidney through the hilus. Visceral sensory neurons innervate the capsule and renal pelvis, while sympathetic vasomotor neurons terminate on the walls of blood vessels.

Excretory passages (calyces, renal pelvis, ureter, and urinary bladder)

Minor calyces form double-walled cups over the ends of the renal papillae for collecting urine. Their inner epithelial wall lines both the papillae and papillary ducts (see above). These minor calyces are continuous with the larger and fewer (two to three) *major calyces*, which are branches of the *renal pelvis*. The renal pelvis is the funnel-shaped, expanded upper end of the *ureter* (**Plate 7, Fig. 1**) which conveys urine to the *urinary bladder* (**Plate 7, Fig. 2**). The histologic organization of these excretory passages is similar, but the major difference is that the walls become thicker in going from the upper to the lower levels. The wall is composed of three coats: (1) *mucosa*, lining the lumen; (2) *muscularis*, peripheral to the mucosa; (3) *adventitia*, peripheral to the muscularis. A submucosal layer is lacking.

Mucosa. This is composed of transitional epithelium lying on a lamina propria of loose connective tissue containing a network of collagen and elastic fibers; a thin basement is usually not seen. The lamina propria is less dense at its periphery and

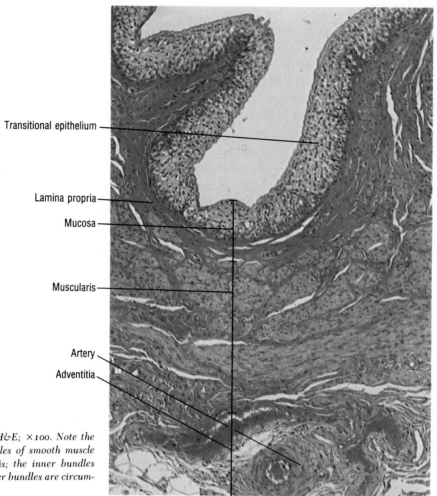

Transitional epithelium

Lamina propria

Mucosa

Muscularis

Artery

Adventitia

FIGURE 1.
Ureter; rabbit; H&E; ×100. Note the
interlacing bundles of smooth muscle
in the muscularis; the inner bundles
are long; the outer bundles are circum-
ferential.

may contain some lymphoid tissue. In the relaxed, nondistended condition the surface epithelial cells are ovoid and the thickness of the epithelium varies according to the specific organ (approximately two to four layers in calyces, five to six layers in the renal pelvis and ureter, and seven or more in the bladder). When an organ is stretched or distended, the epithelium is quite thin and the surface cells flattened (see Chap. 2). A few mucous glands are present near the urethral orifice of the bladder as tubular evaginations of epithelium extending into the lamina propria.

Muscularis. At the upper levels (calyces, renal pelvis, and upper portions of the ureter) the muscularis is composed of two layers of smooth muscle: inner longitudinal and outer circumferential. The urinary bladder and the lower levels of the ureter have an additional third layer of longitudinal muscle, just peripheral to the outer

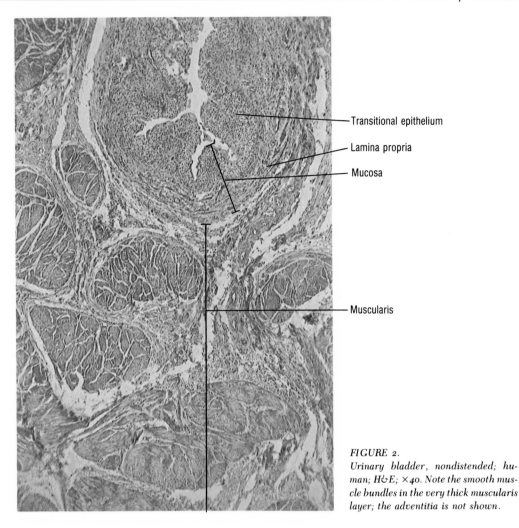

Transitional epithelium

Lamina propria

Mucosa

Muscularis

FIGURE 2.
Urinary bladder, nondistended; human; H&E; ×40. Note the smooth muscle bundles in the very thick muscularis layer; the adventitia is not shown.

circumferential layer. The muscle is divided into many bundles by connective tissue, and in the urinary bladder the bundles interlace so well that it usually is difficult to observe the longitudinal and circular patterns of distribution. The muscularis forms sphincter muscles at various urinary orifices and therefore can regulate their diameters. The muscularis also functions to move urine along the excretory passages by peristaltic contractions.

Adventitia. This is an outer coat of loose connective tissue which blends with the connective tissue of adjacent structures. On the superior region of the bladder, however, the connective tissue is covered by a mesothelium (simple squamous epithelium). This complex forms a protective *serosa*.

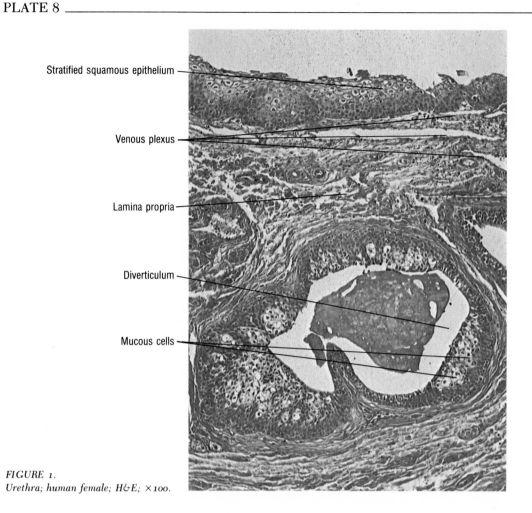

Stratified squamous epithelium

Venous plexus

Lamina propria

Diverticulum

Mucous cells

FIGURE 1.
Urethra; human female; H&E; ×100.

Urethra

The urethra transports urine from the urinary bladder to the exterior of the body, and also carries sperm in the male. It is a tube extending from the bladder to the penis (male) or vestibule (female). Although the urethra shows some histologic similarities in both sexes (both have a mucosa and muscularis but lack a well-defined submucosa and adventitia), there are considerable anatomic differences between them.

FEMALE URETHRA. This is a short tube, about 3.7 cm in length, extending from the bladder and opening into the vestibule just anterior to the vaginal orifice. **Plate 8, Fig. 1.**

Mucosa. This layer lines the lumen of the urethra and is composed of an epithelium lying on a connective tissue bed, the lamina propria; the basement membrane is usually not seen. The epithelium is transitional near the bladder, but distally it is predominately stratified squamous nonkeratinized epithelium interspersed with patches of pseudostratified or stratified columnar epithelium. The epithelium may have small glandlike diverticula extending into the lamina propria. The lining of these diverticula contain some mucous cells, and their cavities may be filled with an acidophilic colloidal substance. The lamina propria is composed of loose connective tissue with many elastic fibers and a prominent venous plexus.

Muscularis. This more peripheral layer of tissue is composed of an inner longitudinal and an outer circumferential layer of smooth muscle. The outer layer is continuous with the muscularis of the bladder, and at the neck of the bladder it forms a thickened *involuntary internal sphincter muscle*. As the urethra passes through the urogenital diaphragm on the floor of the pelvic canal, bundles of skeletal muscle are added to the periphery of the muscularis and form the *voluntary external sphincter muscle*, the sphincter urethrae. See below for innervation of the sphincter muscles.

MALE URETHRA. The male urethra is a tube, about 20 cm long, extending from the urinary bladder to an external opening, the meatus, at the end of the penis. The urethra has three anatomic regions:

1 *Prostatic urethra*. This uppermost portion, about 3.7 cm long, leads from the bladder through the prostate gland. The mucosal lining forms a median longitudinal ridge on its posterior wall. This elevation is the urethral crest, which receives the paired ejaculatory ducts and openings of the prostate gland. In cross section the lumen appears as a U-shaped slit.

2 *Membranous urethra*. This is distal to the prostatic urethra. It is about 1.3 cm long and extends through the urogenital and pelvic diaphragms, which form the pelvic floor behind the pubic symphysis. Its lumen appears as a stellate slit in cross section.

3 *Spongiosa (cavernosa) urethra*. This is distal to the membranous urethra. It is about 15 cm long, lies within the penis, and terminates at the meatus. The lumen is a transverse slit surrounded by vascular erectile tissue of the penis (corpus spongiosum).

Mucosa. The epithelium of the mucosa varies in type along the length of the urethra. Near the bladder the epithelium of the prostatic urethra is transitional; at the urethral orifice it is stratified squamous nonkeratinized; and between these two regions the membranous and spongiosa urethrae may be pseudostratified or stratified columnar. Numerous irregular pockets, *lacunae of Morgagni*, are formed by the epithelium and extend into the lamina propria. They are continuous with the deeper, branched tubular *mucous glands of Littre*, which are most abundant along the spongiosa urethra. Nests of mucous secreting cells may also be found within the epithelial lining of the lacunae of Morgagni. The lamina propria is highly vascularized, containing many elastic fibers in a loose connective tissue bed. **Plate 8, Fig. 2.**

Muscularis. The muscularis is present along the entire urethra but is more prominent in the prostatic, membranous, and proximal portions of the spongiosa urethra. In these regions it is composed of an inner longitudinal and an outer circular layer of smooth muscle, but at the lower levels the muscularis contains only longitudinal muscle. Like the female, the male has internal and external sphincter muscles with a similar type of innervation. The *internal sphincter* is a thickened layer of circumferential smooth muscle. It is derived from the muscularis of the upper portion of the prostatic urethra, near the bladder. The internal sphincter muscle is innervated by sympathetic and parasympathetic fibers coming from the vesicle plexus of the autonomic nervous system. It regulates the diameter of the neck of the

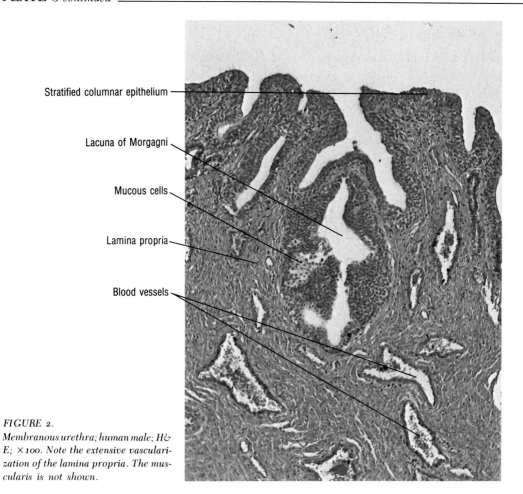

Stratified columnar epithelium

Lacuna of Morgagni

Mucous cells

Lamina propria

Blood vessels

FIGURE 2.
Membranous urethra; human male; H&
E; ×100. Note the extensive vasculari-
zation of the lamina propria. The mus-
cularis is not shown.

bladder and upper portion of the prostatic urethra. The *external sphincter* (sphincter urethrae) is a concentric mass of skeletal muscle fibers. These fibers are added to the surface of the muscularis as the membranous urethra passes through the tissues of the pelvic floor. The external sphincter is innervated by the perineal branch of the pudendal nerve and is under voluntary control.

BLOOD AND LYMPHATIC VESSELS OF THE EXCRETORY PASSAGES (calyces, renal pelvis, ureter, urinary bladder, and urethra). Arteries extend into the wall of these organs and form extensive capillary networks within the muscularis, deeper regions of the lamina propria, and just below the epithelium. Comparable veins drain the same regions.

Lymphatic vessels accompany the blood vessels and are present in all of the excretory passages. They are abundant in the deeper regions of the lamina propria and muscularis, but in the bladder lymphatic vessels occur only in the muscularis.

NERVES OF THE EXCRETORY PASSAGES (calyces, renal pelvis, ureter, urinary bladder, and urethra). Ganglia and networks of sympathetic and parasympathetic nerve fibers are located in the adventitia or loose connective tissue peripheral to the muscularis. Visceral sensory fibers terminate in the mucosal epithelium.

Female Reproductive System 15

The reproductive system of the female is composed of internal organs, external genitalia, and mammary glands. The latter are integumentary structures but may be considered with the reproductive system. The external genitalia and internal organs form a continuous system of tubes leading from the pubic region to within the pelvic cavity. These structures are illustrated in **Plate 1**, **Fig. 1**, and listed below in their anatomical order. Going from the exterior to the interior of the body they are the: *vulva* (clitoris, labia majora, and minora surrounding a cavity, the vestibule), *vagina*, *cervix*, *uterus*, *paired fallopian tubes* (with three regions—isthmus, ampulla, and infundibulum), and paired *ovaries*.

A *broad ligament* forms an important anchor for the uterus and other internal reproductive structures. It also carries blood vessels, lymphatics, and nerves to these organs. The broad ligament is a wide, vertical septum with a free superior edge. It divides the lower pelvic canal into anterior and posterior regions as it extends from one wall of the canal to the other. The broad ligament is composed of two fused layers of peritoneum. These layers are split by the uterus, so that one layer covers the anterior and the other covers the posterior surface of the uterus. At the margins of the uterus, the two layers are fused as they continue toward the pelvic wall. The fallopian tubes extend from the body of the uterus to the ovaries. They are embedded within the free superior edge of the broad ligament. That portion of the broad ligament between a fallopian tube and ovary is the *mesosalpinx*. The ovaries are suspended from the posterosuperior region of the broad ligament, just lateral to the uterus, by a small fold of the broad ligament, the *mesovarium*. At the junction between the uterus and fallopian tube, the medial region of the ovary is attached to the body of the uterus by the *ovarian ligament*. This cordlike structure is contained within the broad ligament and contains some smooth muscle tissue from the myometrium of the uterus (see below). The ovary is anchored laterally to the pelvic wall by a *suspensory ligament*, another fold of the broad ligament. **Plate 1, Fig. 1.**

In the mature human female there are reoccurring periodic ovarian cycles which will control the menstrual and, to some degree, mammary cycles. These cycles are characterized by changes in concentrations of sex hormones, changes in the structure and physiology of reproductive organs, and to some degree, changes in behavior. The average cycle is 28 days long, but can vary by several days. The

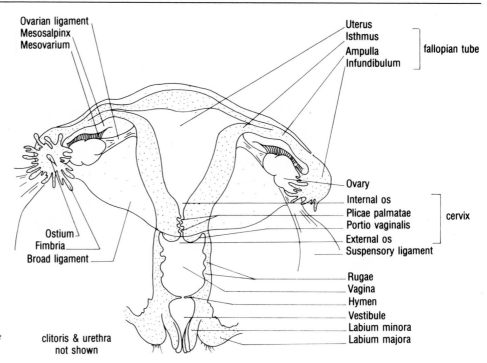

Ovarian ligament
Mesosalpinx
Mesovarium

Uterus
Isthmus
Ampulla
Infundibulum

fallopian tube

Ovary
Internal os
Plicae palmatae
Portio vaginalis
External os
Suspensory ligament

cervix

Ostium
Fimbria
Broad ligament

Rugae
Vagina
Hymen
Vestibule
Labium minora
Labium majora

clitoris & urethra
not shown

FIGURE 1.
Drawing of the female reproductive
system, posterosuperior view.

ovarian cycles are regulated by reciprocal relationships between pituitary gonadotropic hormones, ovarian sex hormones, and chorionic gonadotropic hormones
(during a pregnancy).

Ovaries

The ovary is an oval-shaped structure, about 4 cm long, 2 cm wide, and 1 cm in
thickness. The margin of the ovary, where the mesovarium is attached, is designated
as the *hilum*. It is through this region that vessels and nerves enter the ovary. The
surface of the ovary is covered with a simple squamous or cuboidal epithelium, the
germinal epithelium, which is continuous with the mesothelium covering the
mesovarium. The germinal epithelium rests on a thin basement membrane. A
prominent layer of dense, irregular collagenous connective tissue, the *tunica
albuginea*, is present just below the germinal epithelium. Both the tunica albuginea
and germinal epithelium are discontinuous at the hilum. The ovary is organized into
two major regions: an outer *cortex* surrounding an inner *medulla*. Although the
cortex is composed of dense connective tissue and the medulla has loose connective
tissue, the boundary between the two regions are indistinct. The connective tissue
of the cortex and medullary regions is designated as the *stroma*. The dense stroma
of the cortex is composed of reticular fibers and many packed, fusiform cells with

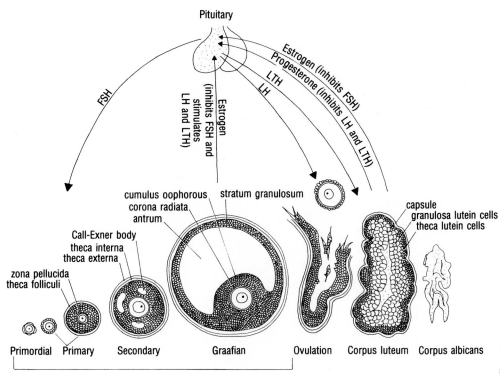

FIGURE 2.
Diagram of ovarian cycle, showing the interrelationship between the ovary and pituitary, and their hormones.

elongate nuclei. These are multipotential cells. They are capable of differentiating into *interstitial cells*, which are important in forming theca layers around developing follicles (see below). In the medulla, the stroma contains loose connective tissue with many elastic fibers, fibroblasts, and some scattered smooth muscle cells. Vessels and nerves are embedded within the stroma and follow a spiral course from the hilus to deep within the medulla. Gonadotropic hormones, produced by the anterior pituitary, influence the ovary to produce a sequence of histologic stages that accompany the maturation of sex cells and the secretion of steroid sex hormones, estrogen and progesterone. One sequence of these stages is an *ovarian cycle*, the hormones of which influence the menstrual cycle, and to some degree the mammary cycle. Unless there is a pregnancy, the ovarian cycle repeats about every 28 days. The histologic stages of the ovarian cycle are confined to the cortex but may encroach onto the medulla. **Plate 1, Fig. 2; Plate 2, Fig. 1.** Although the stages of one ovarian cycle, starting from the earliest to the latest, are taken in order, all may appear randomly scattered throughout the cortex. This is possible because several oogonia may start the maturation process during one cycle. Usually only one gamete will ovulate, and all the rest disintegrate.

Germinal epithelium—

Tunica albuginea—

Primordial follicle —

Primary follicle (growing)—

Stroma —

Corpus albicans —

Oöcyte —

Secondary follicle (early)—

Antrum —

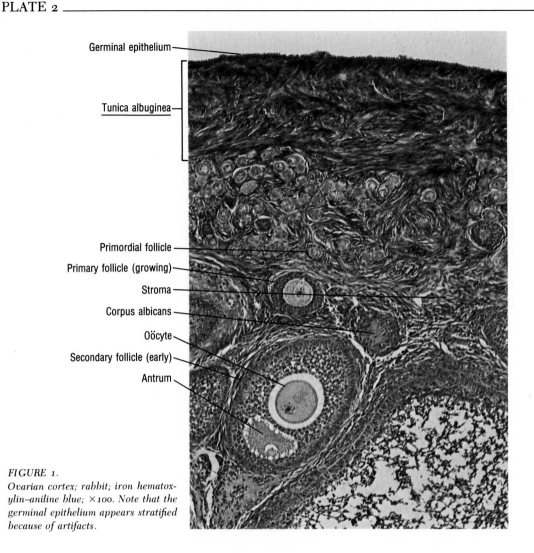

FIGURE 1.
Ovarian cortex; rabbit; iron hematoxylin–aniline blue; ×100. Note that the germinal epithelium appears stratified because of artifacts.

1 *Primordial follicle.* These are the immature resting follicles. They are located in the cortex, just under the tunica albuginea, as spheres of cells. Each follicle contains a large, spherical primary oocyte surrounded by a single layer of flattened follicular cells. The oocyte has a large, pale, vesicular nucleus containing one or more prominent nucleoli. In the embryo, primordial sex cells, oogonia, are derived from entoderm tissue of the yolk sac. These cells migrate into the developing gonad and multiply in the cortex. The oogonia then proceed through the early stages of meiosis but become arrested as primary oocytes. The first meiotic division may be completed at puberty or later, when the oocyte is stimulated by gonadotropins to continue its maturation. The follicle cells are derived from the germinal epithelium and surround the primary oocyte. At birth, the female infant has about 350,000 primordial follicles in the resting state. During her lifetime the numbers of follicles will decline by atresia (degeneration) and ovulation; only about 450 follicles ever undergo ovulation. Primordial follicles are usually absent from the ovarian cortex of a woman who is in her menopause. **Plate 1, Fig. 2; Plate 2, Figs. 1 and 2.**

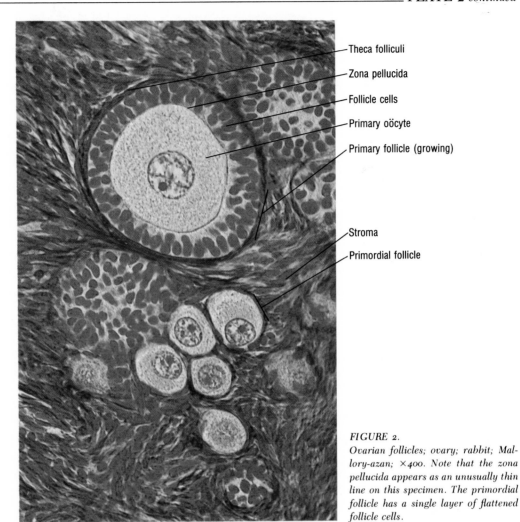

Theca folliculi
Zona pellucida
Follicle cells
Primary oöcyte
Primary follicle (growing)

Stroma
Primordial follicle

FIGURE 2.
Ovarian follicles; ovary; rabbit; Mallory-azan; ×400. Note that the zona pellucida appears as an unusually thin line on this specimen. The primordial follicle has a single layer of flattened follicle cells.

2 *Primary follicle (early).* At puberty, or at the onset of a menstrual cycle in a mature woman, follicle-stimulating hormone (FSH) is produced by the anterior pituitary and carried by the blood to the ovaries. It stimulates several primordial follicles to mature into primary follicles. This process marks the onset of an ovarian cycle. Usually only one follicle will mature and release its sex cell, while the others undergo atresia. The primary follicle contains a larger primary oocyte, and the single layer of follicle cells become cuboidal or low columnar. **Plate 1, Fig. 2.**

3 *Primary follicle (growing).* The primary oocyte continues to enlarge under the influence of FSH as the follicle cells become mitotically active. Two to six layers of cuboidal follicle cells form a stratified epithelium resting on a thin basement membrane. With an H&E–stained specimen, a prominent, bright pink, homogeneous layer, the *zona pellucida*, can be seen between the primary oocyte and inner layer of follicle cells. The zona pellucida is composed of glycoprotein, probably secreted by the oocyte and follicle cells. The large follicle is surrounded by a thin sheath of stromal cells, the *theca folliculi*, lying just outside the follicle cells. In older and larger primary follicles the theca folliculi will differentiate into a *theca interna*, immediately surrounding the follicle cells, and a more peripheral *theca externa* (see below). **Plate 1, Fig. 2; Plate 2, Figs. 1 and 2.**

4 *Secondary follicle* (vesicular follicle). This larger follicle has from 6 to 12 layers of follicle cells surrounding the primary oocyte. In the early secondary follicle, small, irregular interstitial pools of follicular fluid collect among the follicle cells. These pools are designated as the *Call-Exner bodies*, and in the later follicle they eventually coalesce to form a single prominent, fluid-filled cavity, the *antrum*. The follicular fluid filling the antrum is designated as the *liquor folliculi*. It contains high concentrations of hyaluronic acid. In routine sections the follicular fluid may appear as a granular substance. At this stage of the ovarian cycle, the primary oocyte attains its largest size, which is about six times its original diameter; it does not enlarge any further.

As the antrum forms, follicular fluid displaces the follicle cells to the periphery of the follicle, forming a stratified cuboidal epithelium, the *stratum granulosum*. The oocyte lies within an eccentric mound of follicle cells, the *cumulus oophorus*, which projects into the antrum. The single layer of follicle cells immediately surrounding the oocyte is the *corona radiata*. It remains in place as the gamete passes down the fallopian tube. The *thecae interna* and *externa* are similar to those described for the primary follicle. The theca interna, lying next to the follicle cells, contains many capillary plexuses and large, fusiform secretory cells. The cells have pale, oval nuclei and vacuoles of estrogen in the cytoplasm. The more peripheral theca externa is composed of connective tissue, fibroblasts, and many collagen fibers. It is more fibrous than the theca interna and lacks secretory cells and capillary plexuses. **Plate 1, Fig. 2; Plate 2, Fig. 1; Plate 3, Figs. 1 and 2.**

5 *Graafian follicle* (mature follicle). This is an enlarged version of a late secondary follicle and may reach 10 mm or more in diameter. The secondary follicle will develop into the larger Graafian follicle as much follicular fluid (liquor folliculi) accumulates within the antrum and the stratum granulosum increases in thickness. These are big, baglike structures covering the entire width of the cortex. They may encroach onto the medulla and also elevate the surface of the ovary. The primary oocyte now proceeds through its first maturation division, becoming a secondary oocyte with the formation of the first polar body. The vascular theca interna is well developed; its many large cells, which are fusiform or ovoid, contain pale, oval nuclei and droplets of estrogen in their cytoplasm. The theca externa remains as a prominent fibrous layer. It contains spindle-shaped nonsecretory cells and collagen fibers which blend with the surrounding ovarian stroma. **Plate 1, Fig. 2.**

As estrogen is produced, it is carried by the blood to the uterus, increasing its muscular tone and vascularization. This activity prepares the uterus for a possible implantation of an embryo if a gamete has been fertilized. Second, estrogen is carried to the anterior pituitary, inhibiting the synthesis of FSH, so a new ovarian cycle cannot start and new primordial follicles will not ripen. Third, estrogen stimulates the production of luteinizing hormone (LH) and prolactin or luteotropic hormone (LTH) by the anterior pituitary. Finally, estrogen stimulates the growth and development of the mammary glands.

The increasing titers of LH and decreasing FSH may possibly stimulate the rupture or ovulation of the Graafian follicle. Thus, the liquor folliculi, fragmented pieces of the cumulus oophorus, and the secondary oocyte, surrounded by the corona radiata, are released at the ruptured surface of the ovary. Immediately on its release, the oocyte is swept into the ostium of the fallopian tube by the ciliated fimbria. If sperm are present, fertilization occurs in the upper one-third of the fallopian tube, and only then will the secondary oocytes go through their second meiotic division to become ootids. The ootids then develop into mature ova.

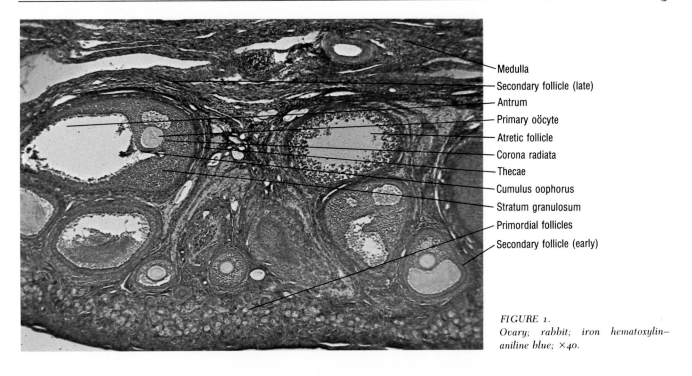

Medulla
Secondary follicle (late)
Antrum
Primary oöcyte
Atretic follicle
Corona radiata
Thecae
Cumulus oophorus
Stratum granulosum
Primordial follicles
Secondary follicle (early)

FIGURE 1.
Ovary; rabbit; iron hematoxylin–aniline blue; ×40.

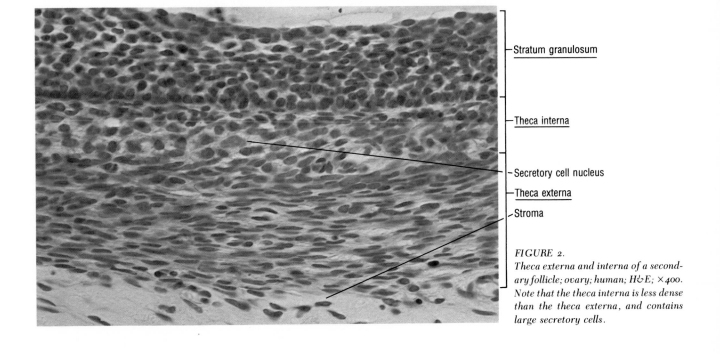

Stratum granulosum

Theca interna

Secretory cell nucleus
Theca externa
Stroma

FIGURE 2.
Theca externa and interna of a secondary follicle; ovary; human; H&E; ×400. Note that the theca interna is less dense than the theca externa, and contains large secretory cells.

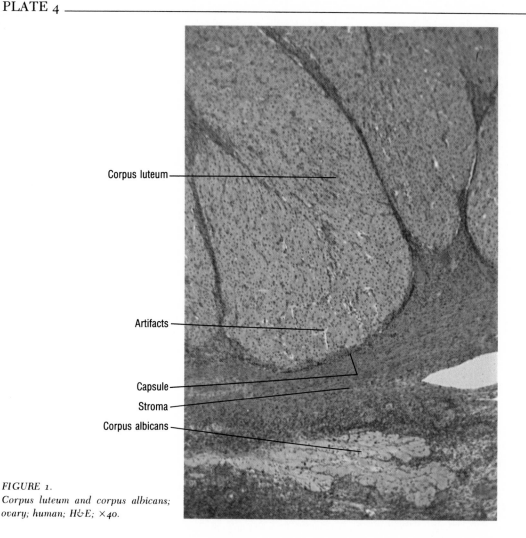

Corpus luteum

Artifacts

Capsule

Stroma

Corpus albicans

FIGURE 1.
Corpus luteum and corpus albicans;
ovary; human; H&E; ×40.

6 *Corpus luteum.* The luteinizing hormone is instrumental in organizing the tissues of the ovulated Graafian follicle into a *corpus luteum.* This is a large, pale, solid, plicated, vascularized glandular structure lying within the ovarian stroma. The granulosum cells differentiate into *granulosa lutein cells* located within the interior of the corpus luteum. These are large, pale cells, usually with a vacuolated cytoplasm. The pale, vesicular nuclei are relatively large and contain a nucleolus. The periphery of the corpus luteum is lined by *theca lutein cells*, derived from the glandular cells of the theca interna. The theca lutein cells are smaller and darker than the granulosa lutein cells, and have smaller and darker nuclei. The theca externa persists as a fibrous connective tissue *capsule* containing collagen fibers and fibroblasts. Capillaries of the theca interna, and connective tissue of both interna and externa, grow into the lutein tissues. They form extensive vascular plexuses and a delicate reticular network which supports the lutein cells. In addition, fibroblasts line the old follicular cavity and proceed to absorb and convert any coagulated blood produced during ovulation into a small, fibrous core. LTH stimulates the granulosa lutein cells to secrete progesterone and the theca lutein cells to secrete some estrogen. Also, LTH maintains the corpus luteum and supplements estrogen in stimulating lactation.

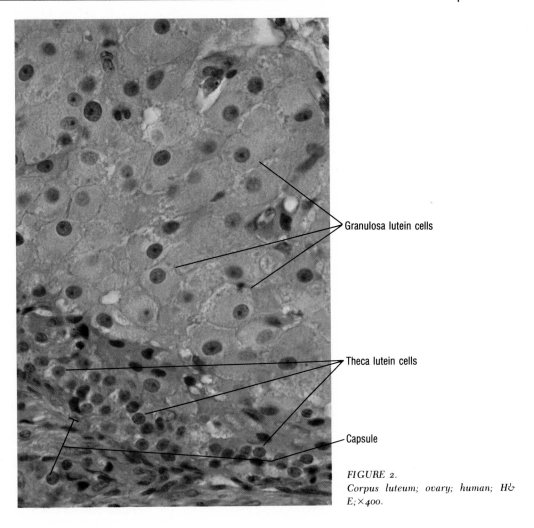

Granulosa lutein cells

Theca lutein cells

Capsule

FIGURE 2.
Corpus luteum; ovary; human; H&
E; ×400.

As progesterone increases in concentration, it is carried by the blood to the uterus. Here, it reduces muscular activity and increases vascularization and glandular development, all of which are optimal conditions for the implantation of an embryo within the uterine mucosa. Second, progesterone is carried to the anterior pituitary where it inhibits further production of LH and LTH. Third, progesterone, like estrogen, contributes to the development of the mammary glands. Even though estrogen is produced by the corpus luteum, and its physiologic influence is in some ways antagonistic to that of progesterone, it is overshadowed by the high progesterone titers. Estrogen, however, will continue to inhibit FSH production. **Plate 1, Fig. 2; Plate 4, Figs. 1 and 2.**

7 *Corpus albicans.* This is an irregular mass of connective tissue, disintegrating cells, and hyalinized intercellular substances, which is formed from a disintegrating corpus luteum. It is a nonfunctional white scar in the ovary which eventually disappears. The disappearance of the corpus albicans marks the end of one ovarian cycle. **Plate 1, Fig. 2; Plate 2, Fig. 1; Plate 4, Fig. 1.**

As progesterone inhibits LH and LTH, the corpus luteum of menstruation can no longer be maintained and degenerates to become the corpus albicans. With the regression of the corpus luteum, estrogen levels drop and no longer inhibit the production of FSH by the pituitary. This allows a new ovarian cycle to begin. If there is a pregnancy, the embryonic membranes produce chorionic gonadotropins, which are *similar* to LH and LTH, so that a corpus luteum of pregnancy is maintained even though pituitary LH and LTH are not present. The corpus luteum of pregnancy ensures a supply of estrogen and progesterone to maintain the uterus in a pregnant condition and to inhibit FSH. In the latter stages of pregnancy, the chorionic gonadotropins are no longer produced and the corpus luteum of pregnancy degenerates. As this occurs the placenta secretes estrogen, chorionic LTH (prolactin), and progesterone; it is the only source of these hormones to maintain pregnancy. At birth, with the removal of the placenta, FSH is no longer inhibited by estrogen, and in a period of time a new ovarian cycle begins.

ATRETIC FOLLICLES. Although several follicles may start to mature during an ovarian cycle, only one usually ovulates. The rest, for one reason or another, become atretic and degenerate. The atretic follicle has one or more of the following traits: (1) degenerating oocyte, (2) degenerating follicle cells; and (3) heavily thickened zona pellucida and or basement membrane of the stratum granulosum. In the latter, the basement membrane appears as a thick, homogeneous, somewhat scalloped structure, designated as the *glassy membrane*. **Plate 3, Fig. 1.**

BLOOD AND LYMPHATIC VESSELS OF THE OVARY. The ovarian arteries are the main vessels supplying the ovaries with arterial blood. They originate from the dorsal aorta. These arteries are carried through the suspensory and broad ligaments, and then extend into the mesovarium where they enter the hilum of the ovary. The vessels branch and form spiral helicine arteries within the medulla. The helicine arteries form plexuses at the corticomedullary junctions which send branches into the cortex. These branch vessels supply capillary plexuses within the cortex, and the theca interna of growing follicles. Venules and veins drain these plexuses, following the approximate pattern of distribution as the arteries. At the hilum, however, the veins form a large network, the pampiniform plexus, which gives rise to the ovarian vein.

Lymphatic capillaries are present around developing follicles, and extend into the theca layers. They are also quite numerous in the corpora lutea. Lymphatic vessels drain the capillaries toward the medulla and then the hilum.

NERVES OF THE OVARY. The autonomic ovarian plexus and the uterine nerves supply mainly unmyelinated and some myelinated fibers to the ovary. Many unmyelinated postganglionic sympathetic, some unmyelinated postganglionic parasympathetic, and some visceral afferent nerve fibers have been described in the stroma of the ovary; some form plexuses around developing follicles. The sympathetic fibers innervate smooth muscle tissue in the arterioles.

Fallopian tubes (oviducts, uterine tubes)

The paired fallopian tubes extend medially from the ovaries to enter the upper lateral margins of the uterus. Each tube is about 13 cm long and is divided into four regions: the *intramural region*, passing through the uterine wall; the *isthmus*, the narrow, lower one-third of the tube which extends laterally from the intramural region to the ampulla; the *ampulla*, the expanded, upper two-thirds of the tube which is continuous with the isthmus; the *infundibulum*, the large, trumpet-shaped

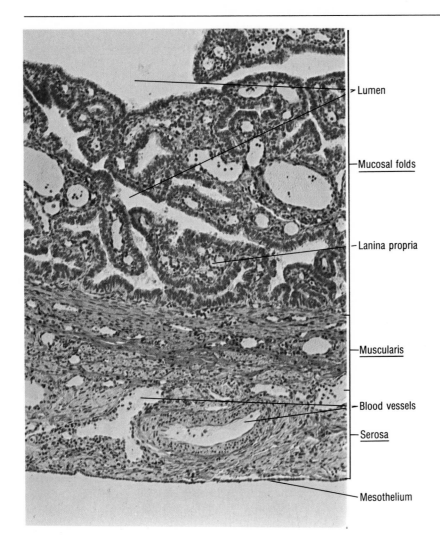

Lumen

Mucosal folds

Lanina propria

Muscularis

Blood vessels

Serosa

Mesothelium

FIGURE 1.
Ampulla of fallopian tube (cross section); human; Masson's trichrome stain; ×100. Note that the muscle bundles of the prominent muscularis are extensively separated by bundles of connective tissue.

end of the tube lying near the ovary and open to the peritoneal cavity by an *abdominal ostium*. The infundibulum has many long ciliated processes, the *fimbriae*, surrounding the ostium. The fimbriae sweep the surface of the ovary. The fallopian tube is embedded within the free superior border of the broad ligament, the *mesosalpinx*. The function of the tubes is to provide a passage for the ovulated secondary oocytes from the surface of the ovaries to the uterine cavity. The fallopian tubes are composed of three distinct histologic layers: an inner *mucosa*, a middle *muscularis*, and an outer *serosa*. **Plate 1, Fig. 1; Plate 5, Fig. 1.**

Mucosa. The mucosa forms an elaborate system of interconnected, highly branched longitudinal folds in the ampulla, so that its lumen appears much like a labyrinth of spaces. In the lower region of the tubes, the folds are fewer in number, lower, and nonbranched. A *simple columnar epithelium* lines the mucosa and is composed of two types of cells lying on a delicate basement membrane: columnar ciliated cells and columnar nonciliated secretory cells. The ciliated cells are more numerous toward the ovarian end than the uterine end of the tube, and their ciliary beat is toward the uterus. Although ciliary beat is important for moving the secondary oocyte into the infundibulum, peristaltic activity is probably more important for moving the sex cell along the fallopian tube toward the uterus. The secretory cells produce a mucoid substance which may have nutritive values. The height of the epithelium is influenced by sex hormones produced by the ovary. The epithelium is tall during high estrogen levels, and low when progesterone concentrations are greatest. The *lamina propria* is composed of a thin vascular layer of loose connective tissue containing reticular fibers and numerous fusiform cells. Mucoid secretions are dependent on the secretory cells, since glands are absent in the lamina propria.

Muscularis. The prominent muscularis is composed of an inner circular and outer longitudinal layers of smooth muscle. Both layers appear somewhat discontinuous because their muscle bundles are separated by much loose connective tissue. Near the uterus the circular layer becomes thicker, and another layer of longitudinal muscle is present between it and the lamina propria. These three layers of muscle are not well separated, and because they tend to intermingle, distinct borders cannot be determined.

Serosa. This outer layer is continuous with the mesosalpinx. It is a prominent layer of loose connective tissue, with a mesothelium covering its surface. Bundles of longitudinal muscle fibers from the underlying muscularis intermingle with the inner connective tissue layers of the serosa.

BLOOD AND LYMPHATIC VESSELS OF THE FALLOPIAN TUBES. Branches of the ovarian and uterine arteries supply the fallopian tubes directly and indirectly from anastomotic complexes. Arterioles carry blood to capillary plexuses in the lamina propria, muscularis, and serosa. The lamina propria and serosa have a more extensive pattern of vascularization than the muscularis. The venous drainage pattern is comparable to the arterial pattern. *Lymphatic* capillaries form extensive plexuses in the lamina propria and serosa. They are drained by larger lymphatic vessels which follow the blood vessels.

NERVES OF THE FALLOPIAN TUBES. Myelinated and unmyelinated nerve fibers of the autonomic nervous system, and visceral sensory fibers are carried in branches of the uterine and ovarian nerves. These nerves accompany the tubal blood vessels and have a similar pattern of distribution. While postganglionic sympathetic, postganglionic parasympathetic, and visceral sensory fibers in the fallopian tube have been described, parasympathetic ganglia have not been found. It is possible that the parasympathetic relay may occur within paracervical ganglia located in a plexus near the cervix.

Uterus

The uterus is a single, hollow, pear-shaped organ which is flattened anteroposteriorly. It is about 7 cm long by 5 cm at its widest part in the nonpregnant adult. The uterus has thick, muscular walls and a reduced lumen. It is located in the lower part of the pelvic canal and supported by the broad ligament. The uterus separates the anterior urinary bladder from the more posterior rectum. The rounded upper end of the uterus, where the fallopian tubes enter, is the *fundus*. Below the fundus, the remaining expanded part of the uterus is the *corpus or body*. The tapered lower end of the uterus is the *cervix*; it is separated from the body by a narrow constriction, the *isthmus*. The cervix protrudes a short distance into the vagina as a rounded collarlike *portio vaginalis*; its opening to the vaginal lumen is the *external os*. The walls of the body and fundus have a similar histologic organization. They are composed of an inner *endometrium* (mucosa), middle *myometrium* (muscularis), and outer *perimetrium* (serosa). **Plate 1, Fig. 1.**

ENDOMETRIUM. Of all three uterine layers, the endometrium undergoes extensive changes during the menstrual cycle and pregnancy. In the early to middle part of the menstrual cycle the upper portion of the endometrium thickens; it becomes glandular and vascular. The significance of these changes is the preparation of the endometrium for a possible implantation of an embryo. If there is no implantation, there will be a subsequent degeneration of the thickened tissue. It will be sloughed from the uterine wall and lost as the menses. These changes are correlated with the ovarian cycle and are influenced by the ovarian hormones estrogen and progesterone. The menstrual cycle is characterized by five sequential histologic stages that occur over about 28 days: *menstrual* (bleeding, 1st to 5th day); *resurfacing* (repair, 6th day); *proliferative* (follicular growth, 7th to 15th day); *secretory* (luteal, progravid, 16th to 27th day); *ischemic* (arteriole constriction, 28th day).

Proliferative stage. The endometrium increases progressively in thickness from 0.5 to 3 mm. The growth of the endometrial tissues coincides with the growth of the ovarian follicles, and is influenced by increasing concentrations of estrogens. The tall simple columnar epithelium has scattered groups of ciliated cells, all of which lie on a thin basement membrane. The deepest portion of the endometrium, next to the myometrium, is the *stratum basalis*; it is never shed during menstruation. The upper level of the endometrium, the *stratum functionalis*, is periodically shed and restored. The lamina propria or stroma of the endometrium is a very thick layer. It is composed of loose connective tissue with abundant ground substance. This tissue may appear somewhat similar to mesenchyme connective tissue (see Chap. 3). The stellate cells have large, oval, pale nuclei and form a delicate framework on reticular fibers. Lymphocytes, granular leucocytes, and macrophages are also present. Long, straight, or slightly coiled, simple tubular glands extend from the endometrial surface almost to the myometrium. The glands may be slightly branched in the stratum basalis. In the latter portion of this stage the glands become more numerous and more highly coiled. The glandular cells are similar to those on the surface of the mucosa. At first they produce thin mucoid secretions, but later, glycogen accumulates in their cytoplasm. Spiral arteries, growing up from the branches of the arcuate artery (see below), extend into the lower half of the endometrium. **Plate 5, Fig. 2.**

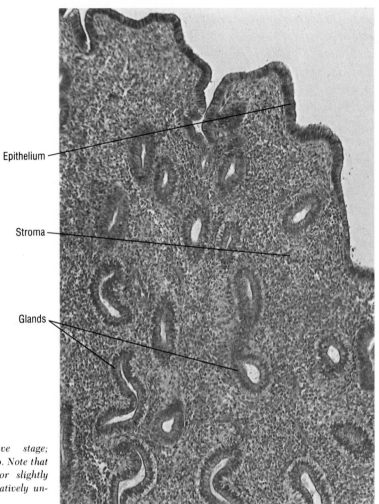

Epithelium

Stroma

Glands

FIGURE 2.
Endometrium, proliferative stage; uterus; human; H&E; ×100. Note that the glands are straight or slightly coiled. The lumina are relatively undilated.

Secretory stage. The endometrium will develop to its maximum thickness, 4 to 6 mm, mainly by an accumulation of interstitial fluids and secretions, and hypertrophy of tissues. This stage of the menstrual cycle is coincident with the formation of the corpus luteum, and its development is directly influenced by estrogen and mainly progesterone. The glands no longer proliferate but become highly coiled and enlarged. They have dilated lumina, and some have saclike outpocketings. The glands secrete a thick mucoid substance rich in glycogen. The connective tissue cells of the stroma become quite large, and their cytoplasm contains glycogen. The endometrium becomes very vascular as the spiral arteries (see below) become more numerous and compact. The arteries extend to the upper two-thirds of the mucosa where they supply capillary plexuses. The stratum basalis is supplied by straight arteries coming from branches of the arcuate arteries. During this stage of the menstrual cycle, the endometrium appears somewhat stratifed. The stratum basalis is unchanged and contains the blind ends of the uterine glands, but the stratum functionalis forms an upper *compact* and lower *spongy layer*. The compact layer is thin and contains the straight portions of the uterine glands, while the spongy layer is thicker and contains the enlarged, tortuous portions. During menstruation or

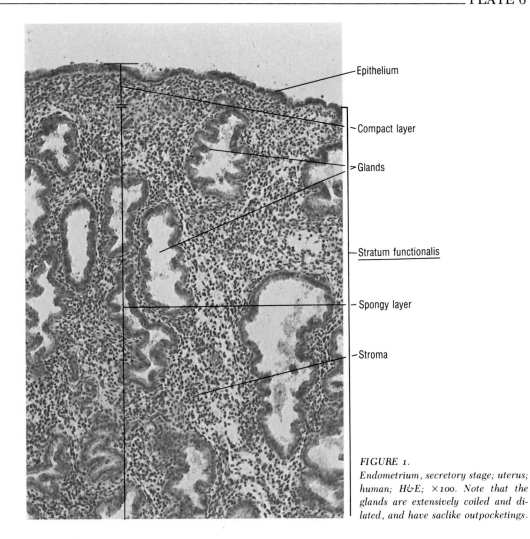

Epithelium

Compact layer

Glands

Stratum functionalis

Spongy layer

Stroma

FIGURE 1.
Endometrium, secretory stage; uterus;
human; H&E; ×100. Note that the
glands are extensively coiled and di-
lated, and have saclike outpocketings.

parturition, only the stratum functionalis is sloughed from the endometrium and expelled from the uterus. **Plate 6, Fig. 1.**

Ischemic stage. As the corpus luteum degenerates, toward the end of the ovarian cycle, estrogen and progesterone concentrations decrease. The low concentrations of these sex hormones influence the spiral arteries to undergo periodic constrictions, which intermittently interrupt the flow of blood to the stratum functionalis. This process, *ischemia*, begins about one day before menstruation and lasts for several hours. Eventually the bases of spiral arteries become permanently constricted and so the stratum functionalis becomes anemic; the glands become nonsecretory; and the stroma loses fluids to become a dense mass of connective tissue containing many leucocytes. The endometrium shrinks down to about 3 to 4 mm in thickness as the stratum functionalis becomes necrotic.

Menstrual stage. Menstruation is the stage when bleeding from the uterus occurs. At this time the necrotic stratum functionalis, which formed during the ischemic stage, sloughes off the endometrium and is shed from the uterus. The bases of the spiral arteries relax periodically and, along with ruptured veins and capillaries, soak

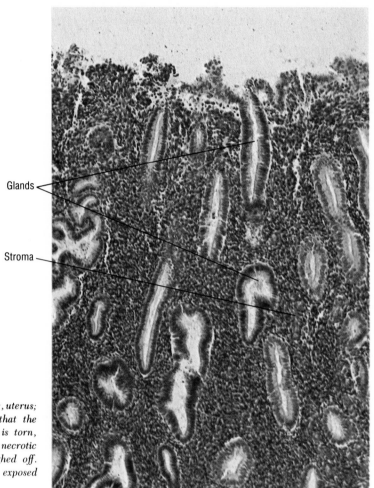

Glands

Stroma

FIGURE 2.
Endometrium, menstrual stage, uterus;
human; H&E; ×100. Note that the
surface of the endometrium is torn,
broken, and fragmented as the necrotic
stratum functionalis is sloughed off.
Glands and blood vessels are exposed
as ragged, raw surfaces.

the sloughing stratum functionalis with uncoagulated blood. This bloody mass of tissue, the *menses*, contains glands, broken blood vessels (including upper portions of spiral arteries), and stroma. The menses leave the uterine cavity and flow through the vagina. Bleeding lasts for about 5 days. Eventually the functionalis is lost, leaving the raw stratum basalis with exposed spiral arteries, veins, and ends of uterine glands. **Plate 6, Fig. 2.**

Resurfacing stage. Before the bleeding has ceased, repair of the raw endometrial surface begins and usually lasts one day. This process is regulated by estrogen produced by the growing follicles. The torn glands, deep in the stratum basalis, provide epithelial cells which migrate over the raw surface of the endometrium and differentiate into a new simple columnar epithelium. The spreading of these nonmitotic cells characterizes early wound healing.

MYOMETRIUM. The myometrium is relatively constant throughout the menstrual cycle and does not undergo any changes. It is a very thick muscular layer, about 1.25 cm in thickness. It is composed of three layers of smooth muscle: a thin inner longitudinal layer, the *stratum submucosum;* a thick middle layer of spiral to circular muscle, the *stratum vasculare;* and a thin outer longitudinal layer, the *stratum supravasculare*. The unusually long (40 to 90 μm) muscle fibers form bundles, somewhat separated by connective tissue. Since the bundles are interconnected, distinct boundary lines separating the three layers are not apparent. The stratum vasculare appears as a spongy network of muscle fibers because of the many large blood and lymphatic vessels located there. The stratum supravasculare sends muscle fibers into the round ligament, ovarian ligament, broad ligament, and fallopian tubes.

PERIMETRIUM. This outermost layer is a typical serosa covering most of the uterus. It is composed of a loose connective tissue layer covered with mesothelium. The perimetrium is technically a part of the broad ligament which encloses the uterus (see above). The perimetrium appears as an adventitial layer where the bladder lies on the anterior and inferior surface of the uterus.

BLOOD AND LYMPHATIC VESSELS OF THE UTERUS. Branches of the uterine arteries are carried in the broad ligament. They pass through the perimetrium and into the stratum vasculare of the myometrium. Here they branch into several *arcuate* arteries, which run circumferentially around the uterus. Each arcuate artery has several radial branches extending toward the endometrium. Before the radial arteries enter the endometrium they send branches into the myometrium to supply extensive capillary plexuses. As the radial arteries reach the endometrium, they branch into *straight arteries* supplying the stratum basalis and *spiral arteries* supplying capillary plexuses in the stratum functionalis. The capillaries are drained by a network of venules, sinusoids, and veins into venous plexuses of vessels located between the endometrium and myometrium. The venous plexuses are then drained into the stratum vasculare by larger veins, and from this point the veins approximate the arteries in their distribution.

Lymphatic plexuses are prominent in the perimetrium and myometrium, but are only present in the lower regions of the endometrium. The plexuses are drained by larger lymphatic vessels carrying lymph to several nodes (superficial inguinal, external iliac, lateral aortic, and preaortic).

NERVES OF THE UTERUS. Branches of the uterine nerves, carrying sympathetic and parasympathetic fibers, enter the perimetrium and generally follow blood vessels in the myometrium and endometrium. Most of the fibers innervate smooth muscle tissue of the uterine wall and blood vessels, while some surround glands in the endometrium. It is generally believed that the sympathetic fibers can produce uterine contractions and vasoconstriction of the blood vessels, while the parasympathetic fibers prevent contractions and bring about vasodilation. The autonomic nerves, of course, work in concert with the sex hormones.

Cervix

The cervix is about 3 cm long and forms the tapered, tubelike lower portion of the uterus. The upper one-third of the cervix, the *isthmus*, resembles the body of the uterus and undergoes some cyclic menstrual changes. The lower two-thirds is histologically quite distinct from the body and does not show cyclic changes. The cervix extends into the upper anterior region of the vagina as a rounded prominence, the *portio vaginalis*, which contains an opening, the *external os*. The cervical canal is continuous with the uterine cavity by a constricted area, the *internal os*, and the vaginal cavity by the external os. **Plate 1, Fig. 1.** The walls of the cervix are composed of a *mucosa*, *muscularis*, and *adventitia*. Of the three layers, only the mucosa shows a histologic difference between the superior and inferior levels. **Plate 7, Fig. 1.**

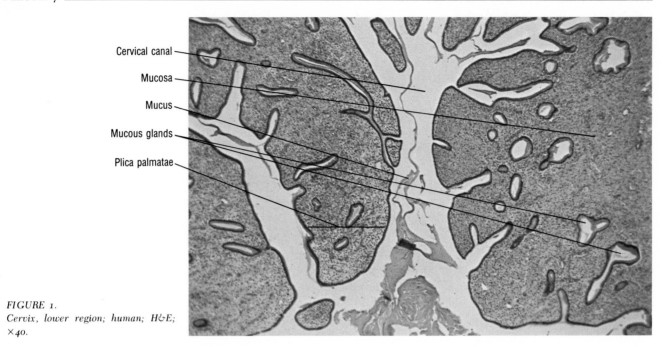

Cervical canal —
Mucosa —
Mucus —
Mucous glands —
Plica palmatae —

FIGURE 1.
Cervix, lower region; human; H&E;
×40.

Mucosa. In the *upper one-third* of the cervix, the mucosa is somewhat similar to that in the body of the uterus, except that it is thinner and lacks spiral arteries, and its tubular glands are fewer in number and nonbranched. Although this portion of the cervix does not bleed, it produces some reduced histologic changes during the menstrual cycle.

The lower *two-thirds* of the cervical mucosa is about 4 mm in thickness and forms deep, branching longitudinal folds, the *plicae palmatae*, which interdigitate so as to almost obliterate the cervical canal. The mucosa is lined by a simple columnar epithelium composed of tall mucous cells and a few scattered ciliated cells. The thick lamina propria is composed of a moderately dense connective tissue (less cellular than the stroma of the endometrium) containing many large, extensively branched tubular mucous glands. The epithelium of the glands is the same as that lining the mucosa. Occasionally the glands form large, mucous-filled spherical cysts, *Nabothian cysts*, as the result of plugged ducts. **Plate 7, Fig. 1.**

Muscularis. This is a poorly developed layer of irregular bundles of smooth muscle scattered through a bed of dense fibroelastic connective tissue. In the outer region of the muscularis, some bundles of longitudinal muscle fibers extend into the vaginal walls.

Serosa. Except for its anterior surface, which abuts against the bladder, the cervix is surrounded by a serosa. The serosa is continuous with the perimetrium of the uterine body. It is a thin layer of loose connective tissue covered by mesothelium. On the anterior surface of the cervix the serosa is replaced by an adventitial layer of loose connective tissue.

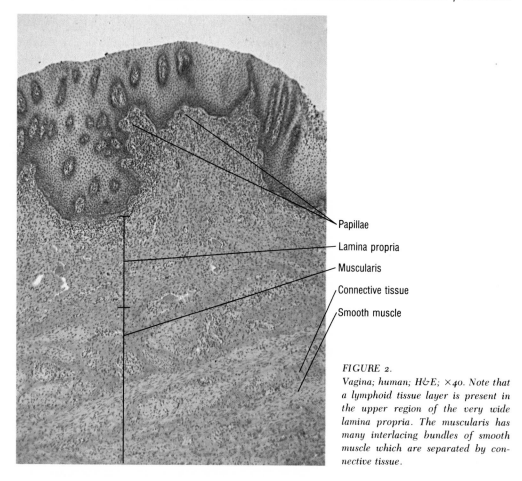

Papillae

Lamina propria

Muscularis

Connective tissue

Smooth muscle

FIGURE 2.
Vagina; human; H&E; ×40. Note that a lymphoid tissue layer is present in the upper region of the very wide lamina propria. The muscularis has many interlacing bundles of smooth muscle which are separated by connective tissue.

Vagina

This is the most inferior of the internal reproductive organs. It is a somewhat flattened tube extending from the vulva to the internal portio vaginalis of the cervix. It is about 8 cm long and located between the bladder and rectum. The vagina serves as a copulatory organ, a passage through which menses pass, and a birth canal. Its walls are quite distensible and composed of three distinct histologic layers: an inner *mucosa*, middle *muscularis*, and outer *adventitia*. **Plate 1, Fig. 1; Plate 7, Fig. 2.**

Mucosa. This relatively thick layer is formed into a number of transverse folds, or *rugae*. At its upper level it is continuous over the surface of the portio vaginalis of the cervix and extends into the external os. At the lower level of the virginal vagina the mucosa forms a perforated membrane, the *hymen*. The hymen extends transversely across the vaginal canal and separates the vagina from the vestibule (see below). Just inside the external os there is an abrupt change from simple columnar cervical epithelium to the thick stratifed nonkeratinized epithelium of the vagina.

The vaginal epithelium is nonkeratinized, but the cells may have keratohyalin granules in their cytoplasm. Even though the epithelium in the human does not undergo marked cyclic changes during menstruation, the cells contain much cytoplasmic glycogen at midcycle, when the estrogen levels are greatest. Lymphocytes are usually found in the epithelium. They migrate from lymphoid tissue located in the upper regions of the lamina propria. The lamina propria is a relatively wide layer of fibroelastic tissue composed of collagen and elastic fibers. Under the epithelium it is quite dense and forms papillae, but near the muscularis it is less dense and contains many large vessels and nerves. Since glands are absent in the lamina propria, the vaginal canal must be lubricated by mucus from the cervical glands.

Muscularis. This is divided into two layers of smooth muscle. The inner layer is thin and circular and the outer layer is thick and longitudinal. At their interface, the layers are not well separated and form interlacing bundles. At the upper end of the vagina the longitudinal bundles are continuous with those in the muscularis of the cervix. At the lower end, an additional layer of striated muscle, the bulbospongiosus, surrounds the muscularis and forms a sphincter muscle around the vaginal orifice.

Adventitia. The inner portion of the adventitia is a thin layer of dense collagenous connective tissue containing some elastic fibers. At its periphery, where the adventitia blends with the loose connective tissue of adjacent organs, it is less dense and contains large vessels, venous plexuses, and nerves.

BLOOD AND LYMPHATIC VESSELS OF THE VAGINA Arteries of the vagina are derived from several sources: uterine, vaginal, and internal pudendal arteries, and rectal branches of the internal iliac arteries. Branches of these arteries enter the adventitia and supply networks of capillaries, mainly in the mucosa and adventitia. The capillaries are drained by a network of venules and veins, which form extensive plexuses in the outer mucosa and adventitia. The plexuses are similar to erectile tissue both in appearance and function. They are drained by vaginal veins, and the blood is then dumped into the internal iliac veins. *Lymphatic plexuses* and vessels are present in the vaginal walls. They are distributed in approximately the same pattern as the veins. As the larger lymphatic vessels leave the vagina, they become confluent with lymphatics draining the cervix, rectum, and vulva.

NERVES OF THE VAGINA. Myelinated and unmyelinated somatic and visceral afferent fibers are present in the vaginal wall, along with sympathetic and parasympathetic fibers of the autonomic nervous system. The efferent fibers innervate the smooth muscle tissue of the muscularis and blood vessels, while afferent fibers are abundant in the mucosa and terminate in special sensory endings. Also, parasympathetic ganglia and their accompanying plexuses of fibers are present in the adventitia. All these fibers, which innervate the vagina, are carried by several different nerves: splanchnic nerves, pudendal nerves, and nerves from the vaginal plexuses.

Vulva (external genitalia)

The vulva contains several components: (1) the *vestibule*, a cavity into which opens the vaginal canal and the urethra; (2) two pairs of lips, which surround the vestibule, the inner *labia minora*, and the outer *labia majora*; (3) the *clitoris*, a small tubercle of erectile tissue located at the anterior end of the vestibule. **Plate 1, Fig. 1.**

VESTIBULE. The floor of this cavity is lined with a stratified squamous epithelium and contains many small mucous glands. The lateral walls of the vestibule have a pair of large, tubuloalveolar *Bartholin glands*. These glands secrete a lubricating mucus, and are analogous to the male bulbourethral glands. **Plate 1, Fig. 1.**

CLITORIS. The clitoris is homologous to the penis. It is composed of erectile tissue which is organized into a pair of corpora cavernosa bodies and terminates as a free rudimentary glans clitordis. The corpora bodies are surrounded by dense layers of collagenous connective tissue. A thin stratified squamous epithelium covers the glans clitordis. The epithelium is indented by many papillae composed of vascular connective tissue. The papillae contain sensory receptors, such as Meissner's and Pacinian corpuscles, and Krause's end bulbs.

LABIA MINORA. These are the inner or lesser lips of the vulva, forming the lateral walls of the vestibule. They partially ensheath the clitoris at the anterior end of the vulva. One labium is a fold of mucosa lined on both surfaces by a lightly keratinized stratified squamous epithelium. The epithelium is usually pigmented in its basal layer, and indented by tall papillae of the lamina propria. The lamina propria is composed of highly vascularized loose connective tissue containing many sensory receptors. Although hair follicles and adipose tissue are not present, sebaceous glands are prominent on both surfaces. **Plate 1, Fig. 1.**

LABIA MAJORA. The labia majora are the external or outer lips of the vulva and cover the labia minora. They are homologous to the scrotum of the male. A labium is a fold of skin with a core of loose connective tissue. The connective tissue contains many fat cells, some smooth muscle, vessels, nerves, and sensory receptors. The inner surface of the labium majora is lined with a mucosa similar to that lining the labia minora, except it contains sweat glands. The outer surface is typical thin skin containing hair follicles and sebaceous and sweat glands. The epidermis is stratified squamous and keratinized. **Plate 1, Fig. 1.**

Mammary glands

The mammary glands (breasts, mammae) are modified sweat glands derived from the integument. Since they are influenced by sex hormones and gonadotropins to undergo cyclic changes, they are treated here rather than with integumentary structures (see Chap. 11). Mammary glands develop in both the prepuberty male and female. At puberty they develop slowly in the male, but cease development at about 20 years. In the female, they enlarge rapidly, mainly by accumulations of adipose and connective tissues, but remain incompletely developed until a pregnancy occurs. Usually the mammary glands of a matron will show cyclic changes which are correlated with the ovarian and menstrual cycles. After menopause, the glands undergo regression and become atrophied.

The mammary glands in the mature female are rounded elevations lying anterior to the pectoralis major, external oblique, and serratus anterior muscles. They are separated from these muscles by loose connective tissue, which allows them some degree of movement. The mammary glands are covered with skin and lie within the subcutaneous layer. Just below the center of the anterior surface of the mammary gland the skin is formed into an elevated, pigmented *nipple*. The base of the nipple is surrounded by a circular, pigmented, textured area of skin, the *areola*.

The mammary gland is composed of 15 to 20 tubuloalveolar glands or lobes. The lobes are separated from each other by interlobar septa of dense connective tissue, usually containing much fat. Each lobe is subdivided into tiny lobules by dense interlobular connective tissue, usually lacking fat. The lobules are composed of *intralobular ducts (alveolar ducts)* and *alveoli,* embedded in a delicate stroma of intralobular loose connective tissue. The secretory alveoli are drained by many secretory *intralobular ducts;* these ducts are drained by fewer and larger *interlobular ducts;* the interlobular ducts converge to form a single large *lactiferous duct.* Each lobe is drained by its own lactiferous duct toward the nipple. As the lactiferous duct approaches the base of the nipple, it enlarges to become the *lactiferous sinus.* The duct narrows once again as it continues toward the surface of the nipple. The surface of the nipple is usually perforated by fewer openings than there are lactiferous ducts because of fusions between some of the ducts at their upper levels.

In the matron, the mammary glands usually undergo cyclic histologic changes as a direct response to sex hormones produced during the ovarian cycle. Increasing concentrations of estrogen stimulate growth of the duct system, while progesterone and estrogen result in increased but limited proliferation of the secretory end pieces. A decrease of these hormones in the last phases of the ovarian cycle is accompanied by a regression of the mammary tissues. If the woman is pregnant, the mammary glands become highly developed under the influence of chorionic LTH (chorionic prolactin). At parturition, with the loss of the placenta, the inhibiting influence of progesterone on pituitary LTH (pituitary prolactin) is removed. This is important, because the suckling of the infant stimulates LTH production by the anterior pituitary. The pituitary LTH keeps the mammary glands in a fully developed secreting condition until weaning. The suckling also stimulates the posterior pituitary to release oxytocin (secreted in the hypothalamus), which is instrumental in the removal of milk from the lactiferous ducts by contraction of the myoepithelial cells.

INACTIVE MAMMARY GLAND. The major histologic characteristics of this nonproliferating, nonlactating gland are listed below. **Plate 8, Fig. 1.**

1 Connective and adipose tissues are abundant, while glandular structures are scarce; lobules are not well defined.

2 The sparse glandular alveoli are small, solid, budlike structures. They are composed of relatively small nonsecretory epithelial cells lying on a basement membrane.

3 Ducts are more prominent and abundant than secretory alveoli. The smallest ducts are lined with a simple cuboidal epithelium lying on a basement membrane. The larger ducts have two layers of cuboidal epithelium, and at the nipple the epithelium is a thick stratified squamous layer. Stellate myoepithelial cells lie between the duct cells and basement membrane (see below).

ACTIVE MAMMARY GLAND. In response to the ovarian hormones during the menstrual cycle, the mammary glands become proliferated but nonlactating in a nonpregnant matron. The glands become highly developed during pregnancy. In the late stages of pregnancy, and just a few days after partuition, the glands become secretory and produce colostrum—a watery fluid rich in lactoproteins and antibodies but low in fat. As colostrum ceases to be produced, the mammary glands secrete milk, which is rich in fat, lactoproteins, casein, and lactose. The histologic characteristics for proliferating, nonlactating glands, and lactating glands are given below.

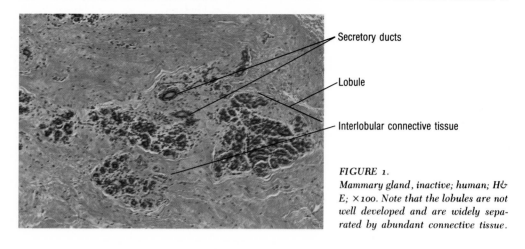

Secretory ducts

Lobule

Interlobular connective tissue

FIGURE 1.
Mammary gland, inactive; human; H&
E; ×100. Note that the lobules are not
well developed and are widely sepa-
rated by abundant connective tissue.

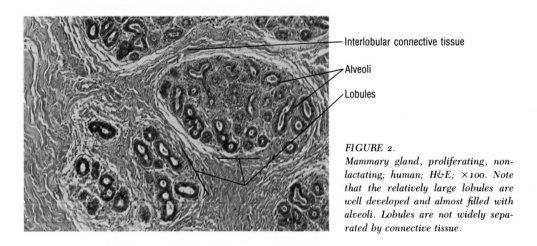

Interlobular connective tissue

Alveoli

Lobules

FIGURE 2.
Mammary gland, proliferating, non-
lactating; human; H&E; ×100. Note
that the relatively large lobules are
well developed and almost filled with
alveoli. Lobules are not widely sepa-
rated by connective tissue.

Proliferating, nonlactating mammary gland. **Plate 8, Fig. 2.**

1 Ducts, secretory alveoli, and lobules are well developed. The alveoli are of moderate
size and do not fill the lobules. They develop from buds formed at the terminal ends
of the extensively branched duct system. The alveoli are hollow and lined with a simple
cuboidal epithelium. Although the gland is nonlactating, secretions may be present in
some alveoli.

2 Interlobular and intralobular adipose and connective tissues are sparse, but more
abundant than in the lactating glands (see below). The intralobular connective tissue
may be infiltrated with lymphocytes.

Secreting alveoli

Connective tissue

Ducts

Secretions

Lobules

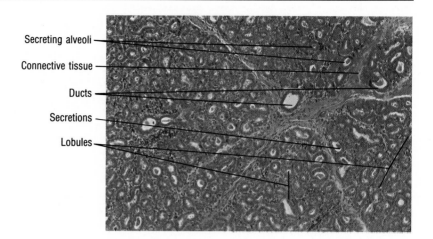

FIGURE 3.
*Mammary gland, lactating; human;
H&E; × 100. Note that lobules are fully
developed and completely filled with
large, saclike secretory alveoli. The
connective tissue separating the lobules
appears as thin septa.*

Lactating mammary gland. **Plate 8, Fig. 3.**

1 Alveoli are large and saclike. They fill the well-developed lobule and usually contain secretions.

2 Interlobular connective tissue appears as thin septa or scattered strands of tissue.

3 The lactating gland has active and resting alveoli within it. The alveoli may be lined with cuboidal or columnar cells. The cytoplasm is acidophilic at the apical ends of the cells, and basophilic near the basal regions. Resting alveoli have small lumina and relatively thick walls, while active alveoli have large lumina and thinner walls. The tall secretory cells gradually become flattened as milk accumulates in the lumen of the alveolus. The cells secrete substances both by apocrine (milk fats) and merocrine (milk proteins, salts, etc.) activities. Myoepithelial cells are located between the secretory cells and the basement membrane. By their contractions, the myoepithelial cells aid in emptying the ducts of their contents. The intralobular ducts are difficult to distinguish from the alveoli, since they also secrete milk.

NIPPLE AND AREOLA. The skin of the nipple and areola has a thin squamous keratinized epithelium which becomes heavily pigmented at puberty. The dermis contains relatively small amounts of adipose tissue, and many tall, vascular papillae indent the epidermis. Only the tip of the nipple is most sensitive. It contains numerous sensory receptors (Meissner's corpuscles and free nerve endings) in the dermal papillae. The nipple has a network of circular and longitudinal smooth muscles distributed within its dermis. The circular muscles are scattered throughout the nipple, while longitudinal muscles are mainly distributed around the lactiferous ducts. The ducts open by pores to the surface of the nipple. The muscles are important in controlling the elevation and rigidity of the nipple. The areola contains large, branched apocrine glands of Montgomery, eccrine sweat glands, and sebaceous glands.

BLOOD AND LYMPHATIC VESSELS OF MAMMARY GLANDS. Arterial branches from the internal mammary, axillary, and intercostal arteries follow the system of ducts. They eventually supply capillary networks surrounding the intralobular ducts and alveoli. The capillaries are drained by venules and veins, which accompany the arterial vessels. *Lymphatic capillaries* form abundant plexuses in the interlobular connective tissue and walls of the lactiferous ducts. These plexuses join those in the subcutaneous layer of the skin and areola of the mammary gland. Larger collecting vessels then drain these plexuses mainly toward the pectoral and axillary lymph nodes.

NERVES OF THE MAMMARY GLAND. Sympathetic nerve fibers are abundant in the mammary gland. They innervate smooth muscle fibers of the blood vessels and nipple. Somatic afferent nerve fibers are also present. They are associated with the many sensory receptors in the nipple. The physiologic activities of the secretory and myoepithelial cells are probably under the influence of only sex hormones and gonadotropic hormones.

Male Reproductive System 16

The male reproductive system, like that of the female, is composed of internal organs and external genitalia. Unlike the female, however, urinary and reproductive organs are united within the pelvic canal. The organs of the male reproductive system are illustrated in **Plate 1, Fig. 1,** and listed below: testes, seminiferous tubules, tubuli recti, rete testis, ductuli efferentes, epididymis, ductus deferens, ampulla, seminal vesicles, ejaculatory duct, prostate gland, bulbourethral glands, and penis. These organs can be placed into two functional categories: (1) *glands* to produce semen, a viscid, white fluid containing spermatozoa, and (2) *excretory ducts* to carry the semen. The glands are the seminiferous tubules of the testes, seminal vesicles, prostate gland, and bulbourethral glands. The remaining organs form a system of excretory ducts.

Testes

The paired testes lie within thin, closed, double-walled serosal sacs, the *tunicae vaginalis*, which are themselves contained within an integumentary sac, the *scrotum*. Actually the tunicae vaginalis surround only about 75 percent of the anterior and lateral portions of the testes. Each sac is divided into an outer parietal layer, closely associated with the scrotum, and an inner visceral layer resting directly on the testis. Each testis is suspended in its sacs by the *spermatic cord*, which extends to the internal inguinal ring and contains the ductus deferens, vessels, nerves, and loose connective tissue. The cord is covered by fascia and bundles of skeletal muscle, the *cremaster muscle*. The testis is a laterally compressed, ovoid gland about 4.5 cm long, 3 cm deep, and 2 cm thick. It is surrounded by a thick capsule of dense collagenous connective tissue containing some elastic fibers, the *tunica albuginea*. Just under the tunica albuginea, a highly vascularized *tunica vasculosa* is present as a loose connective tissue layer. On the posterior surface of the testis, along the midline, the tunica albuginea enlarges as a thickened bed of connective tissue, the *mediastinum testis*. Each testis is subdivided into 200 to 300 small pyramid-shaped *lobuli testi* by thin septa connective tissue, the *septula testis*. These septula radiate from the mediastinum to the tunica albuginea and incompletely separate the lobules.

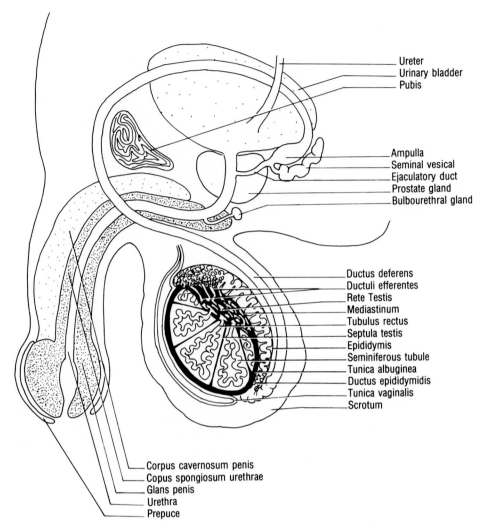

Ureter
Urinary bladder
Pubis

Ampulla
Seminal vesical
Ejaculatory duct
Prostate gland
Bulbourethral gland

Ductus deferens
Ductuli efferentes
Rete Testis
Mediastinum
Tubulus rectus
Septula testis
Epididymis
Seminiferous tubule
Tunica albuginea
Ductus epididymidis
Tunica vaginalis
Scrotum

Corpus cavernosum penis
Copus spongiosum urethrae
Glans penis
Urethra
Prepuce

FIGURE 1.
General drawing of the male repro-
ductive system, sagittal view.

The apex of each lobule joins the mediastinum while its base lies on the tunica albuginea. Each lobule contains a bed of highly vascularized loose connective tissue, the fibers and vessels of which are continuous with those of the tunica vasculosa. The usual cell types (macrophages, fibroblasts, mesenchyme cells, etc.) are found in this connective tissue; in addition, specialized testosterone-producing *interstitial cells* (Leydig cells) are present (see below). Every lobule contains one to four highly convoluted *seminiferous tubules* embedded within the connective tissue. Near the periphery of the lobules the tubules commence as anastomotic loops, or infrequently as blind ends. Close to the mediastinum they lose their convolutions and unite to form straight tubules with a smaller diameter, the *tubuli recti*. The 20 to 30 tubuli recti become confluent with an irregular network of spaces in the mediastinum, the *rete testis*. At the superior region of the mediastinum the rete testis opens into 12 to 20 large ducts, the *ductuli efferentes*. These ducts leave the testis through the tunica albuginea, and each forms a convoluted, conical mass. These masses form the lobules of the epididymis, which collectively represent the head of the epididymis. **Plate 1, Figs. 1 and 2.**

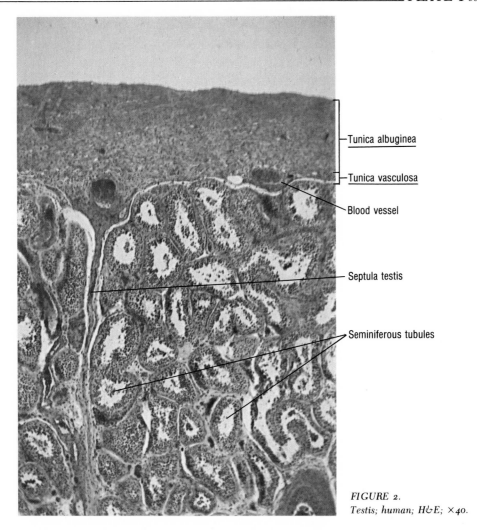

Tunica albuginea

Tunica vasculosa

Blood vessel

Septula testis

Seminiferous tubules

FIGURE 2.
Testis; human; H&E; ×40.

SEMINIFEROUS TUBULES. These tubules are surrounded by several layers of collagen and elastic fibers, and flattened cells. A stratified germinal epithelium lines each tubule and rests on a prominent basement membrane. The process of gamete formation, or spermatogenesis, occurs within the germinal epithelium of the seminiferous tubules. Spermatogenesis is controlled by follicle-stimulating hormone (FSH), a gonadotropin produced by the pars distalis of the pituitary gland. The germinal epithelium is composed of *Sertoli cells* (sustentacular or supporting cells) and *germinal cells*. The outermost peripheral layer of germinal cells are the spermatogonia, and during spermatogenesis they give rise to primary spermatocytes. The primary spermatocytes undergo the first meiotic division to form secondary spermatocytes. The secondary spermatocytes then pass through a second meiotic division to produce spermatids. Eventually the spermatids transform into mature sperm cells by a metamorphic process, spermiogenesis. During the process of spermatogenesis, as the cells mature, they move to successively higher levels in the germinal epithelium. Thus, the spermatids lie closer to the lumen of a seminiferous tubule than primary spermatocytes. **Plate 1, Fig. 2.**

Connective tissue
Interstitial cell
Spermatozoa
Spermatid
Sertoli cell nucleus
Primary spermatocyte
Spermatogonium

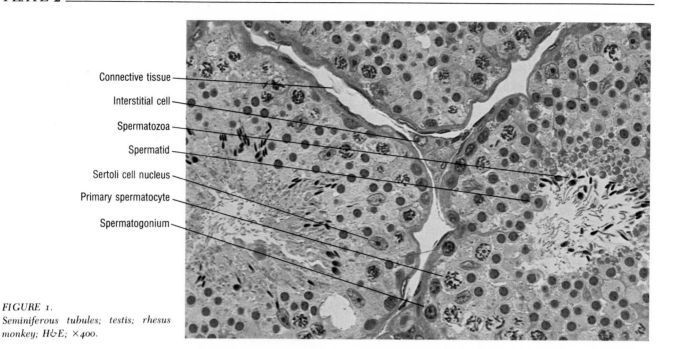

FIGURE 1.
Seminiferous tubules; testis; rhesus monkey; H&E; ×400.

Spermatogonia. These are medium-sized cells, about 12 μm in diameter, lying on the basement membrane. The cytoplasm is pale and may be vacuolated. The round or ovoid nucleus is about one-half the diameter of the cell and contains granulated chromatin with one or more prominent nucleoli. Although two cell types, the A and B spermatogonia, have been distinguished, they are difficult to identify in routine preparations. The type A cell has a pale-staining nuclear vacuole and a dark nucleus. The B type cell lacks the vacuole and its nucleus appears lightly stained. Type A spermatogonia undergo mitosis. Some give rise to more type A stem spermatogonia, while others differentiate into spermatogonia of the B type. The B spermatogonia also undergo several mitotic divisions, but they eventually differentiate into primary spermatocytes. **Plate 2, Fig. 1.**

Primary spermatocytes. These cells lie above the spermatogonia and are closer to the lumen. They are large cells, about 18 μm in diameter, and their nuclei occupy most of the cytoplasm. The chromatin may be granular, netlike, or in coarse clumps. The primary spermatocytes represent the early stages of meiosis. As a cell matures, it prepares for and undergoes the first meiotic division. Every primary spermatocyte gives rise to two secondary spermatocytes, each with a haploid number of chromosomes. **Plate 2, Fig. 1.**

Secondary spermatocytes. These cells lie above the primary spermatocytes. They are about the size of spermatogonia (12 μm), and therefore are much smaller than the primary spermatocytes. The round nucleus is about one-half the diameter of the cell and centrally located in the cytoplasm. The dark-stained chromatin is concentrated and quite dense. Almost as soon as they are formed, secondary spermatocytes undergo the second meiotic division and give rise to spermatids. Because of this activity, secondary spermatocytes are difficult to observe in sections.

Spermatids. The spermatids usually lie near the lumen of the seminiferous tubule. They are about 9 μm in diameter, one-half the size of primary spermatocytes. The young spermatids appear as pale, polygonal cells with a medium-sized, round, pale nucleus which is centrally positioned within the cytoplasm. The chromatin appears as a pale-stained, delicate network. The spermatids do not divide but undergo metamorphic transformations, *spermiogenesis*, where they transform into mature spermatozoa. During spermiogenesis the spermatids become elongate, eventually forming a head, neck, body, and tail (see below). The nucleus becomes oval, smaller, and more condensed, and eccentrically positioned in the cytoplasm. **Plate 2, Fig. 1.**

Spermatozoa. These sexually mature haploid gametes are about 65 μm long. They may be located at the free edge of the germinal epithelium or within the lumen of the seminiferous tubule. Cytologically the cells have a well-developed head, neck, and tail. The *head* contains a condensed, oval, dark-stained nucleus and an anterior acrosomal cap. The acrosomal cap is derived from the golgi apparatus and contains an enzyme, hyaluronidase. This enzyme aids in the penetration of the sperm into the female gamete during fertilization. It digests the intercellular cement of the follicle cells (corona radiata) surrounding the secondary oocyte. The *neck* is the connecting piece between the head and tail; it contains two centrioles. The *tail* (flagellum) is the locomotor organelle of the sperm cell. It is divided into an upper *middle piece*, near the neck, a lower *principal piece*, and a terminal *end piece*. As seen with the electron microscope, the tail contains a core of longitudinal filaments, the axoneme. The axoneme is composed of two single central microtubules surrounded by a peripheral ring of nine doubled microtubules. The *middle piece* contains dense longitudinal fibers which surround the axoneme and also contribute to motor functions. A helix of mitrochondria, lying end to end, forms a sheath just outside the longitudinal fibers and supply the sperm with energy-rich ATP molecules. At the lower end of the middle piece there is a ring of dense material, the *annulus*, which is fused to the plasma membrane. It forms a boundary between the middle and principal pieces. The *principal piece* is a circumferential sheath of dense fibrils surrounding the axoneme. In addition, the longitudinal fibrils from the middle piece also extend into the principal piece. The *end piece* is composed only of the axoneme, and near the end of the tail the doublets of microtubules separate into 18 singles. The entire sperm is surrounded by a plasma membrane, and all but the end piece has a thin layer of peripheral cytoplasm. **Plate 2, Fig. 1; Plate 2, Fig. 2.**

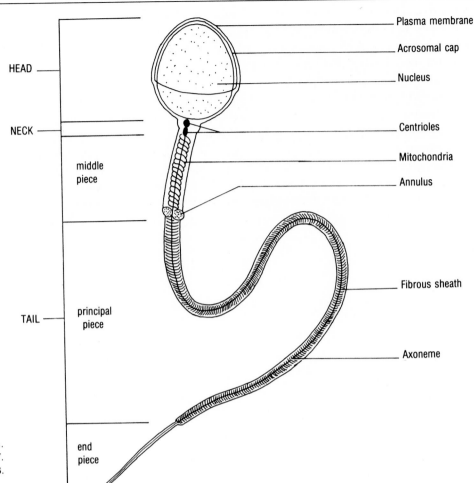

HEAD

NECK

middle
piece

TAIL

principal
piece

end
piece

Plasma membrane

Acrosomal cap

Nucleus

Centrioles

Mitochondria

Annulus

Fibrous sheath

Axoneme

FIGURE 2.
Schematic drawing of a human sperm.
(Adapted from W. Bloom and D. W.
Fawcett, *Textbook of Histology*, W. B.
Saunders Co., Philadelphia, 1975.)

Sertoli cells (sustentacular cells). These are large, tall, irregularly shaped cells extending from the basement membrane to the lumen of the tubule. They are scattered among the more numerous germinal cells. The nucleus usually lies at the base of the cell, near the basement membrane. It is a large, pale, ovoid or irregularly shaped structure containing a prominently stained nucleolus. The nucleolus has an eosinophilic center surrounded by a basophilic rim. The cytoplasm is usually difficult to observe in routine preparations. It may be filled with lipid vacuoles, granules of glycogen, or other substances. Proteinaceous crystalloid structures may be located near the nucleus. These crystalloids are usually elongate with tapered ends. Unlike the germinal cells, Sertoli cells apparently do not divide in the adult testis. They function to provide support and probably nutrition to the developing sperm cell. Although the sperm cells are not attached to the Sertoli cells, they lie in deep recesses of the outer cytoplasm. Immature sperm cells lie along the sides of a Sertoli cell, while the mature sperm are located at its apex. The Sertoli cells may regulate the release of mature sperm into the lumen of the seminiferous tubule. Adjacent Sertoli cells form a blood-testis barrier by a fusion of their plasma membranes near the base of the germinal epithelium. This barrier prevents large macromolecules from being exchanged between the blood and upper epithelium of the seminiferous tubules. **Plate 2, Fig. 1.**

Interstitial cells (cells of Leydig). These cells are located within the loose connective tissue between the seminiferous tubules. They usually appear as clumps of large polyhedral or ovoid cells. The pale acidophilic cytoplasm may contain vacuoles, granules, and protein crystals of Reinke. The dark-stained, round nucleus is filled with coarse clumps of chromatin and contains one or more prominent nucleoli. Smaller, fusiform cells, possibly derived from mesenchyme cells, may also be present in a clump of interstitial cells. These cells are believed to be precursors to the interstitial cells. The interstitial cells are stimulated to secrete testosterone by luteinizing hormone (LH), also known as interstitial cell stimulating hormone (ICSH). ICSH is produced by the pars distalis of the anterior pituitary. Testosterone is a steroid hormone which regulates the maintenance of the reproductive organs. Testosterone also promotes the development of secondary sex characteristics, such as muscle enlargement and hair on the chest. **Plate 2, Fig. 1.**

BLOOD AND LYMPHATIC VESSELS OF THE TESTES. The testicular artery sends branches into the mediastinum, tunica albuginea, and tunica vasculosa. Arterioles extend from the mediastinum and tunica vasculosa to follow the septula testis into the stroma of the testis. Within the stroma, these arterioles supply networks of capillaries surrounding the seminiferous tubules. The plexuses are drained by venules, which in turn are drained by veins toward the mediastinum and tunica albuginea. Veins coming from these regions form the pampiniform plexus in the spermatic cord. *Lymphatic plexuses* are abundant within the loose connective tissue surrounding the seminiferous tubules. They are drained by medium-sized vessels into larger collecting vessels located in the septula testis and tunica albuginea.

NERVES OF THE TESTES. Sympathetic efferent and visceral afferent nerve fibers, derived from the spermatic plexus, form a network in the deeper regions of the tunica albuginea. From this network, fibers extend into the loose connective tissue to form delicate plexuses around seminiferous tubules, interstitial cells, and blood vessels.

Excretory ducts (genital ducts)

These ducts are mainly responsible for the transport of semen, but they also produce a small amount of the seminal fluid. They form a continuous system of excretory sex ducts connecting the seminiferous tubules to the prostatic urethra. The excretory ducts are the *tubuli recti, rete testis, ductuli efferentes, epididymis, ductus deferens,* and *ejaculatory duct*. The ejaculatory duct joins the prostatic urethra.

TUBULI RECTI. At the apex of a lobule several seminiferous tubules lose their convolutions and unite to form a straight, narrow tube, the *tubulus rectus*. About 20 to 30 tubuli recti extend toward the mediastinum where they join the rete testis. At the terminal end of the seminiferous tubule, near the junction of the tubulus rectus, the germ cells gradually disappear, leaving only Sertoli cells. Within the tubulus rectus the Sertoli cells are replaced by a simple cuboidal nonsecretory epithelium lying on a delicate basement membrane. The tubulus rectus is surrounded by loose connective tissue. **Plate 1, Fig. 1; Plate 3, Fig. 1.**

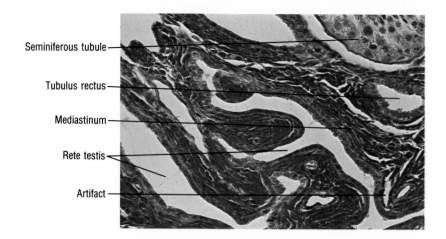

Seminiferous tubule

Tubulus rectus

Mediastinum

Rete testis

Artifact

FIGURE 1.
Tubuli recti and rete testis; testis; hu-
man; iron hematoxylin–aniline blue;
×400; Note that the rete testis appear
as an irregular network of epithelial-
lined channels.

RETE TESTIS. The rete testis is an irregular network of epithelial-lined spaces within the mediastinum. These spaces join the tubuli recti with the ductuli efferentes. The rete testis is lined by a low simple cuboidal or simple squamous nonsecretory epithelium lying on a delicate basement membrane. Occasionally a single flagellum may be seen at the apex of the cuboidal cells, and extend into the lumen. Since the rete testis is enclosed by the dense connective tissue of the mediastinum, it lacks well-organized walls. **Plate 1, Fig. 1; Plate 3, Fig. 1.**

DUCTULI EFFERENTES. The anastomotic spaces of the rete testis are continuous with 12 to 20 tubules of the *ductuli efferentes* at the superior end of the mediastinum. The ductuli efferentes connect the rete testis with the epididymis. Each one of the ductuli is relatively straight as it extends through the tunica albuginea, but just outside the testis it becomes highly convoluted and forms a cone-shaped lobule. These lobules are joined by a vascular connective tissue to form the head of the epididymis. The ductuli efferentes are lined by a scalloped nonsecretory low pseudostratified epithelium lying on a basement membrane. There are alternating patches of superficial columnar and cuboidal cells, which give the epithelium its characteristic scalloped pattern. Some of the cells of both types are ciliated. The cytoplasm is generally pale in the cuboidal cells, and acidophilic in the columnar cells. Nonsecretory granules and pigment may be present in both cell types. Small, polyhedral basal cells appear below the more superficial cells. Simple walls of the ductuli efferentes may be distinguished as a thin layer of circular smooth muscle surrounded by loose connective tissue. Although the ciliated epithelium is instrumental in moving semen towards the epididymis, the muscular coat is most effective in carrying out this function. **Plate 1, Fig. 1; Plate 3, Fig. 2.**

EPIDIDYMIS. This is a cordlike mass of connective tissue containing the duct of the epididymis, vessels, and nerves. It is attached to the posterior border of the testis and is anatomically divided into an upper *head or caput*, middle *body*, and terminal *tail or cauda*. Several lobules, derived from the ductuli efferentes, form the head. At their lower ends, the lobules fuse to form a single duct of the epididymis, the *ductus epididymidis*. The duct extends through the body and tail of the epididymis. It is highly convoluted, and its coils are embedded in the loose connective tissue of the epididymis. The epithelium of the epididymal duct is pseudostratified columnar

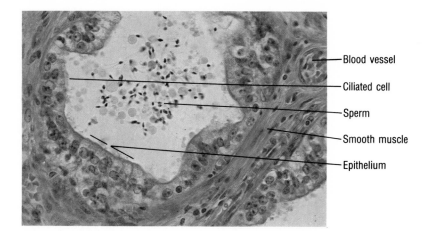

Blood vessel

Ciliated cell

Sperm

Smooth muscle

Epithelium

FIGURE 2.
Ductuli efferentes; human; H&E;
×400. Note that the epithelium is typ-
ically scalloped. The cytoplasm of the
cells is granulated, and some cells are
ciliated.

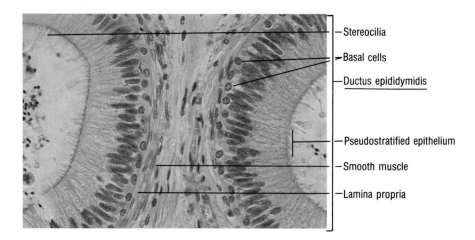

Stereocilia

Basal cells

Ductus epididymidis

Pseudostratified epithelium

Smooth muscle

Lamina propria

FIGURE 3.
Epididymis; human; H&E; ×400.

and rests on a distinct basement membrane. The epithelium is composed of superficial stereociliated columnar cells lying above rounded basal cells (see Chap. 2). The stereocilia are long microvilli which may be both secretory and resorptive in function. The cytoplasm of the cells is usually basophilic and may contain lipid vacuoles and pigment granules. The walls of the ductus epididymidis are more complex than those of the ductuli efferentes, since a thin lamina propria of loose connective tissue is present between the epithelium and a circular layer of smooth muscle. At the upper level of the ductus epididymidis, only a thin layer of circular muscle surrounds the lamina propria; in the body of the ductus, a few longitudinal muscle fibers form an incomplete second layer outside the circular muscle; and in the tail, the outer longitudinal layer becomes very prominent. Loose connective tissue of the epididymis surrounds the smooth muscle an is packed between the coils of the ductus epididymidis. As immobile sperm move passively down the ductus epididymidis, they undergo further maturation. Substances and fluids are absorbed and secreted by the epithelium of the duct, so that the composition of the semen is continually changing. These changes are probably compatible for the further ripening of the spermatozoa. **Plate 1, Fig. 1; Plate 3, Fig. 3.**

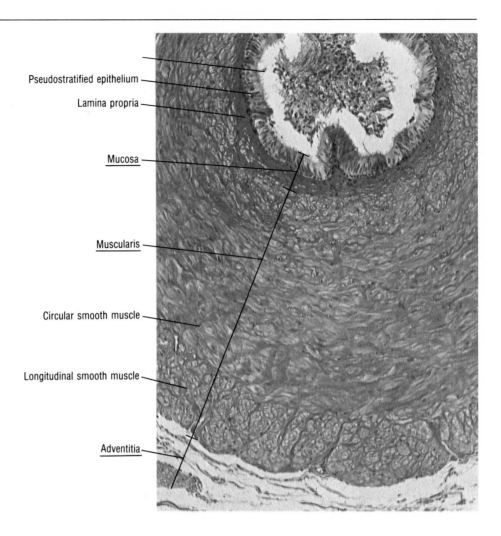

Pseudostratified epithelium

Lamina propria

<u>Mucosa</u>

<u>Muscularis</u>

Circular smooth muscle

Longitudinal smooth muscle

<u>Adventitia</u>

FIGURE 1.
Ductus deferens (cross section); human;
H&E; ×100. Note that three distinct
layers of the muscularis may be seen.
Mucosa is formed into longitudinal
folds.

DUCTUS DEFERENS (vas deferens). This single tube is continuous with the end of the ductus epididymidis. It is coiled at the inferior level of the testis, but soon loses its coils as it extends towards the inguinal canal. At the level of the testis it runs parallel with the epididymis, but above the testis it runs within the spermatic cord. After passing through the inguinal canal and entering the pelvic cavity, the ductus deferens leaves the spermatic cord. It follows a tortuous retroperitoneal path leading to the prostatic urethra. The left and right ducts converge, but do not fuse, at the base of the prostate gland. At this level, each ductus deferens enlarges to form a spindle shaped *ampulla*. Below the ampulla, each ductus deferens is designated as an *ejaculatory duct* as it becomes confluent with the duct of a seminal vesicle. The ejaculatory duct enters the prostatic urethra. The walls of the ductus deferens are more highly developed than those of the ductus epididymidis because they are organized into three distinct histological layers: inner mucosa, middle muscularis, and outer adventitia. **Plate 1, Fig. 1; Plate 4, Fig. 1.**

Mucosa. The mucosa is folded into several longitudinal ridges extending into the lumen of the ductus deferens. In the ampulla, the folds are anastomotic, extensively folded, and highly branched; glandular diverticula may extend into the muscularis. **Plate 4, Fig. 2.** The epithelium in the ductus deferens is a low pseudostratified

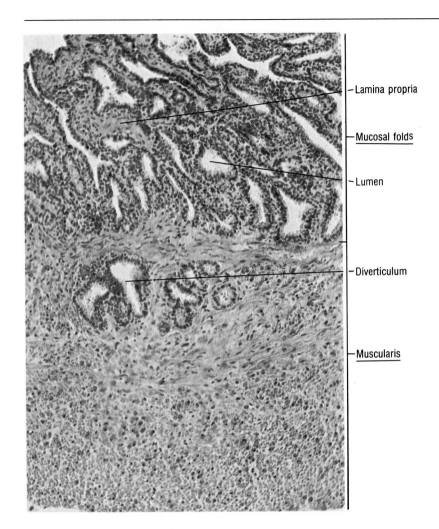

—Lamina propria

—Mucosal folds

—Lumen

—Diverticulum

—Muscularis

FIGURE 2.
Ampulla; human; H&E; ×100. Note that the mucosa forms branched anastomatic folds. The layers of smooth muscle are not as distinctly separated as in the ductus deferens.

columnar sterociliated type, but the ampulla has a simple columnar type of epithelium. **Plate 4, Fig. 2.** In both the ductus deferens and ampulla there is a delicate basement membrane lying above a thin lamina propria. The lamina propria is composed of loose connective tissue containing a dense network of elastic fibers. **Plate 4, Fig. 1.**

Muscularis. This is the thickest (about 1 mm thick) of the three coats making up the walls of the ductus deferens. It is composed of smooth muscle tissue arranged into three layers: thin inner longitudinal; thick middle circular; and thick outer longitudinal. Compared to the ductus deferens, the ampulla has a thinner muscularis of two layers of smooth muscle tissue. The boundary between the inner circular and outer longitudinal layers is not well defined because of intermingling fibers. **Plate 4, Fig. 2.** The main function of the ductus deferens is to move semen toward the urethra, especially during an orgasm, as the muscularis undergoes strong contractions. **Plate 4, Fig. 1.**

Adventitia. This is a layer of loose connective tissue which blends with tissues of adjacent structures. It contains many blood and lymphatic vessels and nerves. **Plate 4, Fig. 1.**

EJACULATORY DUCT. This is the slender terminal end of each ductus deferens, lying below the duct leading to the seminal vesicle. It passes through the prostate gland and enters the posterior aspect of the urethra, where it terminates on a thickened mucosal ridge, the urethral crest. The ejaculatory ducts probably add some secretions to the semen, and, although they are not well endowed with muscle, help move semen into the urethra. The walls are thinner than those of the ampulla, but are also composed of a *mucosa, muscularis*, and *adventitia*.

Mucosa. The mucosa is formed into tall, branched, anastomosing folds. The folds form deep, pocketlike glandular diverticula which may extend into the muscularis. Near the urethral orifice the epithelium is transitional, but in other areas it is simple columnar or pseudostratified columnar. Yellow pigment may be present in the cytoplasm of the epithelial cells. The lamina propria is composed of loose connective tissue and contains many elastic fibers.

Muscularis. This is a thin layer of outer circular and inner longitudinal smooth muscle surrounding the lamina propria. As the ejaculatory duct passes through the prostate gland, the muscle is partially replaced by fibrous tissues from the prostate.

Adventitia. This is a coat of loose connective tissue containing nerves and vessels. It is continuous with connective tissues of adjacent structures, but is lost as the ejaculatory duct enters the prostate gland.

Accessory reproductive glands

The accessory reproductive glands are the seminal vesicles and prostate and bulbourethral glands. They secrete substances which constitute the major fluid component of semen.

SEMINAL VESICLES. The seminal vesicles are paired, saclike, tapered, elongate glands about 5 cm long and 1.5 cm wide. They lie behind the bladder and are lateral to the ampullae. Embryologically, they develop from the ductus deferens, just below the ampullae. Their ducts join those of the ductus deferens to form the ejaculatory duct. The seminal vesicles have a bumpy surface because their walls form bulging, irregular pouches, recesses, and chambers, all of which open onto a common lumen. The walls are organized into three coats of tissue: an inner *mucosa*, middle *muscularis*, and outer *adventitia*. Under the influence of testosterone, the seminal vesicles secrete a large amount of thick, yellowish fluid containing globulin and fructose. This secretion constitutes about 20 percent of the seminal fluid. It possibly provides some nutrition for the spermatozoa, as well as a medium for their transportation. **Plate 1, Fig. 1; Plate 5, Fig. 1.**

Mucosa. The mucosa is formed into many tall, thin primary folds. These folds have secondary and tertiary anastomatic folds which extend well into the lumen of the gland, giving it the appearance of a network of irregular spaces and compartments. These mucosal folds are more extensive than those in the ampulla, and increase the surface area for secretions. The epithelium may be simple columnar or pseudostratified columnar, but the latter type is common in active, healthy seminal vesicles. The pseudostratified epithelium rests on a basement membrane and has tall, columnar secretory cells lying above a layer of rounded basal cells. The secretory cells have an oval-shaped nucleus lying in a vacuolated cytoplasm. The cytoplasm usually contains secretory granules and a yellow lipochrome pigment. The secretions may appear as an adidophilic reticulum filling the lumen of the gland. The *lamina propria* is a thin layer of loose connective tissue containing vessels and nerves.

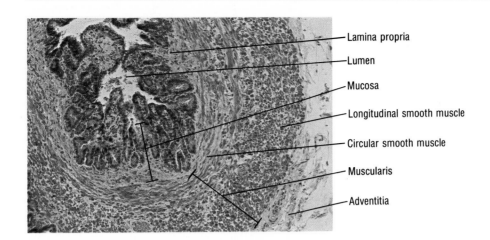

Lamina propria

Lumen

Mucosa

Longitudinal smooth muscle

Circular smooth muscle

Muscularis

Adventitia

FIGURE 1.
Seminal vesicle; human; H&E; ×100.
Note that although the mucosal folds
should be more extensive than those in
the ampullae, the smooth muscle layers
are more distinctly set apart.

Muscularis. This layer of smooth muscle may be used to distinguish seminal vesicles from the ampullae. The muscularis is thinner than the ampullae, and its two layers of muscle are more distinctly set apart. The inner layer is composed of intermixed circular and oblique muscle fibers, while the outer layer contains longitudinal fibers.

Adventitia. This thin, fibrous layer is composed of loose connective tissue containing many elastic fibers, blood and lymphatic vessels, nerve fibers, and parasympathetic ganglia.

BLOOD AND LYMPHATIC VESSELS OF THE SEMINAL VESICLES. Branches of the inferior vesicle and middle rectal arteries enter the adventitial layer of the seminal vesicles and supply capillary networks within the mucosa and muscularis. The capillaries are drained by venules into veins, which generally accompany the arteries. *Lymphatic vessels* are present and run in company with the blood vessels.

NERVES OF THE SEMINAL VESICLES. Plexuses of autonomic nerves and ganglia are located in the adventitia and muscularis of the seminal vesicles. The sympathetic nerves stimulate the musculature of the seminal vesicles and sphincter muscles of the urinary bladder to simultaneously constrict the neck of the bladder and compress the seminal vesicles during an ejaculation. This mechanism prevents a backflow of seminal fluid into the bladder. Visceral afferent nerves are present and innervate tissues within the mucosa.

PROSTATE GLAND. The prostate gland surrounds the upper prostatic portion of the urethra. The ovoid gland is about 4 cm in diameter. It has a fibrous capsule surrounding a bed of fibromuscular tissue containing many glands. Although a section of the ejaculatory duct is present within the prostate gland, the prostatic urethra may be used as a central landmark to establish three somewhat separate histologic regions of the gland. The *mucosa* of the prostate gland immediately surrounds the urethra and contains small glands which open directly into it. Peripheral to the mucosal region is a cresent-shaped *submucosa* lying laterally and posteriorly to the urethra. It contains larger glands, which also empty into the urethra. Peripheral to the submucosal region is the outermost, largest component of the gland, the *principal component*. It also is a cresent-shaped glandular mass of tissue lying laterally and posteriorly to the urethra, but it extends to the capsule.

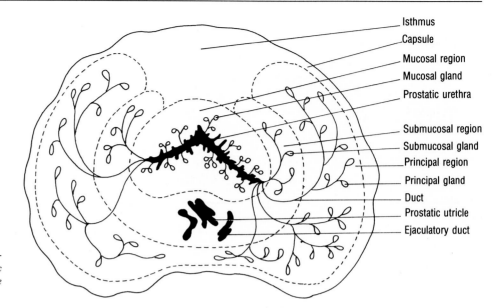

Isthmus
Capsule
Mucosal region
Mucosal gland
Prostatic urethra

Submucosal region
Submucosal gland
Principal region
Principal gland
Duct
Prostatic utricle
Ejaculatory duct

FIGURE 2.
Schematic diagram of the human prostate showing three major histologic divisions: mucosa, submucosa, and the principal component.

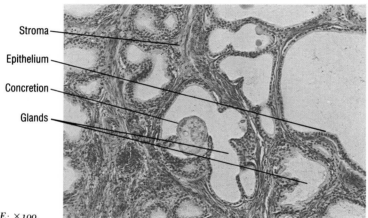

Stroma
Epithelium
Concretion
Glands

FIGURE 3.
Prostate; adult human; H&E; ×100.

This outer region of the prostate gland contains some 30 to 50 compound tubuloalveolar glands organized into five poorly defined lobes. All the glands outside the mucosa empty into the prostatic urethra by some 15 to 30 ducts. The anterior portion of the prostate gland, the *isthmus*, lies between the arms of the crescents. It is a dense fibromuscular area lacking in glands. The three regions described above are more distinct at the upper levels of the gland. The prostate gland secretes about 75 percent of the seminal fluid. The secretion is a white, slightly acid fluid containing several enzymes (e.g., citric acid, acid phosphatase, protease, and diastase). The secreatation coagulates the seminal fluid and may activate the sperm to become motile. **Plate 1, Fig. 1; Plate 5, Figs. 2 and 3.**

Capsule. This is a fibroelastic layer of tissue surrounding the prostate gland. Smooth muscle fibers lie on the inner surface of the capsule and accompany the fibroelastic tissues extending into the underlying stroma.

Stroma. The stroma is continuous with the capsule and is composed of the same fibromuscular tissue. It is a dense bed of collagen and elastic fibers containing many smooth muscle fibers, glands, blood and lymphatic vessels, and nerves. **Plate 5, Fig. 3.**

Glandular parenchyma. All the prostatic glands are of the compound tubuloalveolar type and embedded within the stroma. The glands may appear in one of many morphologic forms, ranging from large, irregular, saclike structures to small, tubelike structures. Thin folds of glandular epithelium with cores of stromal tissue extend deeply into the lumina of many glands. Depending on the functional state of the prostate gland, the epithelium may be simple squamous, cuboidal, columnar, or pseudostratified columnar. The cells may contain secretory granules and droplets in their cytoplasm. The ducts resemble small, tubelike secretory glands, except near the urethra their epithelium is transitional. In the prostate gland of older males, prostatic concretions (corpora amylacea) may be present in the lumina of the glands. These ovoid concretions are about 0.2 to 2 mm in diameter. The larger ones can plug the ducts and cause the gland to become cystic. These acidophilic, sometimes lamellated, concretions are usually calcified. They may be produced as prostatic secretions condense on cellular fragments or desquamated cells. **Plate 5, Fig. 3.**

BLOOD AND LYMPHATIC VESSELS OF THE PROSTATE GLAND. Branches of the internal pudendal, inferior vesicle, and middle rectal arteries extend through the capsule and into the stroma of the prostate gland, where they supply capillaries near the glandular epithelium. Venous blood is drained into a plexus lying anterolateral to the prostate gland. The plexus is then drained into the internal iliac veins. *Lymphatic vessels* are numerous within the stroma and lie close to the blood vessels.

NERVES OF THE PROSTATE GLAND. Sympathetic and parasympathetic fibers, as well as visceral afferent fibers, are present in the stroma of the prostate gland. The nerve fibers are derived from the pelvic and prostatic plexuses. They innervate sensory receptors, possibly the epithelium, and smooth muscle tissue in both the stroma and blood vessels.

BULBOURETHRAL GLANDS (Cowper's glands). These small, round paired glands are about 1 cm in diameter. They lie laterally to the membranous urethra and are surrounded by striated muscle fibers derived from the external sphincter muscle of the urethra. Relatively long ducts connect the glands to the proximal region of the spongiosa urethra. Each gland is covered by a capsule of connective tissue. Many septa extend from the capsule and divide the gland into several lobules. The gland secretes a clear, thick mucoid substance which constitutes a small portion of the seminal fluid. Its function is possibly one of moistening and lubricating the urethra prior to the passage of the ejaculate, since it is quite secretive during sexual foreplay. **Plate 1, Fig. 1.**

Capsule. This is a thin layer of moderately dense fibroelastic connective tissue which contains some striated muscle fibers.

Septa. The septa extend from the capsule, dividing the gland into many lobules. Each septum is composed of fibroelastic connective tissue containing striated muscle, some smooth muscle, vessels, and nerves.

Glandular parenchyma. Compound tubuloalveolar glands are embedded within a moderately dense connective tissue containing some smooth muscle fibers. The secretory end pieces of the glands may be alveolar, saccular, or tubular. The glandular cells appear in various forms, depending on secretory activity. At rest, the cells are cuboidal or columnar, with a spherical nucleus lying within a granular cytoplasm. Active cells have a flattened nucleus lying at the base of a relatively pale cytoplasm filled with acidophilic, spindle-shaped inclusions and mucoid droplets. The secreting cells resemble mucous cells, but they do not produce a true mucus. In completely filled glands the cells may be flattened and appear squamous. Stellate basket cells are present between the secretory cells and basement membrane. Excretory ducts are present in the lobules. They resemble the secretory end pieces of the glands because they also are irregular in size and form, have glandular outpocketings, and patches of secretory epithelium. The larger excretory ducts are lined by a simple columnar epithelium, except near the urethral opening, where the epithelium is pseudostratified columnar. The epithelium of the ducts rests on a basement membrane. It is surrounded by a thin wall of connective tissue and circular smooth muscle. Along the duct, small glandular diverticula extend into the surrounding connective tissue.

Penis

The penis is an excretory and copulatory organ. It is an elongate, cylindrical structure which has an attached *base*, an unattached pendulant portion, the *shaft*, and a terminal *glans penis*. The penis is covered with a thin skin; the subcutaneous layer contains some smooth muscle but is free of adipose tissue. The penis is composed of three longitudinal columns of erectile tissue: two paired dorsal columns, the *corpora cavernosa penis*, and a single ventral column, the *corpus spongiosum urethrae* (corpus cavernosum urethrae), which is smaller than the dorsal columns. The erectile tissue is an extensive anastomosing framework of fibroelastic trabeculae containing some smooth muscle. The trabeculae house an equally extensive labyrinth of blood sinusoids. The trabeculae are lined by endothelium of the sinusoids. At the base of the penis, the corpora cavernosa penis are modified into a pair of elongate swellings, the *crura penis*. Likewise, the corpus spongiosum urethrae has a modified enlargement, the *bulb of the penis*, which encloses the urethra. These enlargements are attached to the pubic arch and lie under the perineum. They can be easily palpated during an erection, when the erectile tissue is engorged with blood. The corpus spongiosum terminates distally as a flattened cone, the *glans penis*, through which the urethra opens to the surface. The paired dorsal corpora cavernosa terminate just proximal to the glans penis, which forms a cap over their distal ends. Throughout the length of the shaft the three corpora are bound together by an outer layer of collagen and elastic fibers, the *tunica albuginea*, which is thick and dense. The inner region of the tunica albuginea has circumferentially organized fibers surrounding each of the three corpora bodies as a tough, dense layer or *albuginea*. Between the paired corpora cavernosa, the fibers of the albuginea jointly form a thick longitudinal median penal septum. The septum is incomplete distally, so that blood sinuses between the two corpora can communicate through openings. This region is designated as the *pectiniform septum*. The albuginea surrounding the corpus spongiosum is thin. It contains some smooth muscle and many elastic fibers. The outer region of the tunica albuginea is composed of longitudinal fibers. It forms a superficial sheath which binds the corpora and provides attachment for the skin of the penis. The skin covering the shaft extends over the glans penis to form a hoodlike prepuce. **Plate 1, Fig. 1; Plate 6, Figs. 1 and 2.**

BLOOD AND LYMPHATIC VESSELS OF THE PENIS. On each side of the inferior pubic ligament the internal pudendal artery forms several branches. One branch, the *deep artery of the penis*, extends into the crus penis. It travels through the center of a corpus cavernosum, sending branches into the trabeculae of the erectile tissue. The small branches terminate either as a capillary network or as spiral *helicine*

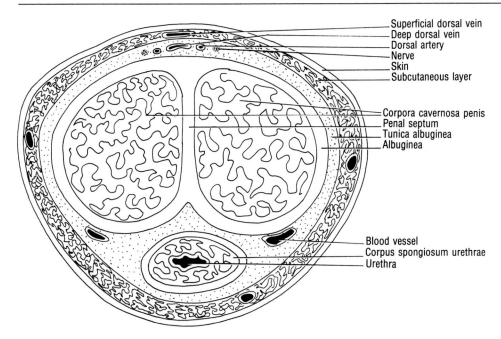

Superficial dorsal vein
Deep dorsal vein
Dorsal artery
Nerve
Skin
Subcutaneous layer

Corpora cavernosa penis
Penal septum
Tunica albuginea
Albuginea

Blood vessel
Corpus spongiosum urethrae
Urethra

FIGURE 1.
Drawing of the penis (cross section).

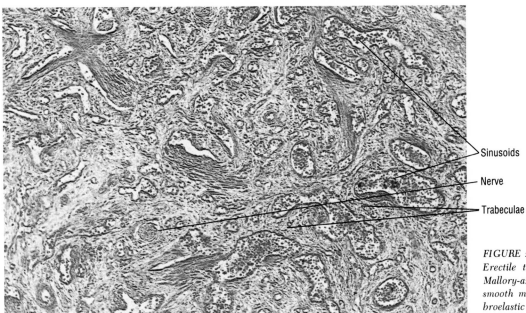

Sinusoids

Nerve

Trabeculae

FIGURE 2.
Erectile tissue, glans penis; human; Mallory-azan. Note that strands of smooth muscle are present in the fibroelastic tissue of the trabeculae. Note the extensive sinusoids.

arteries, both of which supply blood to large sinusoids of the erectile tissue. A second branch of the internal pudendal artery, the *dorsal artery of the penis,* runs along the dorsal aspect of the penis. At the glans, this artery branches; one branch supplies the glans proper while the other extends to the prepuce. Along the shaft, the dorsal artery sends branches through the corpora cavernosa deep into the erectile tissue. In addition, the dorsal artery supplies the skin of the shaft and tissues of the tunica albuginea. A third branch of the internal pudendal artery is the *urethral artery.* It enters the corpus spongiosum and extends all the way to the glans, supplying the urethra and erectile tissue. A fourth branch, the *artery of the bulb of the penis*, supplies erectile tissue of the corpus spongiosum and the bulb. Sinusoids, located under the tunica albuginea, are drained by veins which pass through the tunica albuginea. These veins unite with a deep dorsal vein, running in association with the dorsal arteries. Some of the veins uniting with the deep dorsal vein come from the glans penis, and some come from the upper and lower surfaces of the corpora cavernosa, including anastomotic branches of the corpus spongiosum. Many veins emerge from the tunica albuginea at the base of the penis. They directly enter a prostatic venous plexus, which also drains the deep dorsal vein.

The mechanism of erection is associated mainly with the corpora cavernosa rather than the corpus spongiosum. *At the onset of an erection*, nerve impulses carried by parasympathetic nerves influence the smooth muscle of the arterioles and trabeculae to relax (vasodilation), so that the sinusoids engorge with blood and become rigid. As they increase in size, the sinusoids exert pressure on peripheral venules to close them. This mechanism, by which large volumes of blood enter and small amounts leave the sinusoids, results in rigid erectile tissue, so that an erection can occur and be sustained. During an erection the helicine arteries also become turgid and tend to straighten, which enable large volumes of blood to enter the sinusoids. These arteries have heavy muscular walls with a subendothelial fold of longitudinal muscle. The fold partially occludes the lumen in the flaccid state, but during an erection the muscular walls relax, the fold is reduced in size, and the vessels fill with blood. The process of *detumescence* (return of the penis to the flaccid state) is accomplished by sympathetic nerve impulses influencing the smooth muscles to regain their tonus and contract. This, along with recoil of elastic fibers in the trabeculae and arteries, will compress and empty the vascular spaces.

Lymphatic vessels from the skin of the penis, prepuce, and erectile tissue converge to form a superficial dorsal lymph vessel. This vessel drains lymph into the medial superficial inguinal nodes. The lymphatic vessels from the glans converge to form a dorsal subfacial lymph vessel, which parallels and lies deeper to the superficial vessel. The subfacial vessel drains lymph to the external iliac nodes and to the medial deep inguinal nodes.

NERVES OF THE PENIS. The penis is well innervated, receiving nerves from the sacral and pelvic plexuses. It receives somatic afferent and efferent nerves, as well as visceral sensory, parasympathetic, and sympathetic fibers of the autonomic nervous system. Numerous encapsulated sensory receptors and free nerve endings are present in the penis. The encapsulated receptors are Meissner's corpuscles in the dermal papillae of the skin; Pacinian corpuscles and Krause's end bulbs in the subcutaneous tissue; and genital corpuscles lying within the connective tissue adjacent to the corpora. These sensory receptors are innervated by somatic afferent nerves. Somatic efferent nerves innervate the bulbospongiosus muscle. This muscle may aid in an erection by squeezing the erectile tissue in the bulb of the penis. The sympathetic and parasympathetic nerve fibers innervate the smooth muscle tissue of the trabeculae and blood vessels.

Endocrine Glands 17

Hypophysis

The *hypophysis* (pituitary gland) is a flattened, pea-sized gland, about 1 cm long by 1.5 cm wide by 0.5 cm deep, attached to the hypothalamus by a hollow infundibular stalk. The gland sits in a depression, *sella turcica*, of the sphenoid bone. The dura mater is organized into outer endosteal and inner meningeal layers. The meningeal layer covers the sella turcica, as the diaphragma sellae, and extends over the surface of the gland. Within the sella turcica, the layers of dura mater are firmly united with the capsule of the hypophysis. The infundibular stalk extends through a hole in the diaphragma sellae.

The hypophysis is organized into an anterior glandular *adenohypophysis* and a posterior fibrous *neurohypophysis*. The adenohypophysis is subdivided into a pars distalis, pars intermedia, and pars tuberalis. A remnant of an embryonic structure, *Rathke's pouch*, may be present as a cleft in the infant and separates the pars distalis from the pars intermedia. This cleft usually becomes a discontinuous series of colloid-filled cysts in the adult. The cysts may lie adjacent to, or even extend into, the neurohypophysis. The neurohypophysis is composed of the infundibular stalk, median eminence of the tuber cinereum, and the pars nervosa. Although the hypophysis is highly vascularized, the adenohypophysis has a richer vascular supply than the neurohypophysis. The hypophysis produces nine hormones which maintain a homeostatic condition in the body by a physiologic integration of both the nervous and endocrine systems. **Plate 1, Fig. 1.**

CAPSULE. This rests on the gland and is composed of dense, irregular collagenous connective tissue. At the distal end of the pars tuberalis the capsule gives rise to short trabeculae, carrying blood vessels into the pars distalis. **Plate 1, Fig. 1.**

ADENOHYPOPHYSIS

Pars distalis. This is the largest subdivision of the hypophysis. It is composed of irregular cords of parenchymal tissue drained by an anastomotic network of large capillaries. The parenchymal cells and vascular epithelia sit on basement membranes supported by a light mesh of reticular fibers. Epithelial-lined vesicles, filled with

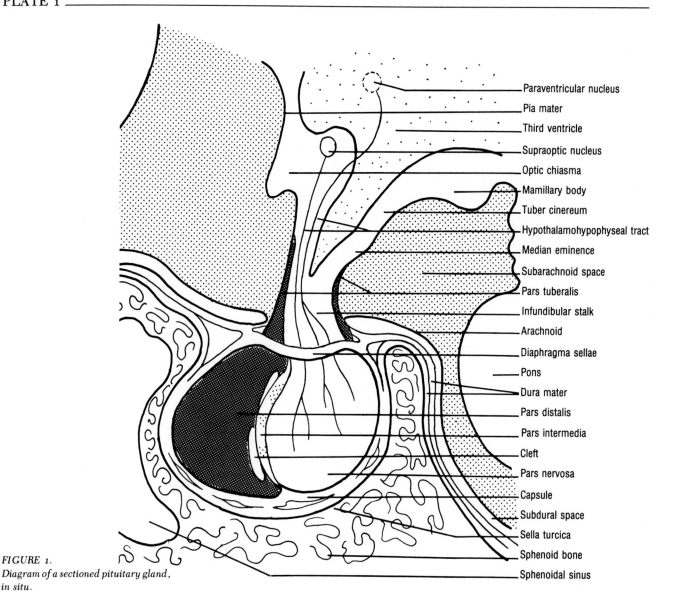

Paraventricular nucleus
Pia mater
Third ventricle
Supraoptic nucleus
Optic chiasma
Mamillary body
Tuber cinereum
Hypothalamohypophyseal tract
Median eminence
Subarachnoid space
Pars tuberalis
Infundibular stalk
Arachnoid
Diaphragma sellae
Pons
Dura mater
Pars distalis
Pars intermedia
Cleft
Pars nervosa
Capsule
Subdural space
Sella turcica
Sphenoid bone
Sphenoidal sinus

FIGURE 1.
Diagram of a sectioned pituitary gland,
in situ.

colloid, may be present; however, their significance is not known. There are three main types of parenchymal cells: basophils, acidophils, and chromophobes. **Plate 1, Figs. 1, 2,** and **3.**

BASOPHIL CELLS (beta cells). These are the least numerous and largest of the three cell types. They have large, round nuclei; granular, basophilic cytoplasm; and are present along the anterior lateral margins of the gland. Although two types of basophils, *thyrotropes* and *gonadotropes*, have been distinguished by electron microscope studies and special staining techniques, they are not easily identified in routine H&E preparations. The thyrotropes secrete thyrotropic stimulating hormone (TSH), while gonadotropes secrete luteinizing hormone (LH), follicle-stimulating hormone (FSH), or interstitial cell stimulating hormone (ICSH). **Plate 1, Figs. 2** and **3.**

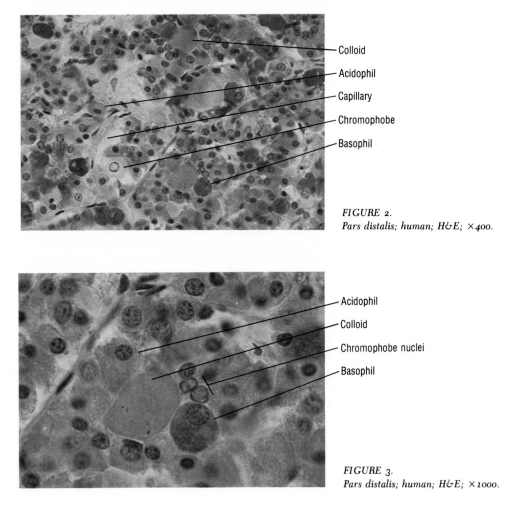

FIGURE 2.
Pars distalis; human; H&E; ×400.

— Colloid
— Acidophil
— Capillary
— Chromophobe
— Basophil

— Acidophil
— Colloid
— Chromophobe nuclei
— Basophil

FIGURE 3.
Pars distalis; human; H&E; ×1000.

ACIDOPHIL CELLS (alpha cells). These cells are smaller and more numerous than the basophils. Their nuclei are darker and smaller than basophil nuclei and they have a granular, acidophilic cytoplasm. They lie in the posterior part of the gland. By using special stains or the electron microscope, two types of acidophils can be identified. These cells, however, cannot be differentiated in H&E preparations. One type, the *somatotrope*, produces somatotropin (STH), while the other, the *mammatrope*, produces prolactin. **Plate 1, Figs. 2 and 3.**

CHROMOPHOBE CELLS. These usually are the smallest and most abundant of the parenchymal cells in the pars distalis. They have a colorless, angular, scanty cytoplasm with pale-stained granules and indistinct plasma membranes. Because of the sparse cytoplasm, the small, round nuclei usually appear clumped in the center of parenchymal cords. Two types of cells exist: the large and small chromophobes. The small chromophobes may be stem cells or a resting phase of granular cells. Stem cells are believed to be precursors to parenchymal cells in the pars distalis. The large chromophobes are stellate, and produce adrenocorticotropic hormone (ACTH). **Plate 1, Figs. 2 and 3.**

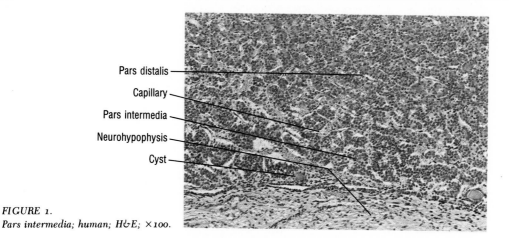

Pars distalis

Capillary

Pars intermedia

Neurohypophysis

Cyst

FIGURE 1.
Pars intermedia; human; H&E; ×100.

Pars intermedia. This is a poorly developed layer of basophil and chromophobe cells lying between the pars distalis and neurohypophysis. In the adult, colloid-filled cysts, remnants of Rathke's pouch, may be found adjacent to the neurohypophysis. **Plate 1, Fig. 1; Plate 2, Fig. 1.**

BASOPHIL CELLS. These cells are smaller than those in the pars distalis, but they also have granules in a basophilic cytoplasm. They may extend into adjacent regions of the pars distalis and pars nervosa. The basophils secrete melanocyte-stimulating hormone (MSH), which influences melanin production in humans. **Plate 2, Fig. 2.**

CHROMOPHOBE CELLS. The cells, with their small, spherical nuclei and sparse, colorless, angular cytoplasm, resemble smaller chromophobes of the pars distalis. The function of these cells is unknown.

CYSTS. The cysts are prominent, colloid-filled, oval or spherical structures lined with a simple epithelium of small, clear cells which may or may not be ciliated. On occasion, basophils may be present in the epithelium. Cysts usually are adjacent to the neurohypophysis, but they may extend into this region. **Plate 2, Figs. 1 and 2.**

Pars tuberalis. This is continuous with the pars distalis, and it forms a collar around the infundibular stalk. It is thickest on the anterior surface but may be incomplete on the posterior surface. The tissue is highly vascularized and organized into short, longitudinal epithelial cords supported by reticular fibers. There are several types of cells, but the most abundant are large cuboidal cells with a pale basophilic cytoplasm. The cytoplasm usually is filled with nonsecretory granules or colloid droplets. These cells may be organized into colloid-filled cysts. Other cell types, such as small acidophils, basophils, undifferentiated cells, and squamous cells, may have migrated into this region from other parts of the hypophysis. **Plate 1, Fig. 1; Plate 2, Fig. 3.**

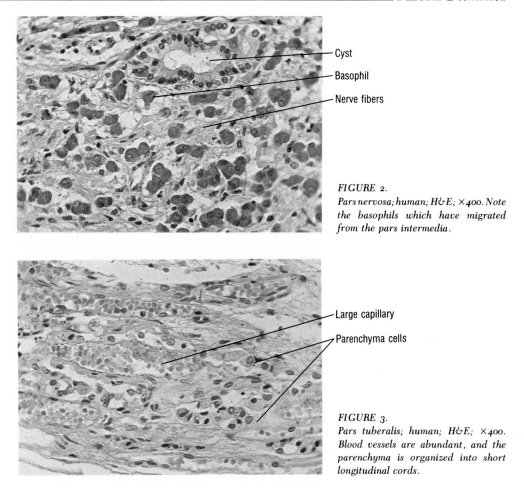

— Cyst

— Basophil

— Nerve fibers

FIGURE 2.
Pars nervosa; human; H&E; ×400. Note
the basophils which have migrated
from the pars intermedia.

—Large capillary

—Parenchyma cells

FIGURE 3.
Pars tuberalis; human; H&E; ×400.
Blood vessels are abundant, and the
parenchyma is organized into short
longitudinal cords.

NEUROHYPOPHYSIS. This posterior region of the hypophysis is a center for storage and release of hormones, oxytocin and vasopressin, produced by neurosecretory neurons in the diencephalon. These hormones are produced in nerve cell bodies located within the supraoptic nuclei of the hypothalamus, the paraventricular nuclei in the thalamus, and other regions. The hormones are carried by unmyelinated axons, the hypothalamohypophyseal tract, through the infundibular stalk and median eminence to terminate on capillaries in the pars nervosa. The pars nervosa is composed of irregular lobules incompletely separated from each other by thin layers of collagen fibers. Each lobule surrounds a branch of the hypothalamohypophyseal tract. Nerve fibers in the tract terminate at the margin of the lobule and form a palisade zone. In addition to axons, vessels, and connective tissue, there are other structures present in the neurohypophysis (see below). **Plate 1, Fig. 1.**

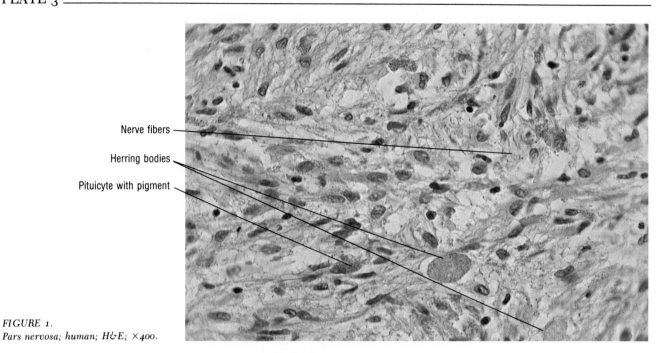

Nerve fibers

Herring bodies

Pituicyte with pigment

FIGURE 1.
Pars nervosa; human; H&E; ×400.

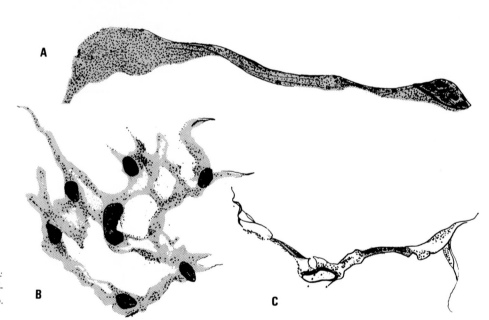

A

B

C

FIGURE 2.
Drawing of three pituicytes, human:
(a) fibropituicyte, ×460; (b) reticulopi-
tuicyte, ×460; (c) micropituicyte, ×260.
(Modified after Romeis.)

Herring bodies. These are spherical structures of various sizes representing axo-plasmic expansions of axons in the hypothalamohypophyseal tract. The bodies may appear either granular or agranular, and contain neurosecretory substances such as oxytocin and vasopressin, an antidiuretic hormone. **Plate 3, Fig. 1.**

Pituicytes. There are four types of pituicytes in the neurohypophysis of humans, but they cannot be readily identified in routine tissue preparations. Pituicytes are modified glial cells. They bind nerve fibers, Herring bodies, and vessels with their cytoplasmic processes. The cells vary in size and shape, and the cytoplasm may be filled with pigment granules. **Plate 3, Figs. 1** and **2.**

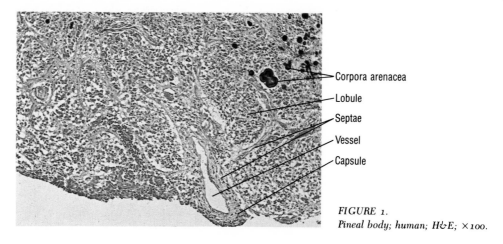

Corpora arenacea
Lobule
Septae
Vessel
Capsule

FIGURE 1.
Pineal body; human; H&E; ×100.

BLOOD AND LYMPHATIC VESSELS. There are two separate arterial patterns supplying the hypophysis. The neurohypophysis receives blood from the inferior hypophyseal arteries, while the adenohypophysis is supplied by superior hypophyseal arteries via the venous portal system in the infundibular stalk. Both the neurohypophysis and adenohypophysis are drained by hypophyseal veins which empty into the cavernous sinus. Lymphatics have not been observed in the hypophysis.

NERVES. Autonomic nerve fibers, believed to be only vasomotor in function, are present in the pars distalis and pars nervosa.

Pineal body

The pineal body is a small, conical, flattened structure, about 7 mm long by 4 mm wide, attached to the epithalamus by a short, hollow stalk. It is surrounded by a thin, vascular, fibrous capsule derived from the pia mater. The capsule gives rise to many septa, subdividing the pineal body into incomplete lobules. The pineal tissue contains parenchymal cells, mast cells, Schwann cells, and axons of autonomic nerves. The pineal body produces melatonin, an amine, which influences the endocrine function of gonads. Melatonin may be involved with the regulation of photoperiodicity in the reproduction of lower vertebrates. Nerve impulses originate in the visual system and are relayed to the pineal body by autonomic nerves. When the nerve impulses reach the parenchymal tissue, melatonin is synthesized from the already present serotonin. **Plate 4, Fig. 1.**

CAPSULE. This is a thin layer of dense, irregular collagenous connective tissue containing some reticular fibers and blood vessels. **Plate 4, Fig. 1.**

SEPTA. These are continuous with the capsule and composed mainly of reticular fibers and blood vessels. **Plate 4, Fig. 1.**

PARENCHYMA. This is composed of two cell types, pinealocytes and interstitial cells, organized into cords and supported on a delicate network of reticular fibers. **Plate 4, Figs. 2** and **3.**

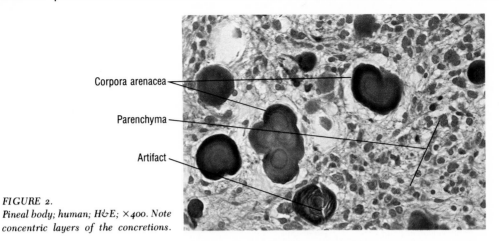

Corpora arenacea

Parenchyma

Artifact

FIGURE 2.
Pineal body; human; H&E; ×400. Note concentric layers of the concretions.

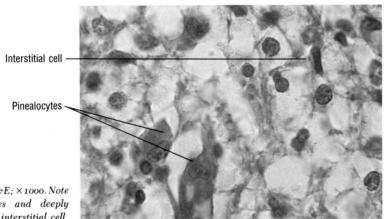

Interstitial cell

Pinealocytes

FIGURE 3.
Pineal body; human; H&E; ×1000. Note the fibrillar processes and deeply stained nucleus of the interstitial cell.

Pinealocyte (chief cell). The pinealocytes are ubiquitously present in the parenchyma. They are large, irregularly shaped cells with narrow processes terminating as bulbous endings. The cytoplasm is basophilic and may contain granules or lipid droplets. The nuclei are large, vesicular, lobulated, oval, and pale, and contain prominent nucleoli. It is believed that pinealocytes secrete melatonin. **Plate 4, Fig. 3.**

Interstitial cells (neuroglia, supporting cells). These cells are less numerous than the pinealocytes. The cytoplasm is drawn out into many fibrillar processes and is more basophilic than that of the pinealocytes. The nuclei are elongate, nonlobulated, and deeply stained. Interstitial cells occur close to blood vessels and between clumps of pinealocytes. They provide an elaborate framework to support the pinealocytes. **Plate 4, Fig. 3.**

CORPORA ARENACEA (brain sand). These are extracellular concretions located in the connective tissue. They are composed of an organic matrix containing hydroxyapatite and calcium carbonate apatite. The concretions are usually formed into concentric layers, they increase in size and numbers from puberty to old age. **Plate 4, Figs. 1** and **2.**

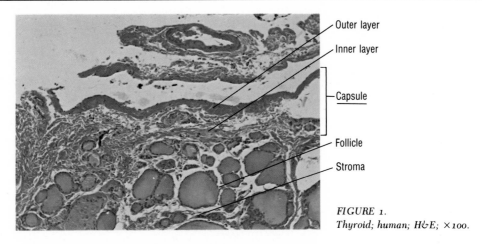

Outer layer

Inner layer

Capsule

Follicle

Stroma

FIGURE 1.
Thyroid; human; H&E; ×100.

BLOOD AND LYMPHATIC VESSELS. Large blood vessels are confined to the capsule and septa, and a rich network of capillaries is found between parenchymal cords. Lymphatic vessels have not been observed in the pineal body. **Plate 4, Fig. 1.**

NERVES. Unmyelinated autonomic nerve fibers, originating in the superior cervical ganglion and carried by the nervi conarii, are more abundant than myelinated nerve fibers. The myelinated fibers originate from the habenular and posterior commissures.

Thyroid gland

The thyroid gland is located in the lower part of the neck at the level of the VIIth cervical vertebra. It may vary in size but usually weighs approximately 25 g. The gland is composed of two lateral lobes connected by a median isthmus and surrounded by a prominent capsule. The capsule is continuous with a deep fascia on its outer surface. The glandular tissue has spherical follicles of various sizes embedded in a vascularized, loose connective tissue stroma. The follicles secrete thyroxine and triiodothyronine hormones, which accelerate the processes of oxidative metabolism and influence growth and maturation. **Plate 5, Fig. 1.**

CAPSULE. The capsule is composed of fibroelastic tissue divided into two layers. The layers are loosely connected with areolar connective tissue. The dense outer layer is continuous with surrounding cervical fascia; the inner layer, which is less dense, rests directly on the surface of the gland. **Plate 5, Fig. 1.**

FOLLICLES. These are thin-walled, oval or round, colloid-filled sacs of parenchymal tissue embedded within a vascular stroma of areolar and reticular connective tissue. Each follicle has the following composition. **Plate 5, Fig. 1.**

Follicular epithelial cells. If the follicle is nonactive, its wall is composed of a simple low cuboidal or squamous epithelium. If it is active, the epithelium is of the simple low columnar type. The cells border the lumen of the follicle and sit on a thin basement membrane. Active cells have large, vesicular nuclei and colloid droplets may be present in a basophilic cytoplasm. **Plate 5, Figs. 2 and 3.**

Blood vessel
Desquamated cell
Colloid
Follicle
Epithelial cell
Stroma

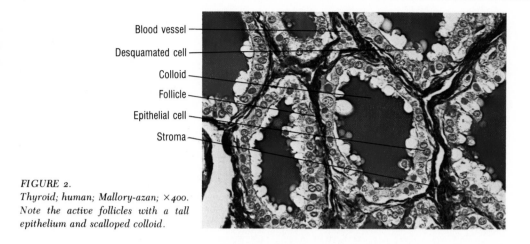

FIGURE 2.
Thyroid; human; Mallory-azan; ×400.
Note the active follicles with a tall
epithelium and scalloped colloid.

Epithelial cell
Colloid
Follicle
Stroma

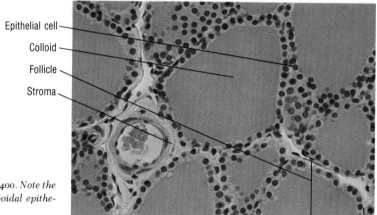

FIGURE 3.
Thyroid; human; H&E; ×400. Note the
inactive follicles with cuboidal epithe-
lium.

Parafollicular cells (light cells, C cells). These are scarce, large, clear, polyhedral cells which lie below the follicular epithelium. In some sections, however, they appear to encroach onto the lumen. The cytoplasm contains no colloid droplets but may have some small argyrophilic granules. The nuclei are larger and more vesicular than the epithelial nuclei. Parafollicular cells are embryonically derived from the ultimobranchial bodies of the fifth pharyngeal pouches. They secrete calcitonin, a hormone which lowers blood calcium and is therefore antagonistic to the function of the parathyroid hormone.

Colloid. The follicle is filled with colloid (thyroglobulin), and depending on the activity of the thyroid gland, it may appear in many forms. In the active gland, colloid is basophilic and usually vacuolated with scalloped edges along its margin. In the inactive gland, colloid is acidophilic and lacks vacuoles or scallped edges. Macrophages or desquamated follicle cells may be found in the usually homogeneous colloid. **Plate 5, Figs. 2 and 3.**

BLOOD AND LYMPHATIC VESSELS. Follicles are surrounded by networks of capillaries and arteriovenous anastomoses, while larger vessels are located in the capsule. *Lymphatic capillary plexuses* occur between the follicles and drain into large vessels beneath the capsule. **Plate 5, Fig. 2.**

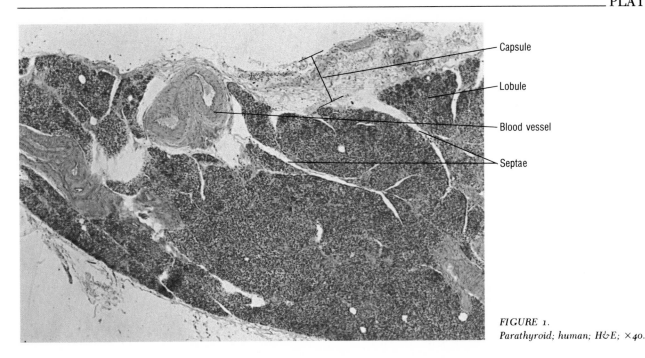

Capsule

Lobule

Blood vessel

Septae

FIGURE 1.
Parathyroid; human; H&E; ×40.

NERVES. Nerve fibers of the sympathetic and parasympathetic nerves are present in the stroma. Some fibers, possibly secretomotor, terminate around follicle cells.

Parathyroid gland

The parathyroid glands usually are four small masses of tissue, each about 7 mm long by 3 mm in diameter, embedded within the fibroelastic capsule or parenchyma of the thyroid gland. They are paired, and each pair is located on the dorsolateral surface of the thyroid. Each parathyroid gland is separated from thyroid tissue by a thin fibroelastic capsule. The parenchyma is divided into poorly defined lobules by thin septa extending from the capsule and carrying blood vessels. Calcium and phosphorus metabolism is regulated by parathormone, which is secreted by the parathyroid glands. **Plate 6, Fig. 1.**

CAPSULE. This is a thin layer of fibroelastic tissue surrounding the parenchyma. **Plate 6, Fig. 1.**

SEPTA. These are thin strands of fibroelastic tissue stretching from the capsule and dividing the parenchyma into irregular lobules. They contain fat cells, blood vessels, lymphatic vessels, and nerves. **Plate 6, Fig. 1.**

LOBULES. These are irregular and imperfectly divided masses of parenchyma further subdivided into cords by vascular tissue. **Plate 6, Fig. 1.**

PARENCHYMA. The parenchyma (glandular tissue) is a mass of epithelial-like cells organized into an irregular network of anastomosing cords and supported by a delicate reticular tissue. There are two main types of cells—chief and oxyphil—although transitionals may exist. **Plate 6, Fig. 1.**

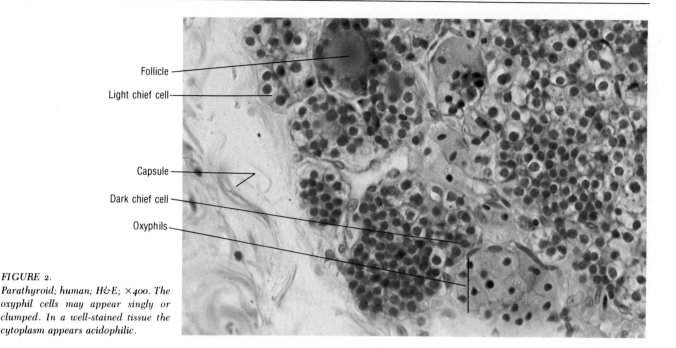

Follicle

Light chief cell

Capsule

Dark chief cell

Oxyphils

FIGURE 2.
Parathyroid; human; H&E; ×400. The oxyphil cells may appear singly or clumped. In a well-stained tissue the cytoplasm appears acidophilic.

Chief cells. There are two types of chief cells: dark cells and light cells. They are identified by stain, size, and presence of granules in the cytoplasm.
DARK CHIEF CELLS. These are small cells with small, dark, round, centrally positioned nuclei. Some glycogen and many small granules may be present in the pale acidophilic cytoplasm if the cells are in a secretory phase. **Plate 6, Fig. 2.**
LIGHT CHIEF CELLS. These cells are more abundant and larger than the dark chief cells, and their nuclei are larger and lighter in color. The cytoplasm is unstained, has much glycogen, and has few or no granules. These cells may represent a resting phase. **Plate 6, Fig. 2.**

Oxyphil cells. These are the largest cells in the parenchyma. They may be singly scattered through the chief cells or may occur in clusters. The cells are polyhedral with a small, dark nucleus surrounded by an abundant, granular, acidophilic cytoplasm. Oxyphils appear at puberty and increase in numbers in older individuals. **Plate 6, Fig. 2.**

Transitional cells. Many of the parenchymal cells are transitional between chief and oxyphil cells. According to electron microscope studies, chief cells may be the only parenchymal cells, and the transitionals and oxyphils are modifications of them.

COLLOID FOLLICLES. Follicles are abundant in the parenchyma of older people. They are small, spherical structures, with a low columnar epithelium surrounding a homogeneous acidophilic colloid. **Plate 6, Fig. 2.**

BLOOD AND LYMPHATIC VESSELS. The parenchyma has many irregular capillaries; these are carried mainly in the reticular tissue, but some anastomose across parenchymal cords. Large blood vessels as well as lymphatics are carried in the septa.

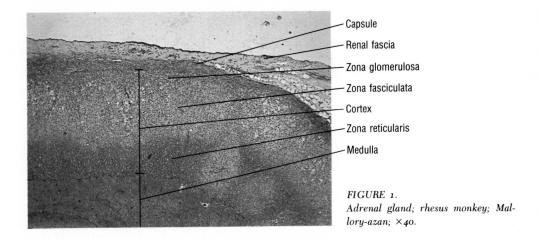

Capsule
Renal fascia
Zona glomerulosa
Zona fasciculata
Cortex
Zona reticularis
Medulla

FIGURE 1.
Adrenal gland; rhesus monkey; Mallory-azan; ×40.

NERVES. Autonomic vasomotor nerve fibers end on vascular tissue and probably do not influence the endocrine function of the parenchymal tissue.

Adrenal gland

The paired adrenal glands are small, flattened, triangular organs, approximately 5 cm long by 3 cm wide by 1 cm thick. They are attached to the cranial end of the kidneys. They have an indented region, the *hilus,* which receives blood vessels, lymphatic vessels, and nerves. A prominent fibroelastic capsule surrounds the gland. It gives rise to delicate trabeculae, carrying vessels and nerves into the parenchyma. The parenchyma is organized into an outer cortex, which is palisadelike, and an inner medulla, which is irregularly shaped. The adrenal gland maintains homeostasis by regulating electrolyte and water balance, protein and carbohydrate metabolism, vasomotor functions, and resistance to stress. **Plate 7, Fig. 1.**

CAPSULE. The outer layer of the capsule is a dense fibroelastic tissue containing some smooth muscle cells. The inner layer is less dense than the outer layer, and has blood vessels, lymphatic vessels, and nerves. **Plate 7, Fig. 1.**

TRABECULAE. These structures are composed of reticular and collagen fibers, and are prominent between columns of parenchymal cells in the cortex. They, like the capsule, give rise to reticular fibers, forming networks around parenchymal cells in the cortex and medulla. **Plate 7, Fig. 3.**

CORTEX. This outer region of the gland has columns of parenchymal cells radiating from the capsule to the medulla. The columns are two cells in thickness throughout most of their length, and each column is bordered by trabeculae and capillaries. The cortex is divided into three ill-defined zones and each is characterized by a special arrangement of the parenchymal cells. The outer zone is the *zona glomerulosa,* the middle is the *zona fasciculata,* and the inner is the *zona reticularis.* **Plate 7, Fig. 1.**

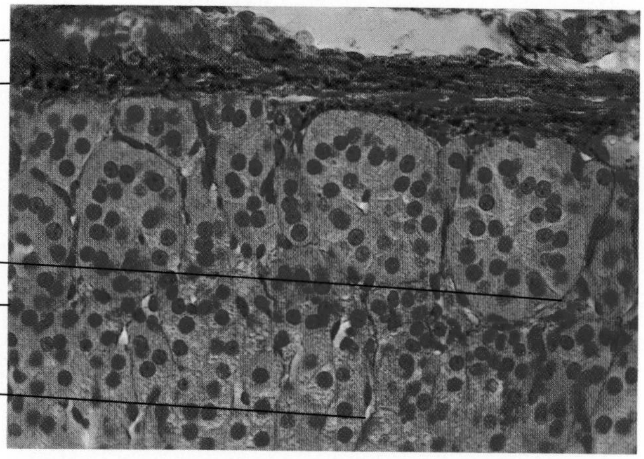

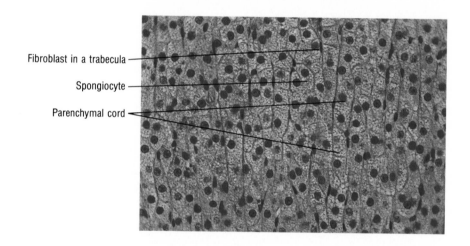

Capsule

Zona glomerulosa

Basement membrane

Zona fasciculata

Capillary

FIGURE 2.
Zona glomerulosa; rhesus monkey;
Mallory-azan; ×400. Note the spherical
arrangement of the cells.

Fibroblast in a trabecula

Spongiocyte

Parenchymal cord

FIGURE 3.
Zona fasciculata; rhesus monkey; Mal-
lory-azan, ×400. Note the parallel
cords and reticulated cytoplasm of the
parenchymal cells.

Zona glomerulosa. This zone is located just below the capsule and constitutes about 15 percent of the cortex. It secretes the mineralocorticoids (desoxycorticosterone and aldosterone), which control water and salt balance. The parenchymal cords form solid, spherical or archlike structures. The cells are small and columnar, with large, deeply stained, spherical nuclei. The cytoplasm stains lightly with acid dyes and contains some lipid droplets. **Plate 7, Figs. 1 and 2.**

Zona fasciculata. This zone is located below the zona glomerulosa, and forms about 78 percent of the cortex. It secretes the glucocorticoids (cortisol, cortisone, and corticosterone), which control the metabolism of carbohydrates, fats, and proteins. The parenchymal cords are relatively straight, parallel structures of one or two cells' thickness, and are separated by capillaries. The cuboidal cells are larger here than in the other two zones. Their nuclei are large, sherical, and vesicular. In the outer region of the zone, the cells normally have numerous lipid droplets of various sizes in an acidophilic cytoplasm. These droplets may be dissolved during the histologic preparation of the tissue so that the cytoplasm will appear reticulated. Cells with this type of cytoplasm are referred to as *spongiocytes.* In the inner region of the zone, the cells have fewer lipid droplets and less reticulation, and will stain darker than the spongiocytes. **Plate 7, Figs. 1 and 3; Plate 8, Fig. 1.**

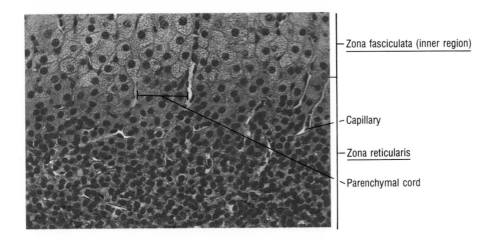

— Zona fasciculata (inner region)

– Capillary

– Zona reticularis

– Parenchymal cord

FIGURE 1.
Zona reticularis; rhesus monkey; Mallory-azan; ×400. Note the irregular cords of the zona reticularis and the transition between it and the zona fasciculata.

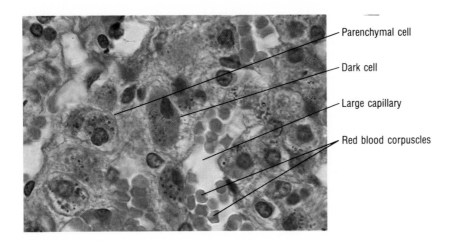

— Parenchymal cell

– Dark cell

– Large capillary

– Red blood corpuscles

FIGURE 2.
Zona reticularis; human; H&E; ×1000. Note the dark cells with lipofuscin granules.

Zona reticularis. This innermost zone accounts for approximately 7 percent of the total cortical area. It also secretes glucocorticoids similar to those produced by the zona fasciculata. The parenchymal cords and capillaries are organized into an irregular network which is continuous with the inner region of the zona fasciculata and the outer region of the medulla. Although the cells are similar to those in the inner region of the zona fasciculata, they are smaller, have less lipid droplets, are darker stained, and may have golden-brown lipofuscin pigment granules in the cytoplasm. Degenerating cells, the *dark cells*, may be found near the medulla. They have dark, shrunken nuclei and dark acidophilic cytoplasm filled with lipofuscin granules. **Plate 7, Fig. 1; Plate 8, Figs. 1 and 2.**

MEDULLA. This region of the adrenal gland is composed of reticular fibers supporting irregular cords and clumps of parenchyma cells, capillaries, venules, ganglion cells, and nerve fibers. The parenchymal cells are large and ovid, columnar, or polyhedral, with vesicular nuclei and basophilic cytoplasm. In primates, the cytoplasm is filled with two types of catecholamine granules, *epinephrine* and *norepinephrine*. In most other mammals there are two types of cells, each with one type of granule. If the cells have been fixed in a fluid containing an oxidizing agent such as potassium bichromate, the catecholamines will be oxidized so that the granules appear as fine

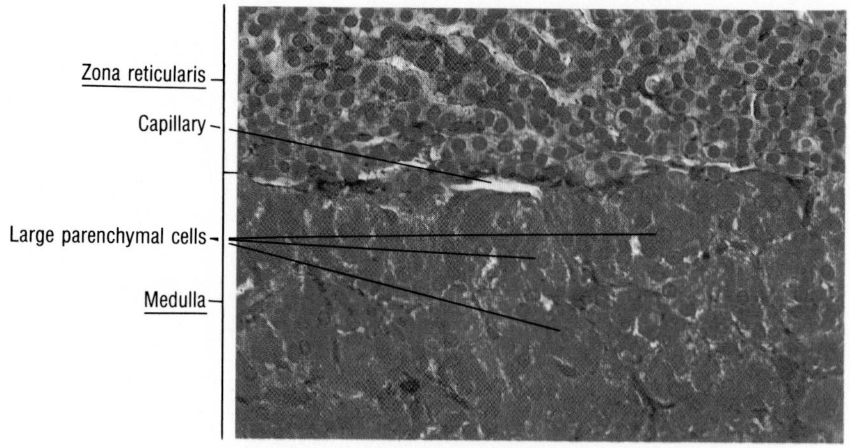

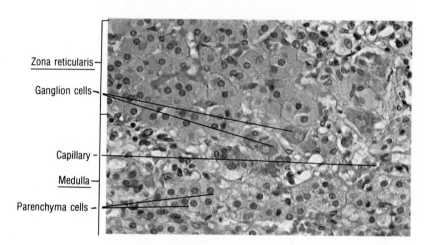

Zona reticularis—
Capillary—
Large parenchymal cells—
Medulla—

FIGURE 3.
Junction between zona reticularis and medulla; rhesus monkey; Mallory-azan; ×400. Note the irregular cords of the zona reticularis and the sharp division between it and the medulla.

Zona reticularis—
Ganglion cells—
Capillary—
Medulla—
Parenchyma cells—

FIGURE 4.
Medulla; human; H&E; ×1000.

brown particles; otherwise they will not be seen. Since these parenchymal cells display this oxidizing chromaffin reaction, they may be designated as *chromaffin cells*. **Plate 7, Fig. 1; Plate 8 Figs. 3 and 4.**

BLOOD AND LYMPHATIC VESSELS. A plexus of large adrenal arteries in the capsule gives rise to smaller vessels which will (1) supply the capsule with capillaries, (2) supply the cortex with an extensive capillary bed draining into the medulla, and (3) supply the medulla, via the trabeculae, with a network of capillaries. Venous blood is drained from the cortical and medullary capillaries by venules in the medulla. These medullary venules become confluent to form the large central vein which is drained by the adrenal vein. The adrenal vein leaves the gland at the hilus and joins the posterior vena cava if it comes from the right adrenal gland. It enters the left renal venin if it comes from the left adrenal gland. *Lymphatic vessels* are associated only with the capsule and large blood vessels.

NERVES. Sympathetic and parasympathetic fibers innervate the gland, but the most significant innervation is that of the sympathetic preganglionic nerve fibers which innervate chromaffin cells. Large autonomic ganglion cells with basophilic cytoplasm and prominent vesicular nuclei are also present in the medulla. **Plate 8, Fig. 4.**

Sense Organs 18

Sense organs are specialized endings of afferent neurons, or complex histologic structures containing sensory cells. They are more sensitive to one type of stimulus than another. Stimulated sense organs initiate nerve impulses which are carried by afferent nerves to specific regions of the brain. Nerve impulses which reach the cerebral cortex are interpreted as sensations. The sensory receptors may be classified as *general* or *specialized*.

The general receptors, both somatic and visceral, are widely distributed throughout the body. They are present in epithelium, muscle, tendon, and general connective tissue. They are sensitive to touch, tissue damage, position of skeletal muscle, temperature, pressure, and visceral stimuli.

The specialized sensory receptors are located in the tongue, eyes, nose, and ears. They are sensitive to light, sound, chemicals (olfaction, taste, and arterial oxygen), and changes in the position and inertia of the body.

General sensory receptors

FREE NERVE ENDINGS. These are bare ends of myelinated or unmyelinated nerve fibers. They may appear as unencapsulated simple or complex branches, or dense networks. They terminate freely among epithelium, muscle, tendon, or general connective tissue. The delicate fibers of the free nerve endings can only be demonstrated with special stains, for example, silver stains or methylene blue. They respond to various somatic and visceral stimuli.

ENCAPSULATED CORPUSCLES. These are the terminal ends of nerve fibers, and are enclosed within a fibrous connective tissue capsule. Only unsheathed nerve fibers extend into the capsule, since their endoneurial sheaths become continuous with the capsule.

Muscle spindles (neuromuscular spindles). The spindles are bundles of 3 to 10 thin, long modified skeletal fibers (intrafusal fibers) surrounded by a collagenous capsule. They are present in skeletal muscle, mainly near its tendon. The muscle spindles

PLATE 1 _____

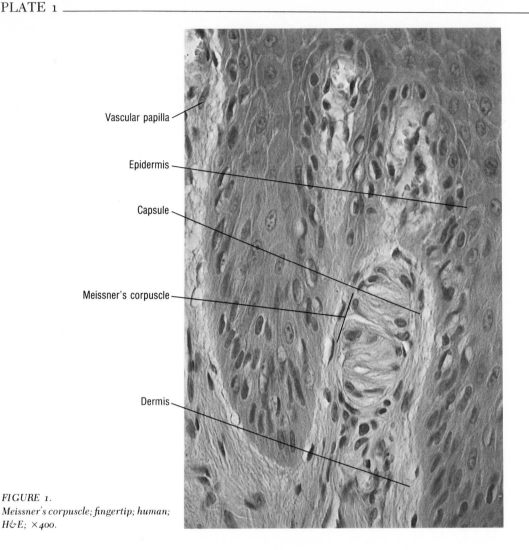

Vascular papilla

Epidermis

Capsule

Meissner's corpuscle

Dermis

FIGURE 1.
Meissner's corpuscle; fingertip; human;
H&E; ×400.

are innervated by somatic afferent and efferent fibers and function as proprioceptors (see Chap. 5).

Tendon spindles (neurotendinous spindles). These are proprioceptors located in the tendon. Each is composed of several collagen fibers encapsulated within a thin fibrous connective tissue and innervated by afferent nerve fibers (see Chap. 5).

Meissner's corpuscle (tactile corpuscle). These are sensory receptors of touch, abundant in the skin of the soles, palms, and fingertips. They are ellipsoidal structures lying parallel to the long axis of the papillae in the pars papillaris. They are approximately 40 to 150 μm in length. The corpuscle has many flattened, horizontally oriented tactile cells forming a central core. The cells are embedded within a ground substance and surrounded by a thin capsule of fibrous connective tissue. The capsule also forms thin horizontal shelves which support the tactile cells. The corpuscle is innervated by one or several myelinated neurons which lose their myelin sheaths as they enter the corpuscle. They extend into the core as a dense spiral of fibers, their branches making contact with the tactile cells. **Plate 1, Fig. 1.**

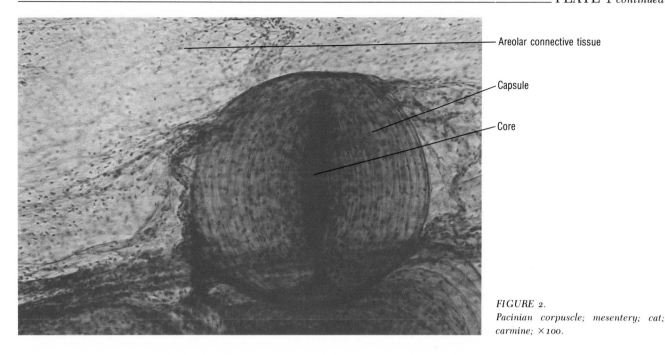

Areolar connective tissue

Capsule

Core

FIGURE 2.
*Pacinian corpuscle; mesentery; cat;
carmine; ×100.*

Cylindrical end bulbs of Krause; terminal cylinders of Ruffini; genital corpuscles.
These are the ends of afferent fibers forming an irregular, dense, bulblike or
cylindrical network. These networks are encapsulated by a thin layer of fibrous
connective tissue. Although some anatomists consider these structures to be tactile
receptors, most believe that the end bulbs of Krause are cold receptors and the
Ruffini cylinders are heat receptors. These sensory receptors are abundant in mucous
membranes and the skin, but they also occur in other tissues and organs.

Pacinian corpuscle (lamellar corpuscle). These are large (about 1 mm in diameter
and 4 mm long), oval pressure receptors located in many areas of the body. They
are most abundant in the subcutaneous layers of the skin. They have a semifluid
central core containing a single branched unmyelinated nerve fiber. The core is
surrounded by a capsule of up to 60 concentric layers of flattened cells and connective
tissue. In section, the Pacinian corpuscle appears as a prominent, pale acidophilic,
lamellated, ovoid body. **Plate 1, Fig. 2; Chap. 11, Plate 1, Fig. 1.**

Special sensory receptors

EAR. Although the ear is anatomically composed of external, middle, and inner
regions, only the inner ear will be considered because it contains the sensory cells
concerned with mechanoreception (sound and changes of body inertia and position).
As these cells are mechanically deformed, they are stimulated to "set up" an impulse.
The inner ear consists of a complex membranous labyrinth housed within a bony
labyrinth. These two labyrinths are contained within the petrous portion of the
temporal bone and are filled with fluid—endolymph in the membranous and
perilymph in the bony labyrinth.

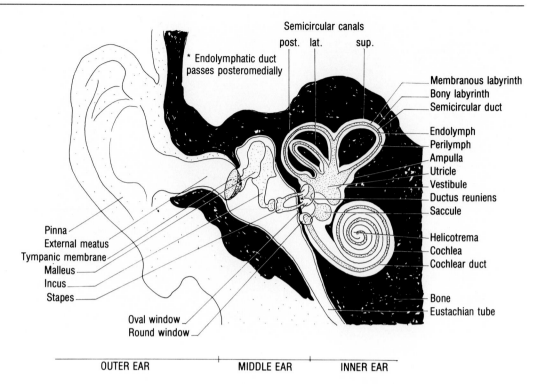

Semicircular canals
post.   lat.   sup.

* Endolymphatic duct
passes posteromedially

Membranous labyrinth
Bony labyrinth
Semicircular duct
Endolymph
Perilymph
Ampulla
Utricle
Vestibule
Ductus reuniens
Saccule
Helicotrema
Cochlea
Cochlear duct
Bone
Eustachian tube

Pinna
External meatus
Tympanic membrane
Malleus
Incus
Stapes

Oval window
Round window

OUTER EAR   MIDDLE EAR   INNER EAR

FIGURE 1.
Drawing of the human ear.

The *bony labyrinth* is composed of a central ovoid *vestibule*, medial to the tympanic cavity; three *semicircular canals* (posterior, superior, and lateral), connected to the posterosuperior region of the vestibule; and a cochlea, attached to the anterior end of the vestibule. The cochlea is a blind tube, broad at the base and narrow at the tip. It is coiled "snakelike" 2.75 turns around a central core of bone, the *modiolus*. The modiolus has a spiral bony shelf, the *spiral lamina*, which follows the cochlear spirals and resembles the thread of a screw. The periosteum on the upper surface of the spiral lamina forms a bulgelike structure, the *spiral limbus*. The limbus has an upper vestibular lip and a lower tympanic lip, forming a notchlike border for an internal spiral tunnel. The spiral limbus and its lower tympanic lip support two membranes that extend across the cochlea, dividing it into an upper *scala vestibuli*, a lower *scala tympani*, and a middle *cochlear duct*. Near the tip of the cochlea the two membranes fuse. This arrangement separates the cavity of the cochlear duct from the scalae and allows the scala tympani and vestibuli to join terminally. This region is named the *helicotrema*. The vestibule, semicircular canals, and cochlea are interconnected and filled with perilymph, a fluid similar to cerebrospinal fluid which is possibly produced by tissues lining the bony labyrinth. At the base of the cochlea, where it joins the vestibule, there are two openings: the *round window* (fenestra cochlea) and *oval window* (fenestra vestibuli). The round window opens to the base of the scala tympani, and the oval window opens to the base of the scala vestibuli; the cochlear duct does not have an opening to the tympanic cavity. These openings are separated from the tympanic cavity of the middle ear by a secondary elastic membrane over the round window, and ligaments of the stapes over the oval window. **Plate 2, Figs. 1 and 2; Plate 3, Figs. 1 and 2.**

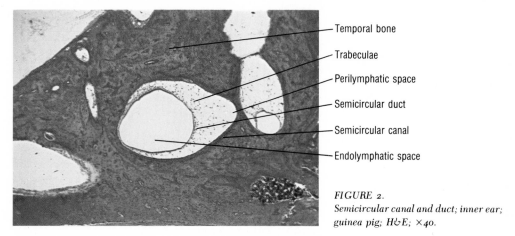

Temporal bone

Trabeculae

Perilymphatic space

Semicircular duct

Semicircular canal

Endolymphatic space

FIGURE 2.
Semicircular canal and duct; inner ear;
guinea pig; H&E; ×40.

The *membranous labyrinth* is composed of interconnected membranous components: utricle, saccule, endolymphatic duct, semicircular ducts, cochlear duct, and ductus reuniens. The *utricle* and *saccule* are interconnected pouches contained within the vestibule. The thin tube connecting these pouches also gives rise to a slender *endolymphatic duct*. This duct terminates as a dilated pouch, the endolymphatic sac, located between the temporal bone and dura mater. The three *semicircular ducts* are set at right angle planes to each other. Each duct lies within a semicircular canal, both ends of which join the utricle. The *cochlear duct* lies within the cochlea and is continuous with the saccule by a slender tube, the *ductus reuniens*. Patches of sensory neuroepithelium (mechanoreceptors) located in the saccule, utricle, and semicircular ducts are stimulated by body movement and concerned with equilibrium, while receptors in the cochlear duct are stimulated by sound waves. The cochlear division of the auditory nerve sends fibers to the receptors in the cochlear duct, while the vestibular division sends fibers to receptors in the saccule, utricle, and semicircular ducts. Except for the cochlear duct, the walls of the membranous labyrinth are histologically similar. They are composed of a vascularized connective tissue. The free inner surface is lined by a layer of simple squamous epithelium, but in special regions (crista and macula, see below) there are localized patches of sensory neuroepithelium. The outer surface of the walls has fibrous trabeculae extending through the perilymph and fusing with the periosteum of the bony labyrinth. The surfaces of the trabeculae and periosteum are lined with a mesothelium. **Plate 2, Fig. 1.**

Semicircular ducts. These ducts are filled with endolymph and each has an enlarged base, the bulblike *ampulla*. An ampulla contains a patch of sensory neuroepithelium, the *crista*, which is stimulated by changes in the inertia of the body. In a cross section a duct appears as a thin-walled, oval tube. One side of the tube is fused to the periosteum of the bony canal. The wall of the duct is composed of vascularized connective tissue lined by a simple squamous epithelium lying on a basement membrane. Delicate fibrous trabecular strands connect the duct to the periosteum, thus forming a network of spaces in the bony canal. The periosteum and trabeculae are lined with mesothelium. In life, these spaces are filled with perilymph and the ducts carry endolymph. **Plate 2, Figs. 1 and 2.**

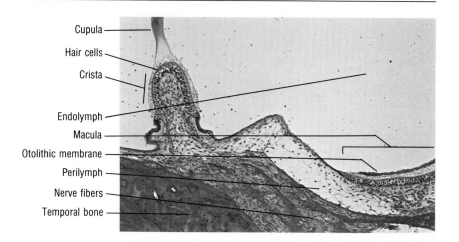

Cupula
Hair cells
Crista
Endolymph
Macula
Otolithic membrane
Perilymph
Nerve fibers
Temporal bone

FIGURE 3.
Crista, and macula in a membranous
labyrinth; inner ear; guinea pig; H&E;
×100.

CRISTA. This is a ridge of connective tissue projecting into the lumen of the ampulla. It is lined by a columnar epithelium containing two major cell types: hair cells and supporting cells. **Plate 2, Fig. 3.**

Hair cells. There are two types of hair cells. One type is flask-shaped and sits on the apex of the crista; these do not reach the basement membrane. They have an apical cilium and many stereocilia (sensory hairs), usually organized into a hair tuft. The second type of hair cell is columnar. These lie below the apex and rest on a basement membrane. They also have a cilium, and many stereocilia organized into a sensory hair tuft. Cells of the first type are innervated by afferent fibers, while cells of the second type are innervated by both afferent and efferent nerves. The nuclei of both types of hair cells occupy a middle level of the epithelium.

Supporting cells. These are columnar cells, randomly mixed with the hair cells to provide support. Although they resemble the columnar hair cells, their nuclei almost sit on the basement membrane.

Cupula. This is a gelatinous, striated, bell-shaped structure lying above the cells; the sensory hair tufts are inserted into the cupula. Any movement in a given plane causes the endolymph to displace the cupula and stimulate the hair cells to set up an impulse.

MACULA. This is a sensory receptor located in the utricle and saccule. It is built on a similar histologic plan as the crista, but with some differences. The macula is a low, elongate patch of hair cells and supporting cells. There is no cupula; instead there is a gelatinous *otolithic membrane* in which crystalline bodies, *otoconia*, are embedded. The otolithic membrane rests on the hair cells and receives their sensory hairs; the function is similar to that described for the cupula (see above). **Plate 2, Fig. 3.**

Cochlear duct. This portion of the membranous labyrinth extends from the base of the cochlea almost to its apex. It separates the scala vestibuli from the scala tympani, except at the apex where the two scalae are continuous; this region is the *helicotrema*. The distal end of the cochlear duct is closed, but the proximal end is continuous with the sacculus by a narrow *ductus reuniens* (see **Plate 2, Fig. 1**). The cochlear duct (**Plate 3, Figs. 1** and **2**) appears somewhat in the shape of a right triangle in cross section, and its walls are formed by the three structures.

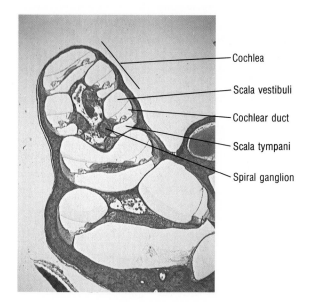

Cochlea

Scala vestibuli

Cochlear duct

Scala tympani

Spiral ganglion

FIGURE 1.
Cochlea; inner ear; guinea pig; H&E;
×20.

1 *Vestibular membrane*. This extends from the spiral limbus to the upper portion of spiral ligament. It forms the roof of the cochlear duct and floor of the scala vestibuli.

2 *Spiral ligament*. This is the thick outer wall of the duct fused with the periosteum of the bony canal.

3 *Basilar membrane*. This stretches from the spiral lamina and tympanic lip to the outer cochlear duct wall. It forms the floor of the cochlear duct and roof of the scala tympani.

VESTIBULAR MEMBRANE (Reissner's membrane). This is a thin membrane composed of two adjacent layers of simple squamous epithelium. The epithelia are separated by a thin layer of ground substance containing few delicate collagen fibers. The epithelial cells lining the scala vestibuli are less attenuated, and easier to observe than those lining the cochlear duct. **Plate 3, Figs. 2** and **3.**

SPIRAL LIGAMENT. This is a highly vascularized, thickened layer of dense, irregular collagenous connective tissue. It forms the outer wall of the cochlear duct. The spiral ligament is composed of tissues from both the cochlear duct and periosteum of the bony cochlea. **Plate 3, Figs. 2** and **3.**

A portion of the spiral ligament is covered by a layer of pseudostratified columnar epithelium, the *stria vascularis*. Both the epithelium and spiral ligament extend the length of the cochlear duct. The epithelium is vascular, since it contains intraepithelial capillaries supplied by the underlying spiral ligament. The stria vascularis is possibly a producer of endolymph, which fills the cochlear duct. **Plate 3, Figs. 2** and **3.**

BASILAR MEMBRANE. The basilar membrane is an extension of the tympanic lip and stretches laterally to fuse with the spiral ligament. It separates the cochlear duct from the scala tympani and supports the cells of the organ of Corti, the sensory receptor for hearing. The basilar membrane is composed of three layers: (1) an upper layer of ground substance, just beneath the organ of Corti; (2) a thin layer of scleroprotein fibers (auditory strings) embedded in ground substance, which lie just below the upper layer and appear as parallel striations; (3) a thin lower layer of delicate collagen fibers facing the scala tympani. **Plate 3, Figs. 2** and **3.**

Organ of Corti (spiral organ). This is a complex of supporting and sensory epithelial cells. Only the supporting cells rest on the basilar membrane. The sensory cells (hair cells) are carried by the supporting cells and do not reach the basilar membrane. The organ of Corti extends the length of the cochlear duct. Below, its cells are listed in order from the spiral lamina to the peripheral spiral ligament. **Plate 3, Figs. 2 and 3.**

1 *Border cells*. Simple columnar cells delimit the inner boundary of the organ of Corti.

2 *Inner hair cells* (sensory cells). This single layer of flask-shaped cells does not extend to the basilar membrane. These cells have many prominent stereocilia on their apical ends. They are innervated by afferent and efferent fibers.

3 *Inner phalangeal cells* (supporting cells). These are tall, thin cells which enclose and support the inner hair cells and nerves. Their nuclei lie close to the basement membrane.

4 *Inner pillar cells* (supporting cells). These are cone-shaped cells with a broad base and a long, tapered apex; the cytoplasm has dark-stained tonofibrils.

5 *Outer pillar cell* (supporting cells). These are similar to the inner pillar cells, but are more elongate. The apical ends of the pillar cells are in intimate contact, forming a large, flat, strong plate to support the hair cells. A space, the inner tunnel, is formed between the bases of the inner and outer pillar cells. The upper portion of the cells, over the tunnel, is joined in a ball-and-socket fashion.

6 *Outer phalangeal cells (Deiter's cells)* (supporting cells). These are tall columnar cells. Each cell has a deep indentation which supports an outer hair cell and nerve fibers.

7 *Outer hair cells* (sensory cells). These are short columnar cells with a rounded base. The cells do not extend to the basilar membrane. They have many prominent apical stereocilia, and are innervated by afferent and efferent nerve fibers. The outer hair cells are supported by the outer phalangeal cells. The innermost hair cell–phalangeal cell combinations are separated from the outer pillar cells by a cavity, *Nuel's space*.

8 *Peripheral cells*. These represent the outer limits of the organ of Corti, and extend from the outer phalangeal cells to the spiral ligament. The peripheral cells, adjacent to the phalangeal cells, are the tall supporting *cells of Hensen*. A small space, the outer tunnel, is located between Hensen's cells and the outer phalangeal cells. Hensen's cells decrease in height as they approach the cuboidal *cells of Claudius*, which extend to the spiral ligament and line a groove, the external spiral sulcus. Small clusters of polyhedral *cells of Boettcher* are present at the base of the cochlea duct. They lie on the basilar membrane, below the cells of Claudius, and are distinguished by a large, spherical nucleus surrounded by a dark-stained cytoplasm. They are possibly secretory cells.

Other structures associated directly or indirectly with the organ of Corti are the following.

Tectorial membrane. This is a thick, elongate, gelatinous structure attached to the vestibular lip of the limbus. It rests on the "hairs" of the sensory hair cells. The tectorial membrane is a cuticular structure secreted by small interdental cells. These cells are located on the upper surface of the limbus and lie under the tectorial membrane. They are partly embedded within the periosteum of the limbus and partly flattened out on the surface of the periosteum. The tectorial membrane may be shrunken and distorted in typical laboratory preparations. **Plate 3, Figs. 2 and 3.**

Internal spiral sulcus. This is a groove bordered by the tectorial membrane and the vestibular and tympanic lips of the spiral limbus. **Plate 3, Figs. 2 and 3.**

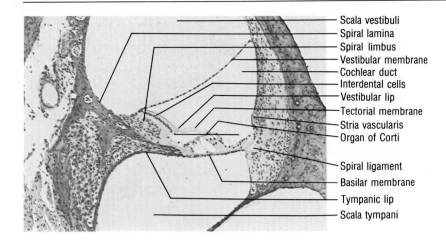

Scala vestibuli
Spiral lamina
Spiral limbus
Vestibular membrane
Cochlear duct
Interdental cells
Vestibular lip
Tectorial membrane
Stria vascularis
Organ of Corti
Spiral ligament
Basilar membrane
Tympanic lip
Scala tympani

FIGURE 2.
*Cochlear duct and organ of Corti;
inner ear; guinea pig; H&E; ×100.*

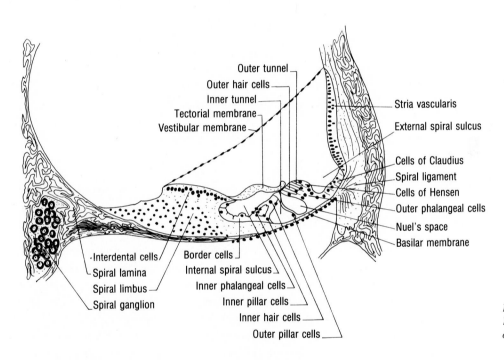

Outer tunnel
Outer hair cells
Inner tunnel
Tectorial membrane
Vestibular membrane

Stria vascularis
External spiral sulcus
Cells of Claudius
Spiral ligament
Cells of Hensen
Outer phalangeal cells
Nuel's space
Basilar membrane

Interdental cells
Spiral lamina
Spiral limbus
Spiral ganglion

Border cells
Internal spiral sulcus
Inner phalangeal cells
Inner pillar cells
Inner hair cells
Outer pillar cells

FIGURE 3.
*Drawing of the organ of Corti based
on the specimen in Plate 3, Fig. 2.*

Auditory nerve. The cochlear division of the auditory nerve extends through the modiolus to innervate the inner and outer hair cells of the organ of Corti. A prominent spiral ganglion is present at the base of the spiral lamina.

As sound waves are transmitted by the stapes through the oval window and into the perilymph of the scala vestibuli, they pass through the endolymph of the cochlear duct and into the perilymph of the scala tympani. These vibrations cause the basilar membrane to move, and as the "hairs" of the hair cells are rubbed against the tectorial membrane, an impulse is initiated. Since fluids are incompressible and the bony labyrinth is a closed space, these vibrations can occur only because a movable elastic membrane covers the round window.

Chemoreceptors

The olfactory epithelium of the nose and the taste buds in the tongue are sensory receptors; they are responsive to chemical stimuli.

TASTE BUDS. These are conspicuous pale, ovoid structures scattered in the epithelium lining the circumvallate, fungiform, and foliate papillae of the tongue. Each bud is open to the epithelial surface by a pore (taste canal). They are composed of taste cells, supporting cells, basal cells, and peripheral cells; the latter two are possibly generative cells. These cells are surrounded by unmyelinated nerve fibers, and only the taste cells are innervated. Refer to Chap. 12 for their morphology.

OLFACTORY EPITHELIUM. This is a pseudostratified columnar epithelium lining the nasal cavity and portions of the nasal septum. It is composed of three types of cells: basal, sustentacular, and olfactory. Of the three, only the olfactory cells are modified receptors, sensitive to olfactory stimuli. Refer to Chap. 13 for their morphology.

Photoreceptors (rods and cones in the eye)

The eye is a spherical structure, about 2.5 cm in diameter, lying within a bony orbit of the skull and surrounded by adipose and areolar connective tissue. It is attached to six ocular muscles. The wall of the eyeball is composed of three layers: an outer *fibrous* layer, middle *vascular* layer, and inner *retina* (nervous layer). For light to stimulate the photoreceptor cells, the rods and cones, it must pass through several structures and substances. Given in the order light passes through them, these are the cornea, aqueous humor, lens, vitreous body, and retina. **Plate 4, Fig. 1.**

FIBROUS LAYER. This outermost coat is composed of a dense, fibrous *sclera* which covers about 83 percent of the posterior region of the eyeball, and a transparent *cornea* which covers about 17 percent of the anterior part.

Sclera. This is a relatively thick (0.3 to 1.0 mm) layer of dense, irregular collagen fibers containing some scattered elastic fibers. Externally, an *episclera* covers the surface of the sclera. It is a thin, highly vascularized loose connective tissue layer which is continuous with a dense connective tissue capsule, *Tenon's capsule.* The inner surface of the sclera is a thin pigmented tissue, the *suprachoroid lamina* (lamina fusca), which loosely binds the sclera to the underlying choroid. The sclera is perforated in a region where optic nerve fibers leave the eye. This perforation is named the *lamina cribosa.* The sclera strengthens and supports the wall of the eye, and provides for the insertion of ocular muscles. **Plate 4, Figs. 1 and 2.**

Cornea. Although the cornea is an anterior continuation of the sclera, it is a modified, transparent, avascular structure composed of five distinct superimposed layers. The border between the cornea and sclera is the limbus, in which is located the circumferential canal of Schlemm (sinus venosus sclerae) and a network of spaces and trabeculae, the *trabecular meshwork.* The canal and meshwork drain aqueous humor from the anterior chamber into a system of ocular veins. The five corneal layers going from the external to the internal surface are listed below. **Plate 4, Figs. 1 and 3.**

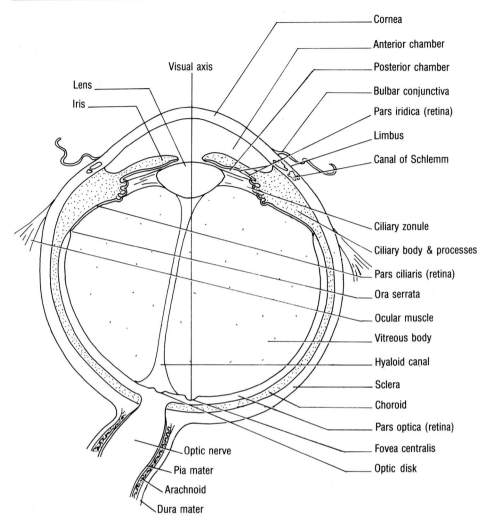

Cornea
Anterior chamber
Posterior chamber
Bulbar conjunctiva
Pars iridica (retina)
Limbus
Canal of Schlemm

Ciliary zonule
Ciliary body & processes
Pars ciliaris (retina)
Ora serrata
Ocular muscle
Vitreous body
Hyaloid canal
Sclera
Choroid
Pars optica (retina)
Fovea centralis
Optic disk

Visual axis
Lens
Iris

Optic nerve
Pia mater
Arachnoid
Dura mater

FIGURE 1.
Drawing of a horizontal section through the human right eye.

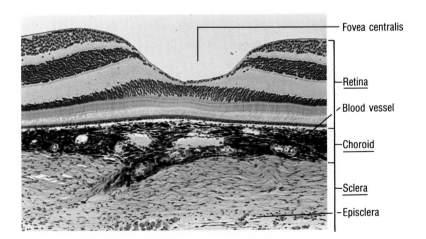

Fovea centralis
Retina
Blood vessel
Choroid
Sclera
Episclera

FIGURE 2.
Sclera, choroid, and retina; eye; rhesus monkey; H&E; ×100. Note that the suprachoroid lamina is a thin pigmented connective tissue lying between the sclera and choroid.

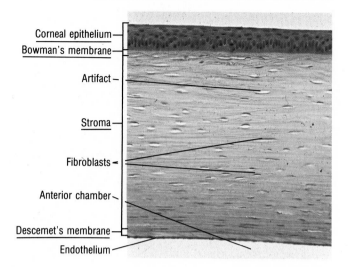

Corneal epithelium
Bowman's membrane
Artifact
Stroma
Fibroblasts
Anterior chamber
Descemet's membrane
Endothelium

FIGURE 3.
Cornea; eye; rabbit; H&E; ×200.

1 *Corneal epithelium.* This is five or six layers of stratified squamous nonkeratinized epithelium.

2 *Bowman's membrane* (anterior limiting layer). This is a thin, delicate fibrous layer lying below the epithelium. It is actually the modified outer region of the stroma (see below) and contains tiny collagen fibers.

3 *Stroma* (substantia propria). This thick layer forms the major part of the cornea. It is composed of bundles of transparent collagen fibers organized into lamellae. The bundles in a lamella are parallel, but lie at angles to those of adjacent lamellae. The fibers and stellate fibroblasts (keratocytes) are embedded in a glycoprotein ground substance.

4 *Descemet's membrane* (posterior limiting membrane). This is a homogeneous, pale acidophilic layer lying below the stroma. It is about the same thickness as Bowman's membrane, approximately 6 to 10 μm. It is composed of collagenlike fibers and represents the basal lamina of endothelial cells lining the membrane.

5 *Endothelium.* This is a simple cuboidal or squamous epithelium. It lines the innermost layer of the cornea, and is bathed by aqueous humor of the anterior chamber.

VASCULAR LAYER (uvea). This middle layer of the wall of the eyeball lies between the sclera and retina. It is a continuous layer with three distinct regions: a posterior *choroid*, a more anterior *ciliary body*, and a most anterior *iris*. **Plate 4, Fig. 1.**

Choroid. The posterior two-thirds of the vascular layer is the choroid. It extends anteriorly to the *ora serrata*, a junction between the retina and ciliary body. The choroid and sclera are firmly united where the optic nerve enters the eye. In other regions, however, they are separated by a narrow perichordial space, but loosely attached to each other by strands of connective tissue, the *suprachoroid lamina* (see above), running through the perichordial space. The lamina is composed of elastic fibers, fibroblasts, and melanophores. The choroid is histologically composed of three layers; going from the suprachoroid lamina to the retina they are the *vessel layer*, the *choriocapillary layer*, and *Bruch's membrane*. **Plate 4, Figs. 1 and 2; Plate 5, Fig. 1.**

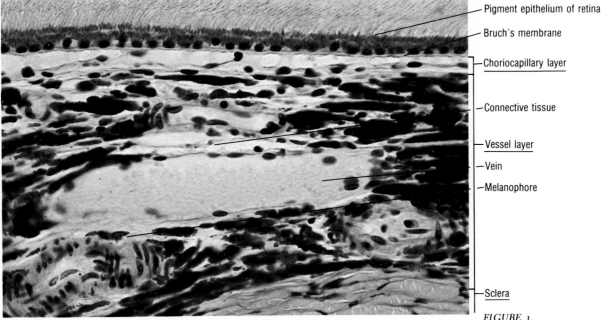

Pigment epithelium of retina
Bruch's membrane
Choriocapillary layer
Connective tissue
Vessel layer
Vein
Melanophore
Sclera

FIGURE 1.
Choroid; eye; rhesus monkey; H&E;
×400.

1 *Vessel layer.* Small branches of ciliary arteries are present in this layer, as are many large veins. The layer also contains stellate melanophores and areolar connective tissue.

2 *Choriocapillary layer.* This is an extensive plexus of large capillaries which nourish the retina. The plexus is quite prominent and appears just below Bruch's membrane, close to the retina. The plexus is supported by a network of collagenous and elastic fibers; fibroblasts are also present.

3 *Bruch's membrane.* This structure appears as a thin (1 to 3 μm), homogeneous layer with the light microscope. It is a composite of delicate elastic and collagen fibers from the choriocapillary layer and the basal lamina of the retinal pigment epithelium. Bruch's membrane may be considered as the basement membrane of the pigment epithelium in the retina.

Ciliary body. This is the thickest region of the vascular layer; it lies between the choroid and iris. It is a prominent ring of smooth muscle tissue which surrounds the lens circumferentially. The muscle fibers run meridionally, longitudinally, and circumferentially. The anterior region of the ciliary body is organized into about 75 radiating folds, the *ciliary processes*. Each process contains a vascular stroma which produces aqueous humor. The posterior portion of the ciliary body lacks ciliary processes and forms a scalloped *ora serrata*, where the pars optica of the retina terminates (see below). Except for the presence of ciliary muscles and lack of a choriocapillary layer, the histology of the ciliary body resembles that of the choroid. Two layers of cuboidal retinal epithelium, the *pars ciliaris*, line the surface of the ciliary body. The superficial inner layer is nonpigmented, and actively secretes substances into the aqueous humor. The deeper outer layer is pigmented and lies on a basal lamina which is continuous with Bruch's membrane.

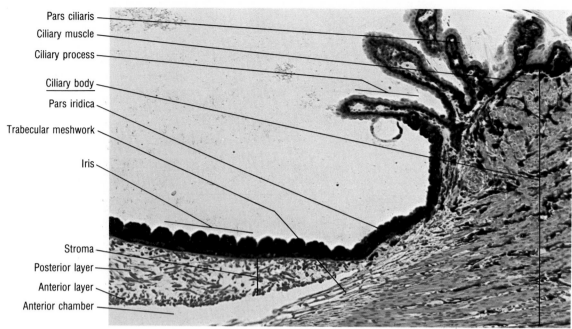

Pars ciliaris —
Ciliary muscle —
Ciliary process —
Ciliary body —
Pars iridica —
Trabecular meshwork —
Iris —
Stroma —
Posterior layer —
Anterior layer —
Anterior chamber —

FIGURE 2.
Ciliary body and iris; eye; rhesus monkey; H&E; ×100. Note that the pars ciliaris is composed of two layers of cuboidal epithelium; the superficial layer is nonpigmented and the deeper layer is pigmented. The pars iridica is composed of two pigmented layers of cuboidal epithelium.

The lens is anchored to the ciliary body by a ring of thin, transparent suspensory ligaments, the *ciliary zonule*. As muscles in the ciliary body contract, tension is exerted on the lens via the ligaments. This tension results in a change of lens shape, thereby changing the focal length of the lens, which allows for accommodation. **Plate 4, Fig. 1; Plate 5, Fig. 2.**

Iris. The most anterior region of the vascular layer is the iris. It is an anterior continuation of the ciliary body, and forms a flat ring of tissue anterior to the lens. Its center is the *pupil*, which can be constricted or dilated by muscular activity. The iris is composed of a loose connective tissue *stroma* organized into *anterior* and *posterior layers*. **Plate 4, Fig. 1; Plate 5, Fig. 2.**

ANTERIOR LAYER. This most anterior portion of the stroma is a thin, dense layer of collagen fibers, fibroblasts, and branched melanophores. The color of the iris is directly related both to the number of melanophores containing brown melanin granules and to the thickness of the anterior layer. Blue eyes have few melanophores and a thin anterior layer, and dark brown eyes have many melanophores and a thick anterior layer.

POSTERIOR LAYER. Most of the iris is composed of this posteior portion of the stroma. It contains loose connective tissue, blood vessels with unusually thick walls, melanophores, fibroblasts, collagen fibers, and some elastic fibers. Large macrophages (about 85 μm in diameter) filled with phagocytized melanin granules are present. These rounded and heavily pigmented cells are designated as *clump cells*. The posterior border of the iris is lined by two layers of heavily pigmented cuboidal cells, the *pars iridica*. These layers are a continuation of the retinal cells which also cover the ciliary body. The most posterior of these two layers, bordering the posterior chamber of the eye, is continuous with the nonpigmented cells lining the ciliary body. Their apical surfaces are covered by a thin basal lamina, or internal limiting membrane, which separates the cells from the chamber. The cuboidal cells in the anterior layer, lying adjacent to the stroma, are modified myoepithelial cells. These cuboidal cells, lying in the epithelial layer, have long, smooth-muscle-like processes which are pigmented and fusiform. These processes extend radially toward the pupil, but terminate near the sphincter muscle surrounding the pupil. Each process, unlike the cuboidal part of the cell, rests on a thin basal lamina. Together, these myofilament-filled processes constitute the *dilator pupillary muscle*, which is three to five layers in thickness. This muscle is innervated by sympathetic nerve fibers, which control the dilation of the pupil. The other set of pupillary muscle, the *sphincter muscle*, is arranged circumferentially around the pupil. Although its muscle fibers are derived from the pigment layer (an ectodermal structure), they are separated from it by connective tissue and appear as typical smooth muscle cells. The sphincter muscle is innervated by parasympathetic fibers and control the constriction of the pupil.

RETINA. Embryonically the retina develops as an optic vesicle of neural ectoderm by an evagination of the prosencephalon wall. The vesicle is attached to the prosencephalon by a hollow optic stalk. In later development, the distal end of the optic vesicle forms a double-walled cup. The inner and outer walls of the cup are separated by a space which eventually disappears as the walls grow together. The posterior portion of the cuplike retina lines the choroid and ciliary body, while the rim of the cup lines the posterior border of the iris. The outer wall of the retina differentiates into an outer *pigment layer*, or *pigment epithelium*. It lines the surface of the vascular layer and gives rise to the pupillary muscles of the iris. The inner wall differentiates into a *nervous layer*. The retina has three anatomical regions, all of which have a pigment layer and a modified nervous layer.

1 *Pars optica*. The nervous layer is modified into a stratified layer of photoreceptive cells lining most of the cup and extending to the ora serrata.

2 *Pars ciliaris*. The nervous layer is reduced to a single layer of secretory cells covering the ciliary processes, and it secretes aqueous humor.

3 *Pars iridica*. The nervous layer covers the posterior border of the iris, and is modified into a single layer of heavily pigmented, nonsensitive cuboidal cells.

Since the pars ciliaris and pars iridica have been considered with the ciliary body and iris, only the pars optica will be discussed. **Plate 4, Fig. 1.**

Pars optica. Except for the fovea centralis and optic disk, the pars optica is composed of ten layers of cells and their processes. The outer layer is the pigment epithelium, and the remaining nine belong to the nervous layer. The nervous layer is composed of photoreceptor cells, association neurons, and supporting cells. In general, light first passes through the inner layers of the pars optica to reach and stimulate the outer photoreceptor cells, the rods and cones. The stimulated cells initiate nerve impulses which travel from the outer to the inner part of the pars optica and converge on the optic disk. The impulses then exit via the optic nerve (**Plate 6, Fig. 1**). A description will be given of the pars optica, going from the outer layer adjacent to the choroid to the innermost layer. **Plate 4, Fig. 2; Plate 6, Figs. 1** and **2.**

1 *Pigment epithelium*. This tissue is a simple cuboidal epithelium lying on Bruch's membrane (see above). The cells have a large, spherical nucleus. Melanin pigment granules are present in the apical cytoplasm and microvilli. The latter extend up between the processes of the rod and cones. The functions of pigment epithelium are varied: it serves to absorb light and prevent backscattering of reflected light; it forms a selective barrier allowing only certain substances in the blood to reach the nervous layer; it is phagocytic; and pigment epithelium may possibly provide nutritive support to the photoreceptor cells.

2 *Rods and cones.* These modified neurons are the photoreceptive cells found in the outer region of the nervous layer. They contain light-sensitive visual pigments in their cytoplasm which decompose on exposure to light. The process of decomposition depolarizes the cell membranes, thereby initiating a nerve impulse. The visual pigment in cones is iodopsin; in rods it is rhodopsin. Rods are very sensitive to light and probably do not discriminate between different wavelengths. Cones are of several types, all of which are less sensitive to light and can discriminate between different wavelengths. Rods, therefore, are stimulated by dim light and cones by bright, colored light.

Rods. These are long, thin cells with thin, tapered ends lying between the microvilli of the pigment epithelial cells. The most distal portion of the tapered end, the *outer segment*, contains rhodopsin and stains only with special stains for phospholipids. The more proximal portion, the *inner segment*, is visible with routine laboratory stains. The region of the cell containing the nucleus lies in the outer nuclear layer (see below).

Cones. The cones, like the rods, also have tapered distal ends lying between the microvilli of pigment cells. The shape of a cone varies according to its location on the retina. Over most of the retina the outer segment of a cone is long and thin, but the inner segment and remainder of the cell body is relatively thick and is cone-shaped. In the fovea centralis, the cones are slender and non-cone-shaped. In general, the staining characteristics of the cones are similar to those of the rods.

3 *External limiting membrane.* This appears as a thin horizontal line just outside the outer nuclear layer (see below). It is a complex of terminal bars formed by contact points between rods, cones, and Müller's cells (supporting cells).

4 *Outer nuclear layer.* This appears as a concentration of rod and cone nuclei, just innermost to the external limiting membrane. Large, oval, pale-stained cone nuclei usually lie near the external limiting membrane. Rod nuclei are round and dark, and located further from the membrane, in staggered layers. In this layer the cytoplasm is usually indistinct for both rods and cones.

5 *Outer plexiform layer.* This layer is just interior to the outer nuclear layer, and appears as a wide, pale-stained fibrous band. It is composed of the terminal ends of rods and cones, which synapse with dendrites of bipolar neurons and horizontal cells in the next layer.

6 *Inner nuclear layer.* The layer is distinguished as a wide, dense band of nuclei lying innermost to the outer plexiform layer. The nuclei belong to association neurons (bipolar neurons, horizontal cells, and amocrine cells), and the supporting Müller cells. The association neurons are important in summation of rod impulses and in the integration of rod and cone impulses.

7 *Inner plexiform layer.* This layer lies inside the inner nuclear layer. It looks like the outer plexiform layer—a wide, pale-stained fibrous band—but it contains some capillaries. It is an area of synapses between axons of the bipolar neurons and dendrites of ganglion cells.

8 *Ganglion cell layer.* The layer appears as a moderately dense band of large multipolar ganglion cells lying just inside the inner plexiform layer. The pale basophilic cytoplasm contains a large vesicular nucleus with a prominent nucleolus. Smaller, denser nuclei of neuroglia cells are also present in this layer.

9 *Nerve fiber layer.* The layer is a pale-stained fibrous region just interior to the ganglion cell layer. It consists of axons of ganglion cells which extend horizontally toward the

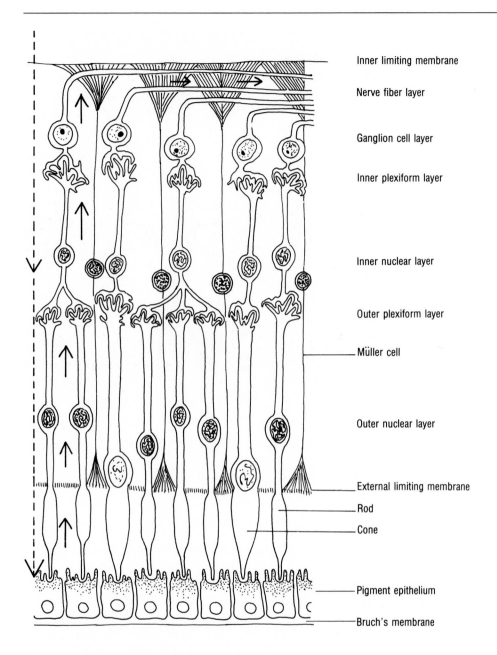

Inner limiting membrane

Nerve fiber layer

Ganglion cell layer

Inner plexiform layer

Inner nuclear layer

Outer plexiform layer

Müller cell

Outer nuclear layer

External limiting membrane

Rod

Cone

Pigment epithelium

Bruch's membrane

light pathway – dotted arrows
nerve impulse – solid arrows

FIGURE 1.
Schematic drawing of the human retina (pars optica). Arrows indicate the direction in which light and nerve impulses pass through the retina.

optic disk and exit as components of the optic nerve. Also within this layer are fibrous processes of Müller's cells, which form a supporting network for the axons, and large blood vessels.

10 *Inner limiting membrane.* This appears as a thin membrane, and represents the innermost boundary of the retina. It is formed as a complex of basal lamina and expanded ends of the fibrous cytoplasmic processes of Müller's cells. It separates the retina from the vitreous body.

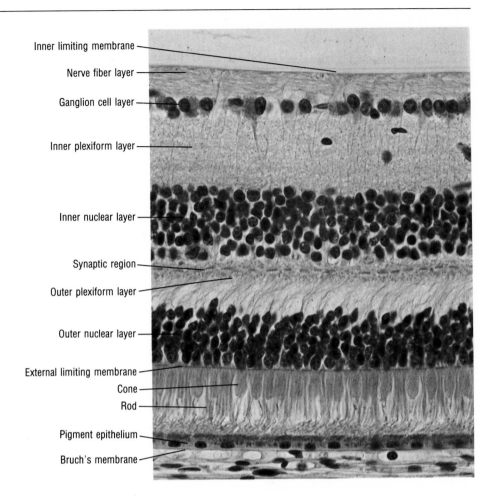

Inner limiting membrane

Nerve fiber layer

Ganglion cell layer

Inner plexiform layer

Inner nuclear layer

Synaptic region

Outer plexiform layer

Outer nuclear layer

External limiting membrane

Cone

Rod

Pigment epithelium

Bruch's membrane

FIGURE 2.
Retina, pars optica; eye; rhesus monkey; H&E; ×400. Note that the dark bodies in the outer plexiform layer indicate synaptic regions between the photoreceptor cells and the bipolar neurons.

Although the nervous layer has the same histologic organization throughout the pars optica, there are two exceptions: the *optic disk* and the *fovea centralis*.

FOVEA CENTRALIS. This region lies at the posterior pole of the eye, directly on the visual axis, and is adapted for greatest visual acuity. Histologically, it appears as a depression or pit (foveola), about 0.4 mm in diameter. It contains a high concentration of long, thin cones and a peripheral aggregation of ganglion cells. The fovea centralis is located within the *macula lutea*, a yellowish region containing carotenoid pigment, which is visible on freshly dissected retinas (see **Plate 4, Fig. 2**).

OPTIC DISK (optic papilla, blind spot). The area is about 1.5 mm in diameter. Axons of ganglion cells converge here to form the optic nerve, which leaves the retina. Since there are no retinal layers in the optic disk, it is insensitive to light.

Blood vessels. A central artery and vein are carried in the optic nerve. They radiate into the nerve fiber layer and extend as small vessels into the inner nuclear layer.

REFRACTIVE STRUCTURES AND SUBSTANCES. As light enters the eye, it must be refracted to fall on the retina so an image can be formed. Refraction is accomplished as light passes through several structures and substances, each with a different refractive index. In addition to the cornea, which has already been described, the remaining refractive components are the aqueous humor, lens, ciliary zonule, and the vitreous body.

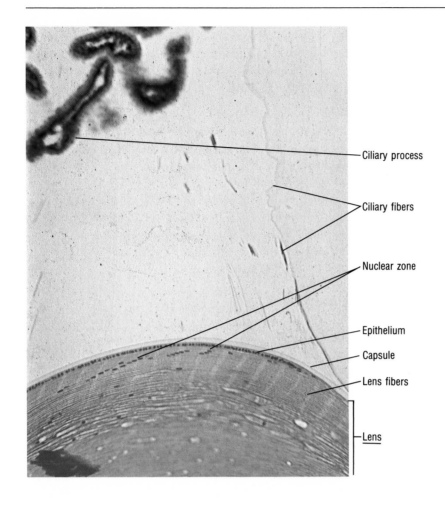

—Ciliary process

—Ciliary fibers

—Nuclear zone

—Epithelium

—Capsule

—Lens fibers

—Lens

FIGURE 1.
Lens; rhesus monkey; H&E; ×100.

Aqueous humor. This is a clear, serumlike fluid. It nourishes and bathes the tissues in the anterior region of the eye, especially the lens and cornea. It will not be seen in a histologic section of the eye because it is a transparent fluid. Aqueous humor is produced by diffusion from the vascular stroma of the ciliary processes, and by active secretion of the nonpigmented ciliary epithelium. It is secreted into the posterior chamber behind the iris; then it flows through the pupil into the anterior chamber, and finally leaves via the canal of Schlemm and intertrabecular spaces in the limbus.

Lens. The lens appears as a biconvex disk with a more convex posterior surface; its peripheral circumference is the equator. It is composed of elongate, transparent prisms, *lens fibers*, which are held together by specialized structures at the ultrastructure level. The lens has an anterior epithelium, and is totally surrounded by a thin, homogeneous elastic capsule. The epithelium is cuboidal, but tends to be columnar toward the equator of the lens. At the equator, the epithelial cells differentiate into new lens fibers by becoming elongate, prismatic, transparent, and enucleate. This process occurs slowly throughout the life of an individual. The outer fibers are arranged in concentric lamellae, and the transitional area from cells to fibers is designated as the *nuclear zone*. The lens is somewhat plastic in the younger person and can change its shape to allow for accommodation (see above). In later years, the lens hardens and loses this ability. **Plate 4, Fig. 1; Plate 7, Fig. 1.**

Ciliary zonule. This is a group of thin, transparent, homogenous fibers extending from the ciliary body to the equator. The fibers insert on the lens capsule, just anterior and posterior to the equator, and function to hold the lens in position. In a stained section the fibers may appear as thin, pale acidophilic strands. As the ciliary muscle contracts, the ciliary body bulges toward the lens. This action decreases the tension on the fibers and lens so that the lens tends to change its shape (bulges). This change in shape also changes the focal length, allowing the lens to accomodate for near vision. **Plate 4, Fig. 1; Plate 7, Fig. 1.**

Vitreous body. In a histologic section the vitreous body may appear as a distorted, shrunken, pale-stained, slightly fibrous structure lying between the lens and retina; or it may be absent. In life, the vitreous body is a transparent, semifluid structure of high viscosity. It is composed mainly of water, some hyaluronic acid molecules, thin collagen fibrils, and a few peripheral cells, *hyalocytes* (fibroblasts and macrophages). The hyalocytes possibly produce fibers and the hyaluronic acid molecules. A hyaloid canal, an embryonic reminant of the hyaloid artery, runs from the lens back to the optic disk. The anterior surface of the vitreous body may have a thin membrane, which is a condensation of fibrils and vitreous substance.

Associated structures (eyelid and lacrimal gland)

EYELID. The eyelid is a thin fold of skin with an outer squamous keratinized epithelium. The inner epithelial surface, the *palpebral conjunctiva*, is continuous with the *bulbar conjunctiva*, which covers the eyeball. The deep folds separating the palpebral and bulbar conjunctiva are the fornices. The palpebral conjunctiva, near the free edge of the lid, is a stratified squamous epithelium containing a few mucous cells. Near the fornix it becomes stratified columnar with many goblet cells. This type of epithelium continues as the bulbar conjunctiva onto the surface of the sclera. The bulbar conjunctiva becomes stratified squamous near the cornea and is continuous with that structure. A dense bed of irregular collagenous connective tissue, the *tarsal plate*, is present within the eyelid. This plate gives strength and form to the eyelid and has many sebaceous glands, *Meibomian glands*, embedded within it. Excretory ducts of these glands open onto the free surface of the lids. The follicles of eyelashes are associated with large sebaceous *glands of Zeis*. Sweat *glands of Moll* are present between the follicles of the eyelashes. Some of the striated orbicularis oculi muscles are present in the eyelids and function to close them. The levator palpebrae muscles, which raise the upper lids, are not present in the lids proper, but insert onto the tarsal plate by an aponeurosis. The orbicularis muscle may be seen in sections. **Plate 4, Fig. 1; Plate 7, Fig. 2.**

LACRIMAL GLAND. This gland is located in the upper lateral region of the orbit above the eyelid. It is divided into a large upper *orbital* and small lower *palpebral* portion. The lower palpebral portion is separated into lobules by loose connective tissue. The gland is tubuloalveolar, and the alveoli resemble serous glands, but the lumina are much larger. The glandular cells are columnar, with a pale acidophilic cytoplasm which is granular or vacuolated. Stellate or flattened myoepithelial cells lie between the basal lamina and bases of the glandular cells. They function to express the secretion (tears) from the gland. The lacrimal gland is drained by approximately 10 to 15 excretory ducts. They open into the conjunctival fornix, where the palpebral and bulbar conjunctiva meet and form a fold. Ducts from the orbital portion of the gland pass through the palpebral portion to terminate on the conjunctiva. The palpebral ducts open directly and independently on the conjunctiva.

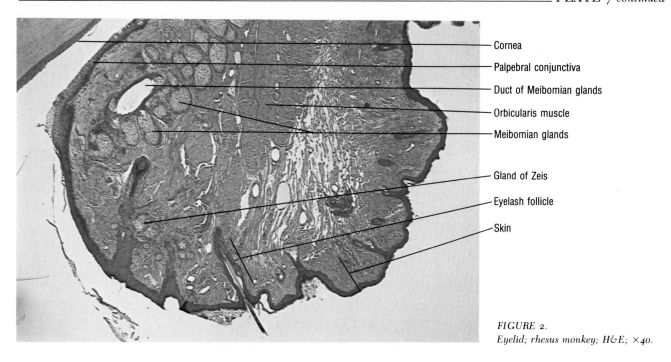

Cornea

Palpebral conjunctiva

Duct of Meibomian glands

Orbicularis muscle

Meibomian glands

Gland of Zeis

Eyelash follicle

Skin

FIGURE 2.
Eyelid; rhesus monkey; H&E; ×40.

The larger ducts are lined by a stratified squamous epithelium, while the smaller, intralobular ducts have stratified cuboidal or simple cuboidal epithelium.

Tears function to lubricate, clean, and moisten the surface of the eyeball and eyelid. In addition to water and salts, the secretion contains *lysozyme*, a bacteriocidal enzyme. As tears are produced, they flush across the surface of the eyeball. They are drained into the nasal cavity through the following structures of the lacrimal apparatus: (1) puncta lacrimalia, (2) lacrimal canaliculi, (3) lacrimal sac, (4) and nasolacrimal duct.

Index

Index

Page references in **boldface** indicate illustrations.

DATE DUE